OPHTHALMIC TERMINOLOGY

SPELLER AND VOCABULARY BUILDER

OPHTHALMIC TERMINOLOGY

SPELLER AND VOCABULARY BUILDER

Harold A. Stein, M.D., M.Sc. (Ophth.), F.R.C.S. (C)

Professor, University of Toronto
President, Joint Commission on Allied Health Personnel
in Ophthalmology, St. Paul, Minnesota;
President, Canadian Ophthalmological Society;
Past President, Contact Lens Association of Ophthalmologists, U.S.A.;
Chief, Department of Ophthalmology,
Scarborough General Hospital, Toronto
Attending Ophthalmologist, Mt. Sinai Hospital, Toronto

Bernard J. Slatt, M.D., F.R.C.S. (C)

Associate Professor, University of Toronto, Ontario, Canada;
Attending Ophthalmologist, Scarborough General Hospital;
Director, Contact Lens Association of Ophthalmologists, U.S.A.;
Attending Ophthalmologist, Mount Sinai Hospital, Toronto, Ontario, Canada;
Advisory Board, Centennial College, Scarborough, Ontario, Canada

Raymond M. Stein, M.D.

Fellow in Cornea, Wills Eye Hospital, Philadelphia, Pennsylvania;
Fellow, Mayo Alumni Association of Ophthalmology
Rochester, Minnesota

SECOND EDITION

with 166 illustrations

The C. V. Mosby Company

ST. LOUIS • WASHINGTON, D.C. • TORONTO 1987

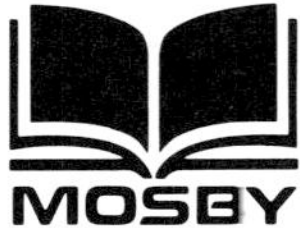

A TRADITION OF PUBLISHING EXCELLENCE

Editor: Eugenia A. Klein
Developmental Editor: Kathryn Falk
Assistant Editor: Beth Campbell
Project Editor: Suzanne Seeley
Design: Rey Umali
Production: Kathy Burmann

SECOND EDITION

Printed in the United States of America

The C.V. Mosby Company
11830 Westline Industrial Drive, St. Louis, Missouri 63146

Library of Congress Cataloging-in-Publication Data

Stein, Harold A. (Harold Aaron)
Ophthalmic terminology.

Rev. ed. of: Manual of ophthalmic terminology. 1982.
Bibliography: p.
Includes indexes.
1. Ophthalmology—Terminology. I. Slatt, Bernard J.
II. Stein, Raymond M. III. Stein, Harold A.
(Harold Aaron). Manual of ophthalmic
terminology. I. Title. [DNLM: 1. Ophthalmology—
terminology. WW 15 S819m]
RE20.S73 1987 617.7′0014 87-7863
ISBN 0-8016-4968-4

GW/VH/VH 9 8 7 6 5 4 3 2 1 02/B/258

To study the phenomena of disease without books is to sail an uncharted sea, while to study books without patients is not to go to sea at all.

Sir William Osler

This book is dedicated to the medical educators who have preceded us.

H.A. Stein, M.D.
B.J. Slatt, M.D.
R.M. Stein, M.D.

FOREWORD

Harold A. Stein, M.D., and Bernard J. Slatt, M.D., continue their indefatigable contributions to the education of allied health personnel in ophthalmology with the preparation of this revised edition of their highly successful *Ophthalmic Terminology: Speller and Vocabulary Builder*. The initial edition was well received by both medical and allied medical personnel in this hemisphere, and it had significant penetration in many foreign countries. This edition has considerably more input in the terminology of the subspecialties. It includes new sections on embryology, genetics, research, and computer terminology. A completely new section on surgical and laser terminology has been added.

The authors have been joined in the preparation of this edition of the text by Raymond M. Stein, M.D., Dr. Stein's son, who recently completed his residency in ophthalmology at the Mayo Clinic in Rochester, Minnesota, and is currently a corneal fellow at the Wills Eye Hospital, Philadelphia. Ray brings his vitality and fresh perspective to all of the new material as well as to much of the revision of the original text. Once again the authors of *Ophthalmic Terminology: Speller and Vocabulary Builder* are to be congratulated for their tireless efforts in support of allied health personnel in ophthalmology.

Whitney G. Sampson, M.D.
Member of the Joint Commission on Allied Health Personnel in Ophthalmology;
Member of the Board of Directors of the American Academy of Ophthalmology;
Past President: Texas Ophthalmological Association, Contact Lens Association of Ophthalmologists, American Academy of Ophthalmology

PREFACE

One ought, every day at least, to hear a little song,
read a good poem, see a fine picture, and, if it were possible,
to speak a few reasonable words.

Johann Wolfgang von Goethe
(1749-1832)

Our first edition arose out of the numerous requests and suggestions made to us from individuals in the ophthalmic field who wished to have a handy reference manual of ophthalmic vocabulary. We attempted to produce a desk-size reference companion that would not only serve as a source book of ophthalmic words but would also serve in developing a vocabulary in one or more specialized divisions of ophthalmology.

The second edition is designed to help several groups of individuals in the ophthalmic professions. It is designed to help the individual just entering the field by presenting words in generalized and specialized areas of ophthalmology with cross-references. The text serves as a reference source for secretaries and ophthalmic technicians and professionals both in the English and non-English speaking world in looking up specific spellings as well as definitions.

This second edition represents a complete reorganization of the first edition. New sections on genetics, embryology, research terms, and computer terms have been added. A greatly expanded surgical terminology section has been added to include laser terminology. While this text is not meant to duplicate a medical dictionary, common medical disorders affecting the eye have been added.

Our terminology is rapidly proliferating with etiological terminology frequently replacing long-standing descriptive terminology and even historical eponymic designations. It is often difficult to identify just when a term has become obsolete and a new term has become common usage.

We have attempted to deal primarily with the more commonly used words. The book is oriented for fast delivery of meanings and definitions with the emphasis on simplicity and practicality. It is definitely not a reference tome to give impressive weight to an ophthalmic bookshelf. Rather than provide an exhaustive list of every ophthalmic word and syndrome in a costly compendium, we have prepared a practical book whose function, at the bottom line, is to assist in communication.

To clarify definitions we have used illustrations from our previous works, *The Ophthalmic Assistant* and *Fitting Guide for Hard and Soft Contact Lenses*, published by The C.V. Mosby Company. Figs. 12-6 and 12-7 are taken from the second edition of Donaldson: *Atlas of External Diseases of the Eye, Volume III. Cornea and Sclera,* published by The C.V. Mosby Company. Figs. 15-4 and 15-5 are taken from the fourth edition of Havener: *Synopsis of Ophthalmology,* also published by Mosby. We would like to thank these authors for their permission to reproduce these figures. New illustrations and diagrams have been added to demonstrate points that clarify a definition.

We are grateful for the contributions to the second edition of Dr. Anthony Vettese and the continuing supervision of Ms. Penny Cook. We would like to express our appreciation to readers of specific sections, namely, Dr. Arthur Keeney, Dr. Melvin Freeman, Dr. Marie Musarella, Mrs. Lynn Maund, and Mr. Keith Harrison. They have critically reviewed portions of the manuscript. We are indebted to Ms. Jill Klintworth for the typing and retyping required. New illustrations by Marie Lehman have been added to those of Mr. Norman Deer.

Harold A. Stein
Bernard J. Slatt
Raymond M. Stein

HOW TO GET THE MOST OUT OF THIS BOOK

This book is divided into sections corresponding to special interest areas. Part of the book is divided into a cross reference in an alphabetical dictionary format. While looking for any particular word, one can look in the dictionary section and refer to the vocabulary-building portion. The text of each chapter introduces the most commonly used words in the section.

One important reason for swiftly learning additional words will be that your attitude toward words will change. You will become enthusiastic about them. You will be curious about them. You will no longer pass over unfamiliar ones. You won't be happy if you do. They will challenge you to discover their meaning. This book is a first step toward forming a new and helpful habit of adding word power to your education. If you form this habit, you will learn words automatically and it will become effortless. It is not true that as you get older it is more difficult to learn. As you grow older you lose nothing in mental power if you keep up active interest. You may however, lose slightly in speed of mastery. The ability of the mind to think and create, barring illness, is with you until the age of 90 and past. Your body may get old, but your mind does not—if you care to use it. The mind never retires.

The sculptor Auguste Rodin did his finest work after 70. Michelangelo was 70 when he painted frescoes on the ceiling of the Sistine Chapel. Verdi composed the opera *Othello* at 75 and *Falstaff* at 80. Thomas Hardy at 88 was in the full flush of his literary career. It is true that 5% of all the works of geniuses have been done after the age of 80.

Everyone can profit by a word study. You can feel more confident by understanding ophthalmic jargon. On the other hand, few things can make you feel more inferior than stammering words that you are using incorrectly. There are a few simple rules to follow.

Good habits

If you are new in the field plan to use this book a short time each day. It really does not matter how fast or how slow you proceed; this depends on you and your time schedule. What is important is the consistency of your efforts. This is not a book that should be read in its entirety but should be read in "bite-sized" portions.

Words

Underline words throughout the book with which you are familiar and hear regularly. When you return to the section, you can then learn new words that have not been underlined with which you are unfamiliar. Write these words down on a separate card and carry them with you for a few days to remind you of these words. Try to recall the definitions. The recall of these words will heighten your working vocabulary. Use the words in an ophthalmic practice. Place the card where you will see it many times during the day so that you can refresh memory. Try to get the correct pronunciation from others you are in contact with. Try to explain the word to others who do not know the term. This is an important test as to whether or not you grasp the essence of its meaning.

Suggested program

The first approach is to read the entire chapter through. Then begin the following day on taking a few of the selected words and writing them as suggested. On the last weekend of each month, test yourself on all the words in the section that you have learned.

Pronunciation

Pronunciation is difficult for most people. The trouble is that our language does not have enough vowels to carry the many different sounds. Consequently, linguists have devised a phonetic system which is rather complicated. It is easier to try to gain pronunciation from staff that are familiar with the words. Develop a phonetic system of writing them down so that you will recall them.

CONTENTS

PART ONE
BASIC SCIENCE

PART TWO
REFRACTION, SPECTACLES, AND CONTACT LENSES

PART THREE
DISORDERS OF THE EYE

PART FOUR
SURGERY OF THE EYE

PART FIVE
OPHTHALMIC TESTS AND DEVICES AND MISCELLANEOUS TERMS

PART ONE

BASIC SCIENCE

CHAPTER 1

ANATOMY

The word *anatomy* is derived from the Greek word *anatome,* a compound of *ana-,* "over," and *-tome,* "to cut." Hippocrates, Galen, and many other ancient authors were familiar with the study of human dissection, and they coined a great number of terms whose use and meaning remain unchanged. Anatomy and its sister science pathology (Greek for "that which happens" plus "knowledge") were revived in 1315, when Modino performed the first documented human dissection since classical times. *Pathology* is the study of changes caused by diseases in the structure and function of the body. *Embryology* is the study of the origin and development of an individual organ.

Eyelids

The globe is covered externally by the eyelids to protect it from injury and excessive light and to spread a thin film of tears over the cornea. From *blepharo,* Greek meaning "eyelid," we derive words such as *blepharoplasty,* referring to any plastic surgery performed on the eyelid, and *blepharoptosis,* drooping eyelids. The muscle that elevates the eyelid is the *levator palpebrae superioris,* from *levator,* "to raise," *palpebra,* Latin meaning "an eyelid," and *superioris* meaning "upper." The triangular spaces at the junction of the upper and lower lids are called *canthi* from the Latin and later Greek *kanthas* meaning "angle." These canthi are denoted by the terms *medial* or *lateral,* the former being close to the nasal bridge (Fig. 1-1).

In the medial angle of the eyelids lies the *caruncle,* from Latin meaning "flesh," because this is a fleshy mound on the eye (Fig. 1-2). Adjacent to it lies a fold, the *plica semilunaris* from *plica* (Latin *plicare,* "to fold") and *semilunaris* (Latin "half moon") because the tissue is folded over in a half-moon shape and was originally a remnant of the third eyelid as found in lower animals.

The eyelids have as part of their structure hard plates called *tarsus* (Greek, "flat"), a term used by the ancient Greeks for various flattened objects such as the wing of a bird, the rudder of a ship, and the blades of oars. Because of the similar fluttering movement of the eyelids, the term *tarsus* was applied to the fibrocartilaginous plate that is found in the eyelid.

Within the tarsal plate of the eyelid lie the *meibomian glands* named after Heinrich Meibom (1638-1700), who published the first accurate description of these secreting glands. A disorder of the glands gives rise to a *chalazion,* a word derived from Greek meaning "hailstones," because of the similarity of these lumps in the eyelid to the appearance of large hailstones.

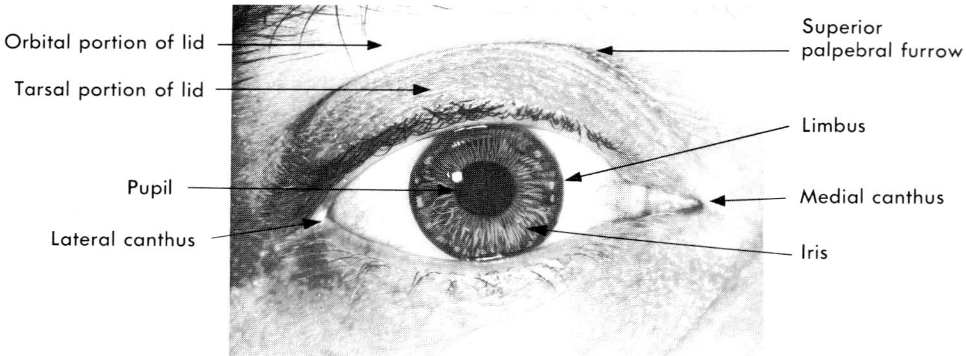

Fig. 1-1. Surface anatomy of the eye.

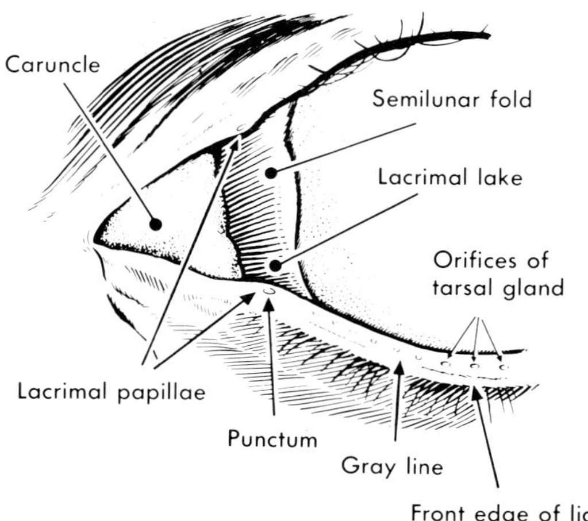

Fig. 1-2. Inner canthus, showing the semilunar fold and the caruncle. Normally the punctum is not visible unless the lower lid is depressed.

Tear duct system

On the medial aspect of the lower lid is a small *papilla,* meaning "elevation." At the apex of this elevation is a small opening, the *punctum* (Latin, "point"), which leads to a small canal called *canaliculus* leading to the *lacrimal sac. Lacrima* is Latin for "tear," and from it *lacrimation, lacrimal gland,* and other words pertaining to tears are derived (Fig. 1-3).

Conjunctiva

Conjunctiva is the filmy, moist membrane that covers the structure of the globe adjacent to the cornea. Conjunctiva covering the eye itself is referred to as the "bulbar conjunctiva," whereas the portion that lines the inner surface of the upper and lower eyelid is called the "palpebral portion." The "junctional bay" created when the two portions of the conjunctiva meet is referred to as the "fornix."

Cornea

The cornea is a clear, transparent structure with a brilliant, shiny surface. *Kerato,* from Greek meaning "hornlike," is the prefix pertaining to the cornea. Ancient Greeks believed the cornea resembled a thinly sliced horn of an animal.

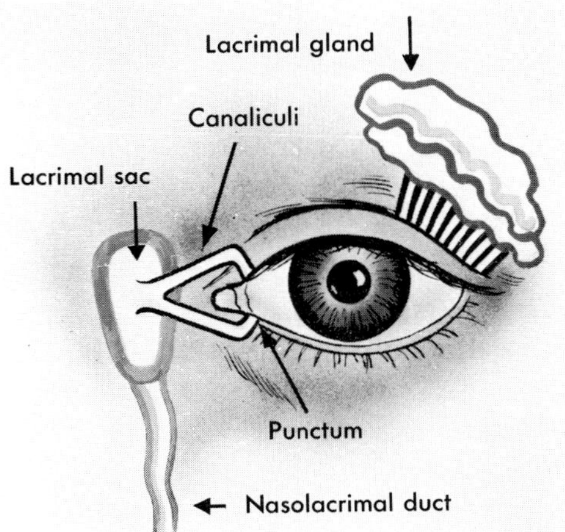

Fig. 1-3. Lacrimal apparatus. Tears produced by the lacrimal gland are drained through the punctum, lacrimal sac, and nasolacrimal duct into the nose.

Sclera

The *sclera* (Greek *scleros,* "hard") is the hard, firm, fibrous outer coat of the eye, which is continuous with the cornea (Fig. 1-4). At its posterior attachment, which is the *optic nerve,* the sclera becomes a thin, sievelike structure called the *lamina cribrosa* (Latin *cribrum,* "sieve"), in which the fine retinal nerve fibers leave the eye to form the optic nerve. The tissue overlying the sclera is the *episclera* (from Greek *epi,* "upon").

Uvea

Uvea was derived in ancient times from the Latin word *uva,* meaning "a grape," because the appearance seemed similar to a grape in which the stalk was torn out leaving a hole in the front, the hole being the pupil. Although at first the term

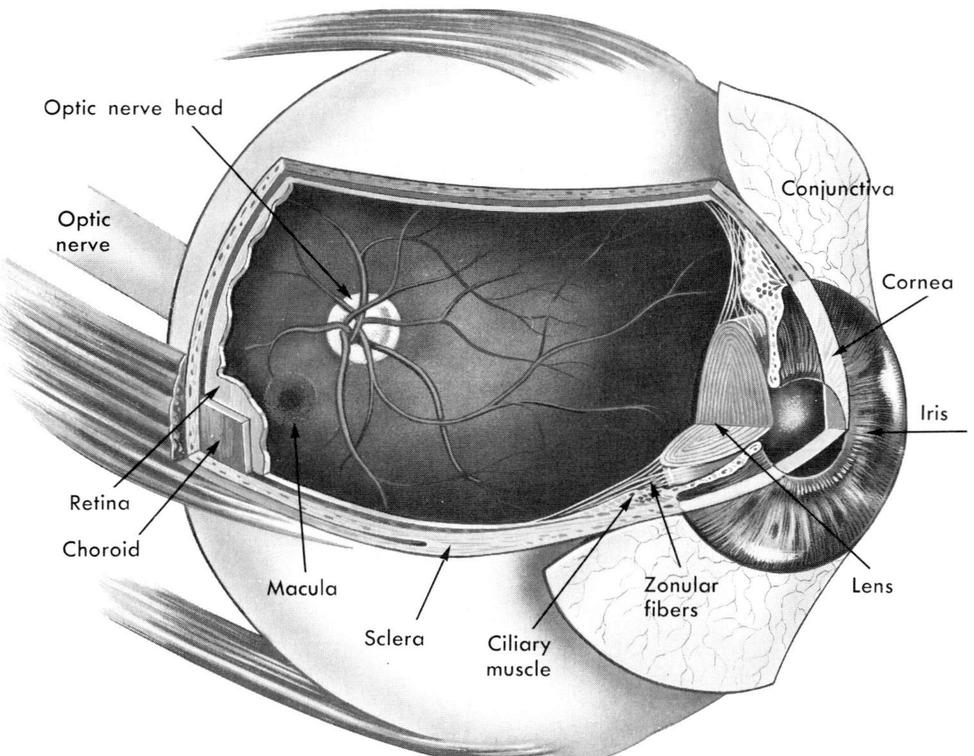

Fig. 1-4. Cutaway section of the eye.

uvea referred to the complete tunics of the eye, its use later was restricted to the inner coats. The uveal tract consists of three structures: the iris, ciliary body, and choroid.

The *iris* is derived from the Greek *iris,* meaning "rainbow," because of the beautiful and abundant colors that were present, particularly in the irises of animals and birds. The Greeks even named one of their goddesses Iris because when they saw a rainbow in the sky, they thought it was their goddess flying through the sky producing a multicolored trail. The central opening, the *pupil,* is derived from the Greek *pupa,* a small doll-like figure that was reflected from the center of the eye when one looked at someone's eyes.

The *ciliary body* is that body of muscle that supports cilia of hairlike processes called *ciliary processes* that are responsible for the major production of aqueous or watery fluid that passes from the *posterior chamber* to the *anterior chamber* of the eye (Fig. 1-5). The lens of the eye is suspended from the ciliary processes by *zonular fibers* (*zonule* being from both Greek and Latin meaning "ring" or "belt"), in which the fibers ring the *equator* of the crystalline lens.

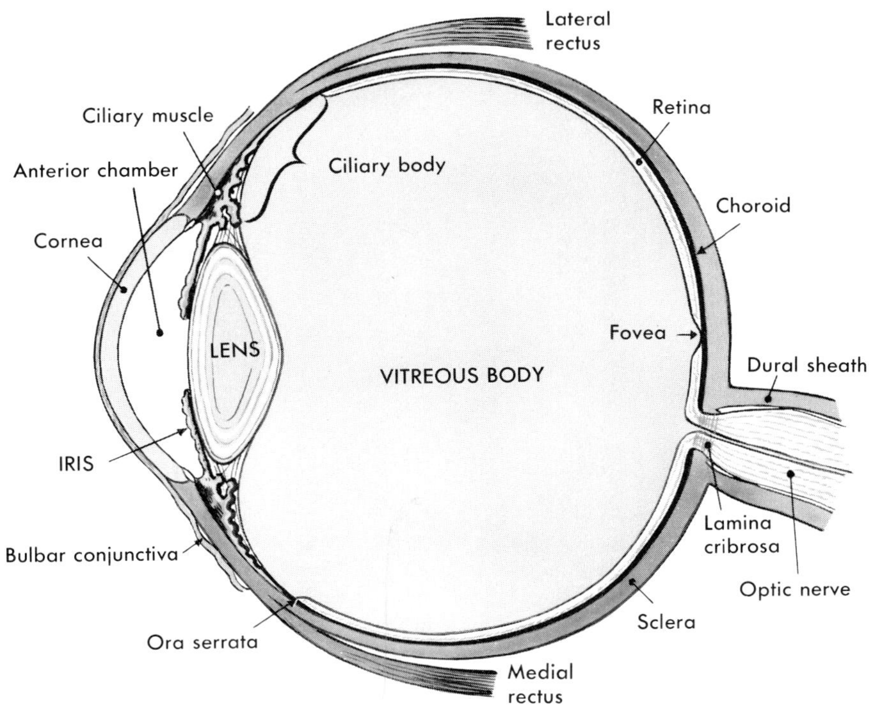

Fig. 1-5. The eye cut in horizontal section.

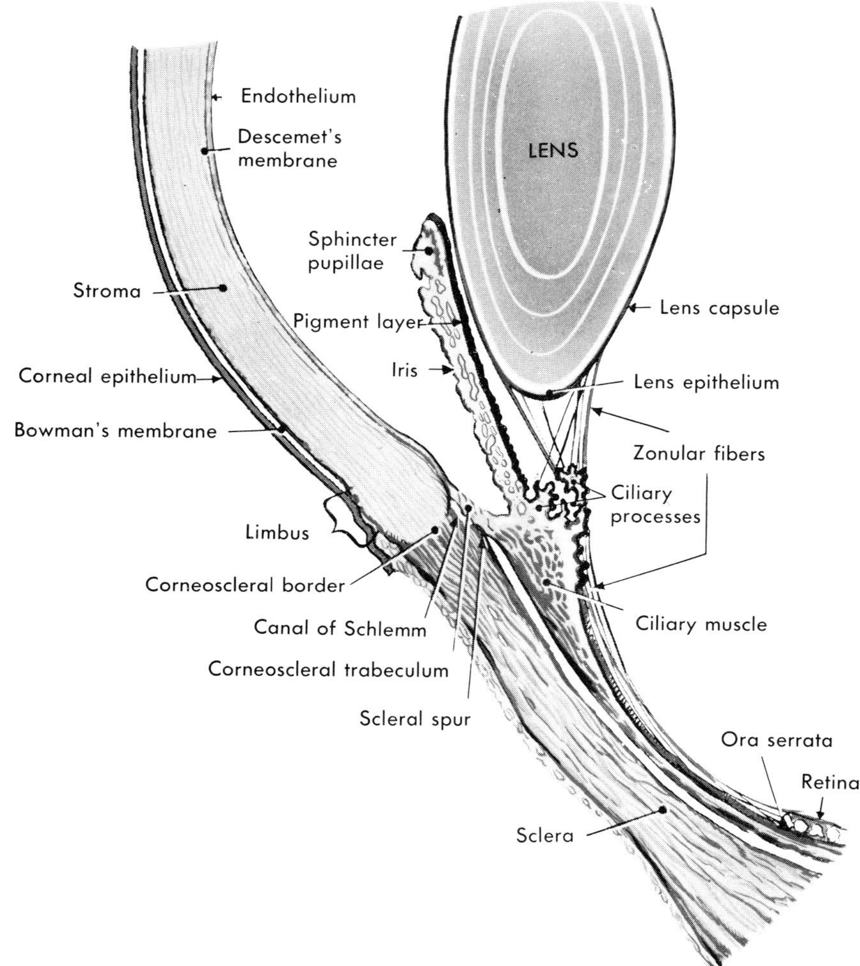

Fig. 1-6. Angle structures of the eye. The angle is formed between the iris and the back surface of the cornea, with aqueous humor of the anterior chamber interposed. The angle structures include corneoscleral trabeculum, canal of Schlemm, scleral spur, a small extension of the ciliary muscle, and the root of the iris.

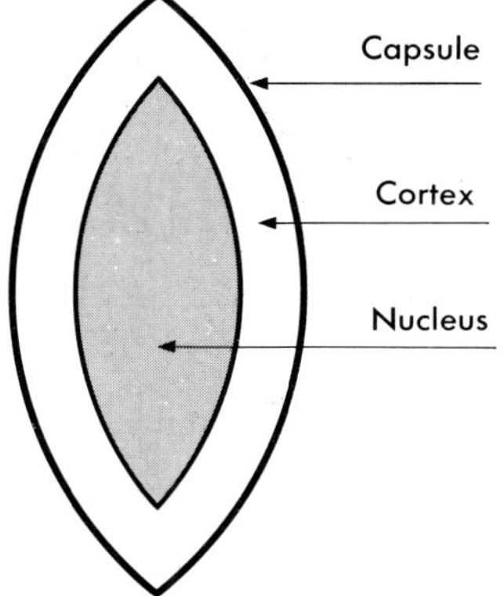

Fig. 1-7. Crystalline lens.

The term *choroid* is derived from the Greek *chorion,* which is the vascular membrane that envelopes the fetus and attaches it to the uterus. The choroid is a highly vascular coat of the eye that nourishes the outer layer of the retina.

Angle structures

The *angle* of the anterior chamber is the angle that lies between the iris and the cornea and through which the aqueous fluid flows out of the eye (Fig. 1-6). The anterior chamber contains this *aqueous* (Latin for "water").

The prefix *gonio-* from the Greek, meaning "corner," refers to the angle of the anterior chamber. Combining it with *scopy,* meaning "examination," results in the word *gonioscopy,* which refers to "examination of the angle of the anterior chamber."

Lens

The *lens* of the eye is a transparent biconvex structure situated between the iris and the vitreous (Fig. 1-7). The lens is covered by a capsule and consists of a central nucleus and an outer cortex.

Vitreous

The *vitreous* is a jellylike substance occupying the posterior concavity of the globe. The term is derived from the Latin *vitreous* meaning "glass," because of its transparent nature. *Vitrectomy* is a surgical procedure to remove a portion of the vitreous from the eye.

Retina

The *retina* is the sensory receptor for light and is composed of *rods* and *cones* whose names represent their physical configurations in the shape of rods and cones. There is a concentration of the cones in an area of the retina known as the *macula lutea* from the Latin *macular* meaning "a spot" and *lutea* meaning "yellow," because this portion of the retina appears as a yellow spot when seen in the stretched-out specimen of the retina. The junction of the retina and ciliary body in the periphery is called the *ora serrata* because of the serrated appearance of the attachment of the retina in the periphery. If the retina is detached at the periphery, it is said to be *disinserted.*

Ocular muscles

Of the six ocular muscles, the *medial, lateral, superior,* and *inferior rectus* muscles are named after their relative position to the globe. The *superior oblique* and *inferior oblique* muscles are also named after their anatomic relationship to the globe and, in addition, after the oblique nature of their mechanical pull on the rotations of the globe when the muscles contract (Fig. 1-8).

Visual pathways

As retinal fibers leave the optic nerves, half of the nasal fibers cross to the opposite side while half pass to the same side of the brain (Fig. 1-9). The place

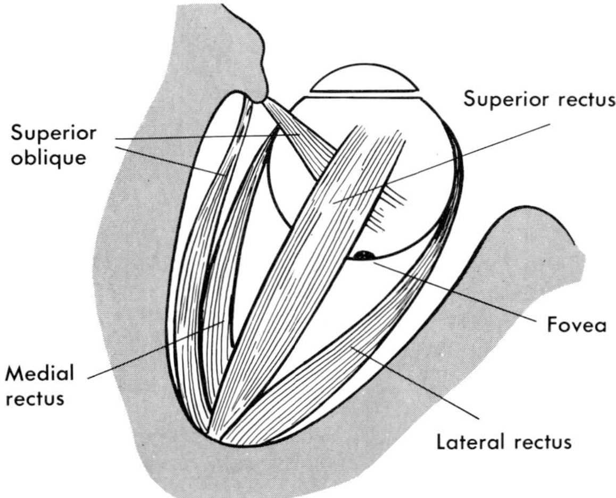

Fig. 1-8. Ocular muscles from above.

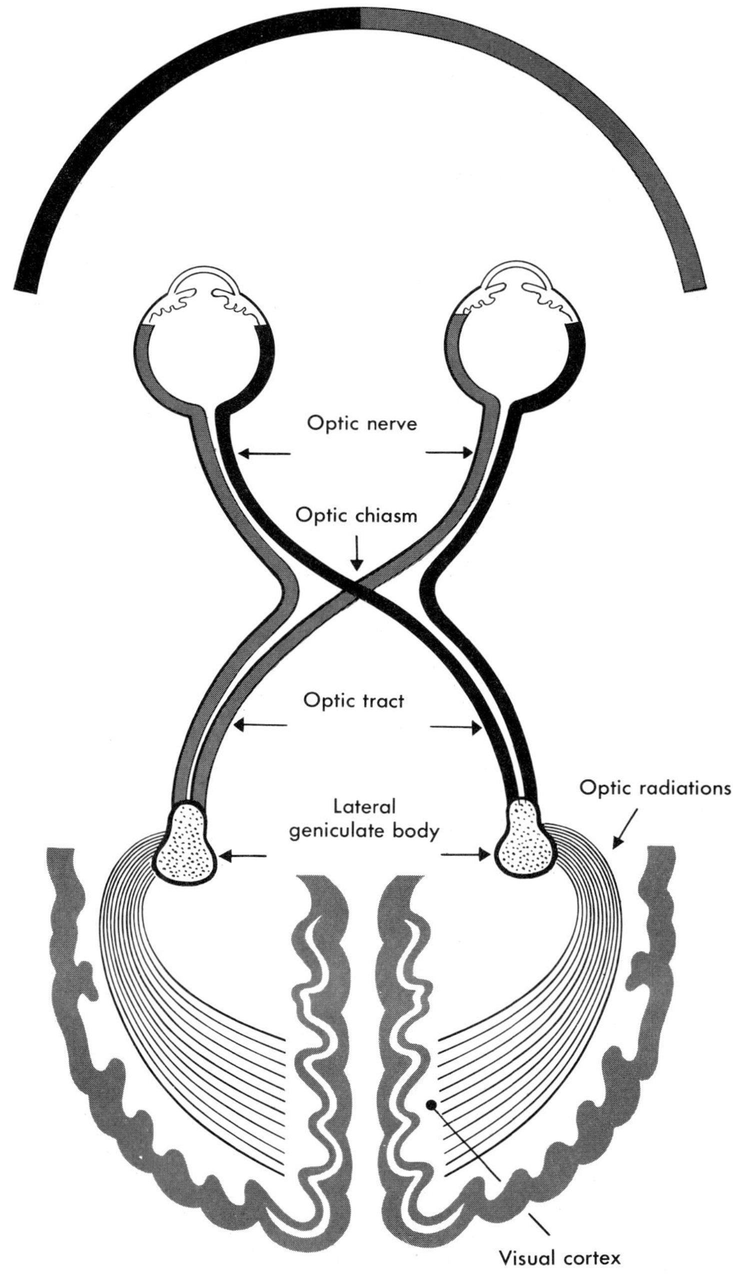

Fig. 1-9. Visual pathway. One half of the visual receptors from each eye extends to one side of the brain. Thus visual impulses from the right visual field of each eye will be transmitted to the left occipital lobe.

of crossing in the brain of the fibers from the two eyes is called the *optic chiasm* after the Greek *chi* or χ, which represents a crossing. The resemblance to the Greek *chi* was first recorded by Galen, the famous Greek physician to the emperor of Rome in 150 AD.

The fibers then form a band called the *optic tract* and pass to the *lateral geniculate body,* so named because this body in the brain is shaped like a knee (Latin *genu,* "knee"). The geniculate body is a relay station. From here fibers spread out in a fan-shaped manner and extend to the parietal and temporal lobes of the brain. From here the fibers continue to their final destination, the posterior segment of the occipital lobe, where the conscious recognition of objects occurs.

A *craniotomy* is a surgical exploration of the brain to identify and localize areas interrupting function. A *lobotomy* is a removal of a lobe of the brain. A *neurectomy* is an excision of a nerve either peripheral or central in origin.

A

abducens: the external rectus muscle.

abducens nerve: the sixth cranial nerve; the nerve that innervates the lateral rectus muscle that abducts the eye.

abduction: the outward rotation of an eye.

aberrant: a deviation from normal.

adductor: a muscle that exerts force toward the midline (for example, medial rectus).

adnexa oculi: accessory structures of the eye, such as the lacrimal apparatus and the eyelids.

anterior: in front.

anterior chamber: the portion of the eye lying between the cornea and the iris-lens and bathed in aqueous.

anterior segment: referring to the front part of the eye.

appendage of the eye: the accessory structures or adnexa of the eye, including the lacrimal apparatus, the conjunctiva, the cilia, the eyelids, and sometimes the extraocular muscles.

B

Bergmeister's papilla: embryologically, a small mass of glial cells that surrounds the hyaloid artery in the center of the optic disc and persists in the adult eye.

blind spot: the natural blind area of the retina where the optic nerve enters the eye.

Bowman's membrane: the thin membrane that lies between the corneal epithelium and the stroma. The second layer of the cornea.

Bruch's membrane: the membrane that lies between the choroid and the retinal pigment epithelium; same as lamina vitrea.

bulbar: pertaining to the globe.

C

canal of Schlemm: see *Schlemm's canal* (see Fig. 2-2).

canaliculi: the two passages from the puncta to the lacrimal sac.

capillaries: the smallest blood vessels, either arterial in function or venous in function.

carotid: refers to the internal carotid artery, one of the major blood vessels supplying the brain, or the carotid artery that serves the neck, face, and side of the head.

caruncle, lacrimal: see *lacrimal caruncle.*

cephalic: pertaining to the head, or the head end of the body.

choroid: vascular, intermediate coat that furnishes nourishment to the other parts of the eyeball.

cilia (plural), **cilium** (singular): eyelashes.

ciliary body: portion of the vascular coat between the iris and the choroid; consists of ciliary processes and the ciliary muscle.

Cloquet's canal: the space in the vitreous that formerly contained the hyaloid artery during development.

collarette: the junction of ciliary and pupillary zones of iris.

cones and rods: two kinds of cells that form a layer of the retina and act as light-receiving media. Cones are concerned with visual acuity and color discrimination; rods are used for motion and vision at low degrees of illumination (night vision).

conjunctiva: mucous membrane that lines the eyelids and wraps around the front part of the eyeball to end at the limbal junction of the cornea.

conjunctival sac: the potential space, lined by conjunctiva, between the eyelids and the eyeball; cul-de-sac.

cornea: clear, transparent portion of the outer coat of the eyeball, forming the covering of the anterior chamber.

corneal endothelium: a single layer of cells that lines the inside of the cornea.

corneal epithelium: multiple layers of cells that form the most superficial layer of the cornea. It rests on Bowman's membrane.

corneal lamella: one of the connective tissue sheets of the corneal stroma.

corneal stroma: multiple sheets of collagen in the center of the cornea, which make up 90% of its thickness.

cortex: the central portion of the crystalline lens.

cryptophthalmus: the congenital absence of eyelids.

crystalline lens: a transparent, colorless body suspended in the front part of the eyeball behind the iris. The function is to bring the rays of light to a focus on the retina.

cul-de-sac: the upper or lower conjunctival recess.

E

elevator muscle: an eye muscle that rotates the eye upward, that is, the superior rectus and inferior oblique muscles.

epicanthus: congenital skin fold that overlies the inner canthus and simulates the appearance of esotropia.

episclera: a loose structure of fibrous and elastic tissue on the outer surface of the sclera, containing a large number of blood vessels in contrast to the sclera, which contains none.

episcleral veins: the small veins on the surface of the sclera that collects aqueous from Schlemm's canal and blood from the anterior superficial portions of the eye.

epithelioid cell: a macrophage that resembles an epithelial cell.

equator: the sagittal midportion of the eye.

eversion of the eyelid: the folding back of the eyelid.

extraocular: pertaining to structures outside the sclerocorneal covering of the eye.

extraocular muscles: the six muscles that cause movement of the eye: medial and lateral recti, superior and inferior recti, and superior and inferior oblique.

eyeball: the globe or ball of the eye.

F

fissure: elliptical space between the open eyelids.

fornix: a loose fold of the conjunctiva, occurring where that part of the eyeball meets the conjunctiva lining the eyelid.

fovea: small glistening depression in retina; the part of the macula adapted for most acute vision and color vision. It consists largely of specialized cone receptors.

fundus: inside of the eye, primarily the retina, the macula, the optic disc, and the retinal vessels that can be seen with an ophthalmoscope.

H

hyaloid artery: an artery that was present during the embryologic period, running from the optic disc to the posterior lens.

I

inferior oblique muscle: muscle that tilts the eyeball up and inward.

inferior rectus muscle: muscle that pulls the eyeball downward.

infraversion: downward rotation of both eyes.

intorsion: rotation of the eye on an anteroposterior axis so that the upper portion of the eye moves inward toward the nose. The right eye rotates clockwise and the left eye counterclockwise.

intraocular: within the eye.

intraocular pressure: the pressure of the fluid within the eye measured in millimeters of mercury.

intrascleral nerve loop: a minute dark spot of uveal tissue on the sclera in which a long ciliary nerve loops in the anterior sclera.

intrinsic ocular muscles: the muscles situated inside the eyeball, consisting of the ciliary muscle, the sphincter pupillae, and the dilator pupillae.

irido-, irid-: pertaining to the iris.

iridodonesis: trembling of the iris on eye movement such as occurs with loss of lens support as in aphakia, dislocated lens, or pseudophakia.

iris coloboma: a notch or defect in the iris.

-itis: inflammation of.

L

lacrimal apparatus: the tear-producing and tear-disposal system of the eye.

lacrimal caruncle: a pink, fleshy, or relatively isolated skin located in the medial canthus area adjacent to the plica semilunaris.

lacrimal gland: a gland that secretes tears; it lies in the upper outer angle of the orbit.

lacrimal sac: the dilated upper end of the lacrimal duct.

lamina cribrosa: a perforated area of the choroid layer through which the optic nerve enters the eye.

lateral rectus muscle: muscle that pulls the eyeball outward.

lenticular: pertaining to (or shaped like) a lens.

limbus: the annular border between the clear cornea and the opaque scleral-conjunctival area.

longitudinal ciliary muscle: the portion of the ciliary body muscle that originates near the scleral equator and passes anteriorly to insert on the scleral spur.

M

meibomian glands: sebaceous glands of the eyelid.

meninges: the three membranes that cover the brain and spinal cord (dura mater, arachnoid, and pia mater).

microaphakia: anomaly in which the crystalline lens of the eye is abnormally small.

Mittendorf dot: opacity of the posterior lens capsule marking the former site of congenital hyaloid artery attachment.

mural cells: pericytes in retinal capillary walls.

N

nasolacrimal duct: the channel connecting the lacrimal sac with the nasal cavity.
neuro-: pertaining to nerves.
neuroepithelium: rods and cones.

O

oculocardiac reflex: see *reflex, oculocardiac.*
oculomotor: pertaining to the movements of the eye.
oculomotor nerve: third cranial nerve.
optic cup: the depression in the optic nerve head, which may be either normal or abnormal.
optic disc: see *optic nerve head.*
optic nerve head: the portion of the optic nerve (the second cranial nerve) that can be seen ophthalmoscopically in the fundus of the eye. It is almost round, pink, and usually has a depression (or cup) in its center.
optic tract: a band of nerve fibers extending from the optic chiasm to the lateral geniculate body and conducting the nasal half of the nerve fibers of the retina of the opposite eye.
orbicularis oculi: the eyelid muscle surrounding the eyelids which closes the eye.
orbit: the bony cavity containing the eye, which is formed by the frontal sphenoid, ethmoid, nasal, lacrimal, and maxillary bones.

P

palpebral fissure: the visible opening between the eyelids.
papilla: head of the optic nerve.
pars plicata: the part of the ciliary body having the ciliary processes.
periorbita: the loose connective tissues lining the inside of the orbit.
phakic: an eye possessing a crystalline lens.
photochemical visual pigment: light-sensitive visual pigment.
photoreceptor: rod or cone cells; the visual receptors of the eye.
pigment epithelium: the most posterior layer of cells in the retina containing pigment granules.
pituitary: a gland attached to the brain that secretes a number of important hormones; it is located near the junction of both optic nerves (the chiasm).
posterior chamber: space between the back of the iris and the front of the lens filled with aqueous.
posterior pole of eye: the center of the posterior curvature of the eyeball.
precorneal tear film: the tear film, composed of three layers, that covers the surface of the eye. The outermost layer consists of the *oily secretion* of the meibomian glands and the accessory, sebaceous glands. The primary function

of this layer is to regulate the evaporation rate. The middle layer of the precorneal tear film is secreted by the lacrimal glands and the accessory glands. This *aqueous layer* contains nutrient and protein materials. Uptake of oxygen through the tear film is essential for normal corneal metabolism. The third layer, *or mucous layer,* adsorbs to the corneal epithelium. Its primary function is to provide the wettable surface that retains the aqueous component of the tear.

pterygium: a triangular fold of growing membrane that may extend over the cornea from the white of the eye. It occurs most frequently in persons exposed to dust or wind over a long period of time.

pupillary reflex: see *reflex, pupillary.*

R

radiation, optic: a band of neural fibers in the temporal and parietal lobe of the brain that carry visual impulses to the occipital lobe of the brain.

rectus muscle: a muscle attached to the eyeball that controls eye movements.

reflex, oculocardiac: a slowing of the rhythm of the heart following compression of the eyes; if ocular compression produces acceleration of the heart, the reflex is called inverted.

reflex, pupillary: constriction of the pupil when stimulated by light and dilation of the pupil when exposed to dim light.

retinal element: any point on the retina.

rhodopsin: light-sensitive pigment contained in the rods.

S

sac: see *conjunctival sac, lacrimal sac.*

Schlemm's canal: a small narrow channel located in the anterior angle of the eye that carries the aqueous from the eye out to the aqueous veins. It lies between the root of the iris and the limbus.

scleral spur: the protrusion of which sclera into the anterior chamber angle, onto which the ciliary body inserts from behind.

second sight: increase in myopia with improved reading ability as occurs in the early stages of cataract.

situs inversus: a mirror reversal of the appearance of the optic disc in which the large vessels run predominantly nasalward from the disc.

socket: the conjunctival-lined orbit that remains after enucleation.

spherophakia: small round lens found in patients with certain mesodermal anomalies (Marchesani's syndrome).

sphincter iridis: the constrictor muscle of the iris.

subcutaneous: beneath the skin.

suprachoroid: outer layer of the choroid.

suture of the lens: junction of the ends of the lens fibers, which results in the formation of Y-shaped and stellate figures within the lens.

synapse: the anatomical junction between nerve fibers.

syndrome: a symptom and sign complex; a group of symptoms and signs that occur together and that may affect the whole body or any of its parts.

T

tarsal plate: the framework of connective tissue that gives shape to the eyelid.

Tenon's capsule: connective tissue layer that envelopes the whole eyeball except the cornea.

trabecular fibers: the fibers that make up the trabeculum or filtering area for the aqueous humor.

trabecular meshwork: multiple sheets of connective tissue with pores covered by endothelium through which the aqueous leaves the anterior chamber.

trabeculum: filtering tissue through which the aqueous humor passes on its way to Schlemm's canal. It lies in the iridocorneal angle.

trochlear nerve: fourth cranial nerve, which innervates the superior oblique muscle, which depresses the eye and produces extorsion.

tunica vasculosa lentis: vascular network that surrounds the fetal lens.

V

Vossius' ring: a ring of pigment visible on the front surface of the lens after trauma to the eye.

Z

zonule of Zinn: the suspensory apparatus of the lens. Numerous fine tissue strands ("ligaments") that stretch from the ciliary processes to the lens equator and support the lens in place.

CHAPTER 2

PHYSIOLOGY

Physiology (from Greek *physis,* "nature," and *logos,* "study"), deals with the vital functions of an organ or organism. The eye, in converting light images into information for the brain, undergoes numerous complex processes.

Light first traverses the cornea by impacting at its sharp, clear surface maintained by a healthy precorneal tear film. The corneal stroma itself is transparent as a result of a state of deturgescence or dehydration maintained by the endothelial pump mechanism. The greatest optical power of the eye is provided by the anterior corneal curvature.

Light must then pass through two optically empty fluids—the aqueous humor anteriorly and the gel-like vitreous further posteriorly. In between is the crystalline lens with its supporting *zonules* and their *ciliary body* attachments. These can alter its shape and therefore its power to focus on near objects. A *cataract* represents an opacity in the usually clear lens.

At the retina light induces *photochemical* processes through which light energy creates chemical reactions in the photoreceptor cells, the rods, and cones. These reactions ultimately result in nerve impulses transmitted through the optic nerve to the brain.

The critical shape of the eyeball results from its intraocular pressure. A normal intraocular pressure is a balance between the production of aqueous humor by the ciliary body and its drainage through the trabecular meshwork and Schlemm's canal. An upset of this balance (usually poor drainage) results in a high pressure and glaucoma.

There are several advantages to having two eyes, including increased *peripheral field* and *stereopsis,* or *depth perception.* Stereopsis requires *binocular vision* and *fusion,* activities in which eye movements are precisely coordinated (Fig. 2-1). Children with strabismus who do not develop binocularity will not have stereopsis.

Other factors maintain eye health. The intact conjunctival and corneal epithelium act as a barrier to infection, and any disruption such as corneal abrasion leaves the eye vulnerable until healed. The constant flow of tears brings fresh oxygen, carries away wastes, and suppresses bacteria through its enzyme component called *lysosyme.*

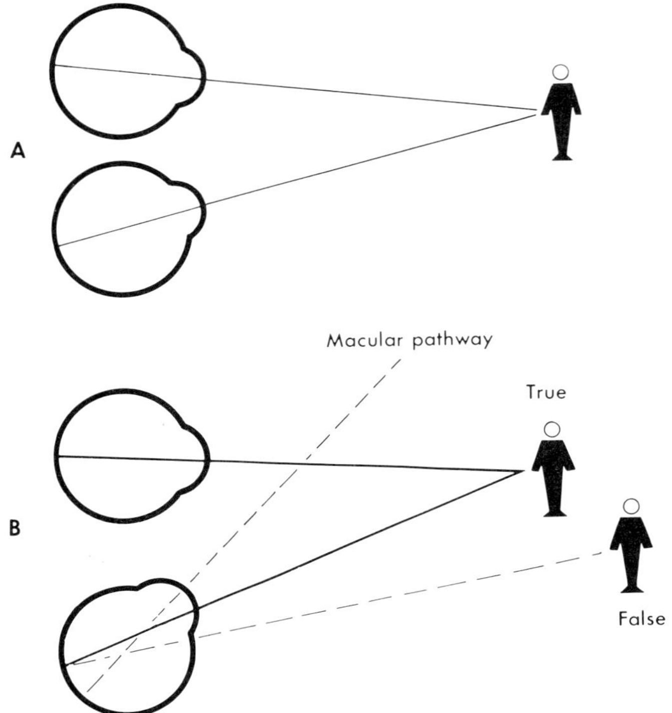

Fig. 2-1. A, Binocular vision (both eyes the same figure). B, One eye is turned in, resulting in double vision. In this case the figure is received by the macula of one eye and a point nasal to the macular of the turned eye. The projection of this nasal point results in the individual seeing two images instead of one of the same figure. This is an example of uncrossed diplopia, as seen in eso deviations. (From Stein, H.A., and Slatt, B.J.: The ophthalmic assistant, ed. 4, St. Louis, 1983, The C.V. Mosby, Co.)

A

abduction: horizontal movement of the eye away from the midline.

accommodation: focusing of the eye on a near object through relaxation of the ciliary muscle and thickening of the lens.

adduction: horizontal movement of the eye toward midline.

amblyopia: diminished vision in one or both eyes usually resulting from lack of proper input during the developmental childhood years.

amplitude of accommodation: the amount of accommodation or near focusing that the eye is capable of as measured in diopters (diminishes with age).

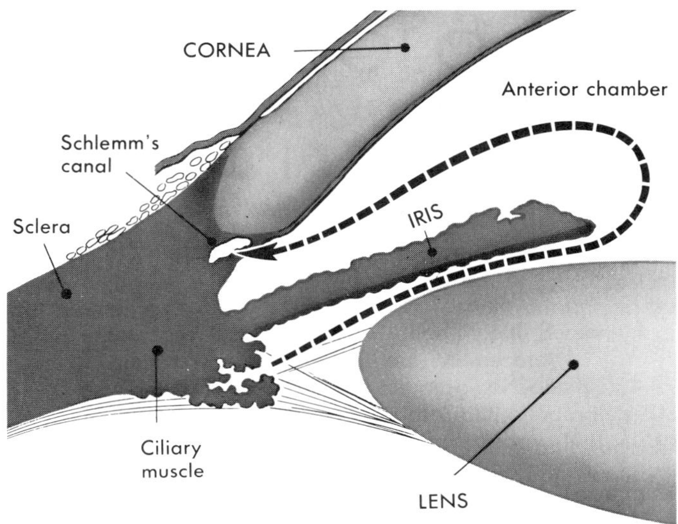

Fig. 2-2. Flow of aqueous humor. Aqueous humor is largely produced by the ciliary processes in the posterior chamber and flows into the anterior chamber and leaves the eye through Schlemm's canal. (From Stein, H.A., and Slatt, B.J.: The ophthalmic assistant, ed. 4, 1983, The C.V. Mosby, Co.)

anterior chamber: the space filled with aqueous humor bounded by the cornea anteriorly and the iris and lens posteriorly.

aqueous humor: the optically clear fluid in the anterior and posterior chambers responsible for intraocular pressure. It is produced at the ciliary processes in the posterior chamber, travels to the anterior chamber through the pupil, and drains through the trabecular meshwork in the iridocorneal angle. (See Fig. 2-2.)

aqueous tear layer: the middle layer of the tear film and major compound of reflex tears produced by the lacrimal gland.

B

basal tear secretion: the constantly present tear production not under any reflex or nervous control.

C

central vision: refers to the fine 20/20 vision, produced at the fovea roughly in the center of the retina by cone cells (also foveal vision).

chamber depth: depth of the anterior chamber. The distance between the cornea and the iris/lens diaphragm, very shallow in narrow-angle glaucoma.

choroidal vessels: the vascular coat surrounding the retina and supplying the outer one third of the retina.

chromophores: pigments, primarily in the lens, that filter out ultraviolet light. These increase with age and ultraviolet exposure.

ciliary body: the group of muscles behind the iris that influence outflow and produce accommodation.

ciliary processes: fingerlike projections from the ciliary body that produce aqueous humor and provide attachment for the zonules.

cones: the retinal photoreceptor cell responsible for color vision and fine central vision.

consensual light reflex: constriction of the pupil in the opposite eye when light is shone into its fellow eye.

convergence: movement of the eyes toward each other and the midline as when focusing on a near object.

D

dark adaptation: adjustment of the eye (retinal photoreceptors mainly) to dark conditions.

deuteranopia: deficiency of one pigment mediating green.

F

fusion: the ability of the two eyes to see an object as a single image.

I

intorsion: a rotational movement of the eye where the 12 o'clock position of the cornea tilts toward the midline.

intraocular pressure: the fluid pressure within the eye measured in millimeters of mercury.

iridocorneal angle: the space containing the drainage structures such as the trabecular meshwork located where the cornea meets the root of the iris.

iris dilator: muscle fibers in the iris that dilate the pupil.

iris sphincter: muscle fibers in the iris surrounding the pupil that constrict the pupil.

L

light adaptation: adjustment of the eye (mainly photoreceptors) to well-lit conditions.

lipid tear layer: the outermost component of the tear film secreted by meibomian glands in the lid and responsible for slowing the evaporation of tears.

lysozyme: the antibacterial enzyme normally in tears.

M

marginal tear strip (tear meniscus): the strip of tears adjacent to the eyelid margin. Its height can be a measure of the tear film adequacy.

miosis: constriction of the pupil by the iris sphincter in response to light or the near reflex.

monochromat: the state of having only one of the three color-sensitive pigments and thus grossly abnormal color vision.

mucous tear layer: the tear layer closest to the cornea, secreted by goblet cells in the conjunctiva and responsible for even wetting of the tear film.

mydriasis: enlargement of the pupil by the iris dilator muscle as occurs in darkness or in response to dilating drops.

N

near reflex (accommodative reflex): through relaxation of the ciliary muscle the lens becomes thicker allowing the eye to focus for near. At the same time the pupils constrict, and the eyes converge.

nerve fiber bundle: refers to the nerve fibers entering the optic nerve from the retina as bundles because of the pattern of their distribution.

O

optically empty: a liquid or material that is optically empty does not scatter or interfere with the transmission of light.

outflow: refers to the drainage of the aqueous humor out of the eye.

P

parasympathetic: the part of the involuntary nervous system mediated by acetylcholine and responsible, for example, for constriction of the pupil and accommodation.

peripheral vision: vision at the extremes of the visual field, grosser than central vision and mediated by the rods.

photochemistry: chemical reactions induced by light, as occurs in the retina.

photopic vision: pertaining to vision in light-adapted conditions—mainly a cone function.

photoreceptors: the cells in the retina (rods and cones) that receive light energy, convert it into chemical processes, and transform the energy into nerve impulses.

posterior chamber: the space containing aqueous humor bounded by the lens, posterior surface of iris, and zonules.

precorneal tear film: the part of the tear film coating the cornea and providing its clarity.

primary action: the major action of an extraocular muscle, e.g., the primary action of the superior rectus is to elevate the eye.

protanope protanomalous: a form of color vision abnormality in which the red color-sensitive pigment is deficient or absent.

pupil block: occurs in acute glaucoma when aqueous cannot pass through the pupil because of iris/lens contact.

R

range of accommodation: the amount of accommodation of which the eye is capable measured in centimeters from the nearest to farthest point of focus.

reflex tear secretion: aqueous tear production in response to physical irritants or emotion.

retinal vessels: the arteries and veins on the surface of the retina feeding the inner two thirds of the retina.

rods: the photoreceptor cells of the retina most important in dim lighting and peripheral vision. They are far more numerous than cones.

S

Schirmer test: a test for tear secretion in which the end of a 5 × 40 mm piece of filter paper is placed in the fornix and its wetting is measured in millimeters after 5 minutes.

scotopic vision: vision under dark-adapted conditions.

secondary action: the second most important action (in moving the eyeball) on an extraocular muscle, e.g., the superior rectus muscle adducts the eye in addition to its primary action of elevating it.

stereopsis (depth perception): a binocular function operating primarily at near, allowing precise judgment of depth or relative distances.

suppression: the input from one eye is relatively ignored by the brain when it would be otherwise confusing, e.g., as in a child with strabismus who would have double vision with one eye deviated.

sympathetic nervous system: the part of the involuntary or autonomic nervous system with norepinephrine and epinephrine as its transmitters, responsible, for example, for dilating the pupil or constricting blood vessels.

T

tear break up time: a measure of the adequacy of the precorneal tear film in which the eye is held open and the time measured for dry spots in the cornea to occur. Sometimes referred to as BUT, or break up time of tears.

tear pump: the hypothetical system involving the eyelid muscles, canaliculi, and lacrimal sac responsible for actively draining tears from the eye.

trabecular meshwork: the drainage network in the iridocorneal angle through which aqueous humor leaves the eye.

trichromat: the normal state of having all three color-sensitive pigments in the cones and thus normal color vision.

trichromatic color theory: the theory of color vision production using a neurological mixing of information from blue-, green-, and red-sensitive pigments in the cones.

V

venous pulsations: the normal pulsation of the central retinal vein, coincident with the heartbeat, visible with the ophthalmoscope.

vergence: movement of the eyes in opposite directions as in convergence or divergence.

version: referring to a binocular eye movement.

Z

zonules: the supporting fibers of the lens attached at their other end to the ciliary body.

CHAPTER 3

OPTICS

Optics may be divided into *physical optics,* which is concerned primarily with the nature and propagation of light; *geometric optics,* which is the branch of optics in which the laws of geometry can be used to design lenses that include spectacles, optical instruments, telescopes, microscopes, cameras, and other lens instruments; and *physiological optics,* which deals with the mechanism of vision and the physiology and psychology of seeing.

Optical terminology is frequently linked with refractive terminology. The latter represents terms used to describe the physiological basis of vision and also the terms related to lens designs to correct those defects in the human eye system in which the rays of light do not focus clearly on the retina.

Physical optics

White light is composed of a number of colors in which the component colors are always found in the same order. Sir Isaac Newton called this arrangement the *spectrum,* and he called the spreading effect caused by a prism, *dispersion.*

When a ray of light passes centrally through a lens or eye, it is said to be *axial,* and the central ray is called the *principal* ray. Rays parallel and just outside the central or principal axial ray are called *paraxial* and those in the periphery called *peripheral or marginal* (Fig. 3-1). On the other hand, a ray may enter from an angle and is called an *oblique* ray.

When light passes from one medium to another, it changes its direction or is *refracted* or bent back because light travels at different speeds in different media. A ray of light entering a medium is called the *incident* ray, and the ray emerging from the media is called the *emergent* ray. The angle that the incident ray makes with the perpendicular surface of the new media is called the *angle of incidence.* The angle the ray makes in the new medium by its change of direction is called the *angle of refraction* (Fig. 3-2). For any given medium, a fundamental law of optics exists, called *Snell's law;* it states that the *index of refraction* is equal to the sine of the angle of incidence divided by the sine of the angle of refraction.

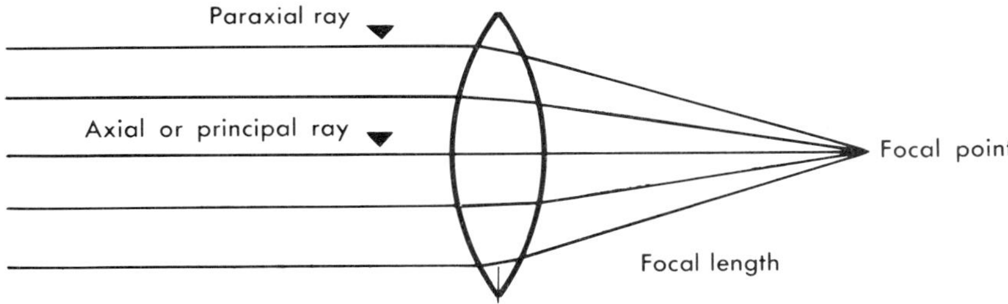

Fig. 3-1. Relationship of the axial and paraxial rays of light. The focal point is the point at which emerging rays come to a focus, and the focal length is the distance from the center of the lens to the focal point.

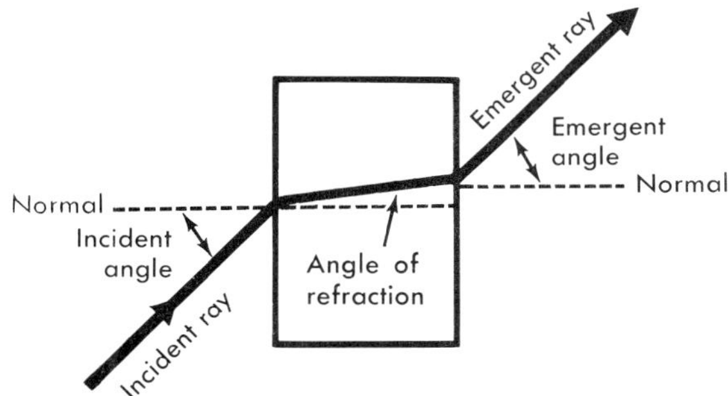

Fig. 3-2. This diagram shows the incident and emergent rays of light through glass. Note the incident angle and the angle of refraction.

Geometric optics

The discovery of the law of refraction in 1621 by Willebrod Snell was the first advance in geometric optics since Euclid. Before this, methods that had been discovered empirically were used to manufacture spectacles and other optical devices. Snell's law combined facts about light and the media through which it passes with geometry to formulate a principle by which a refractive index could be calculated.

A *concave lens* is a lens of plastic or glass in which one or both surfaces are curved inward toward the center of the lens. A *convex lens* is one in which one or both surfaces are curved outward with the thickest part at the center of the lens. When light strikes a concave lens, the emergent rays *diverge* or spread out, whereas in the case of convex lenses the emergent rays *converge* or come together.

These lenses are thus sometimes referred to as *diverging* or *converging lenses.* The former are *minus lenses* used to correct myopia; the latter are *plus lenses* used to correct hyperopia.

Focus is derived from Latin meaning "hearth" or "fireplace," because this was the central point in any room in ancient times. The *focal point* of a lens or mirror is the point in which all the rays emerging from a lens or mirror system come to a common point. The distance this point is from the lens or mirror is the *focal length* (see Fig. 3-1). The point of convergence of the rays is called the *real* focus. For diverging rays, the point at which they would meet if their direction were reversed is called the *virtual* point. A lens must be considered in terms of its focal length. The power or strength of the lens is expressed in *diopters,* a term introduced in 1872 by Felix Monoyer to overcome the cumbersome methods of explaining front and back surfaces of lenses. The *diopter* is the reciprocal of a given lens' focal length in meters. A lens that converges parallel rays of light at a distance of 1 M has a value of 1 D. A focal length of 0.5 M has a value of 2 D. The shorter the focal length, the higher the dioptric value. A *prismatic dioptric* value of 1 is given to a prism that bends a beam of light 1 cm at 1 M.

Aberrations or deviations from ideal optical conditions do occur with lenses. *Spherical* aberration exists when peripheral rays, in striking the lens edge, do not come to the same focal point as the paraxial rays or rays near the center of the lens (Fig. 3-3). *Chromatic aberrations* occur because the edge of a lens behaves like a prism and breaks light up into its spectral components, permitting color fringes to appear.

A *spherical* lens is one in which every point comes to a common focal point. A *cylinder* is a lens with one power in one direction, known as a *meridian,* and with a different power in the opposite *meridian,* set 90 degrees apart. The *axis* or *cylinder axis* is the opposite to the meridian in which the cylinder is oriented. For example, a lens with a stronger curvature meridian at 90 degrees would have its axis at 180 degrees. *Spherocylinders* are combinations of spheres and cylinders. Such a lens system has two focal points. The area between these two focal points is cone shaped and called the *conoid of Sturm.*

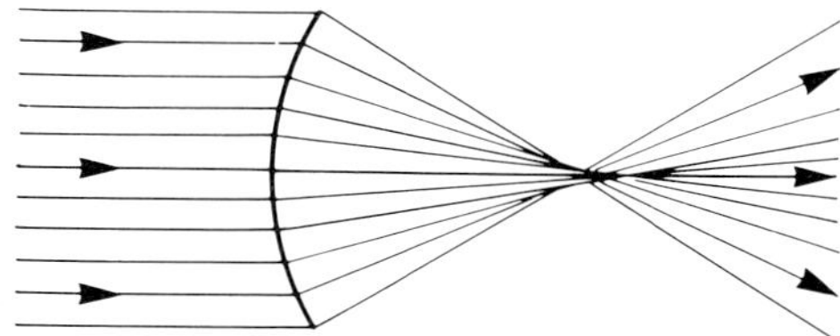

Fig. 3-3. Spherical aberration. The rays of light on refraction by the lens are converged to a meeting area rather than to a single focal point.

A small muscle imbalance or deviation between the two eyes may be corrected by prisms ground in spectacles. A *prism* is a wedge-shaped piece of plastic with an *apex* at its thinnest portion and a *base* at its thickest position.

A

achromatic: a lens that is corrected for color aberration.

angstrom unit: unit of wavelength to one ten-millionth of a millimeter (now preferred: nanometer, or one millionth of a millimeter).

aspheric lens: a lens that corrects for peripheral distortion by having a peripheral ellipsoid shape.

B

bicentric: a lens that is ground with two optical centers.

bioconcave lens: a lens that is bowed inward at the center of the lens.

bioconvex lens: a lens that is bowed outward at the center of the lens.

C

critical angle: the angle beyond which a ray of light passing from a higher to a lesser refractive medium cannot emerge.

D

diffraction: the small amount of spreading of light around an aperture. The larger the aperture, the greater the diffraction.

distortion: an aberration through optical glass that causes objects to appear in other than their true form.

E

electromagnetic spectrum: range of radiant energy that has a variable frequency and wavelength and a constant velocity.

emergent ray: the ray of light leaving a medium.

F

flint glass: glass sometimes used in ophthalmic lenses with a higher index of refraction (1.62) than crown glass. Also used as bifocal segments when fused with main lens of crown glass.

focal point: the point at which distant light comes to a focus after being reflected or refracted.

footcandle: unit of illumination. One footcandle is generated by 1 lumen of light on 1 square foot of surface.

I

incident ray: the ray of light entering a medium.

index of refraction: the ratio of the velocity of light in air to the velocity of light in a given medium. Index of refraction equals speed in air divided by speed in medium.

L

laser: initials stand for light amplification by stimulated emission of radiation; an instrument that transforms an intense beam of light into heat to seal holes in the retina, destroy new blood vessels, and produce iridectomies for glaucoma.

N

n: usually the symbol for index of refraction.

nanometer: unit of wavelength equal to 1 millionth of a millimeter.

O

optical bench: a bar on which are mounted slidable adjustable holders for lights, lenses, mirrors, and screens. It is used for demonstrations of the optical functions of lenses and light.

P

parallax: the apparent displacement or change of position of an object when viewed from different places, such as the alternate use of the right and left eye or the viewing of an object through a moving lens. A plus lens creates an "against" movement of the image. A minus lens creates a "with" movement of the image.

R

radius: the straight-line distance from a point to a curve (for example, from the center of a circle to its boundary).

reflection: the rebounding of light from a surface.

refractive index: the refractive power of a substance in comparison with that of air.

S

schematic eye: a diagrammatic representation of the optical constants of an emmetropic eye.

slab-off: a method of creating a bicentric lens by grinding a prism-shaped slab from one surface of the lens, usually the convex surface.

Snell's law: the law of refraction of light, based on the fact that light travels at different speeds in different media. Snell's law states that the index of refraction is equal to the sine of angle of incidence divided by the sine of the angle of refraction.

Stiles-Crawford effect: light passing through the center of the pupil of the eye is more effective in evoking the sensation of brightness than the same amount of light passing through an equal area near the edge of the pupil.

V

vertex, back: the point from which the neutralizing or back focus of a lens is measured.

vertex, front: the point from which the neutralizing or front focus of a lens is measured.

vertex distance: the distance from the back surface of a lens to the apex of the cornea. For practical purposes the measurement is taken against the closed lid. It is important to measure the vertex distance if the trial lenses are greater than ±4 D, since it can affect the final power of the lens.

visual axis: a line that connects a point in space with the fovea centralis of the retina.

CHAPTER 4

PHARMACOLOGY: OPHTHALMIC DRUGS AND TOXIC SUBSTANCES

Drugs

Most drugs that are used by ophthalmologists are standardized. They are made by commercial drug firms and are uniform in quality. The role of the pharmacist has changed. That person is no longer preparing drugs but is instead explaining to the patient the method of taking the drug, its shelf life, and its side effects. The physician has to be concerned about toxicity, allergic reactions, and normal side effects of each drug taken.

Despite the uniformity of drugs, a knowledge of ophthalmic medications should be present to render the best service to the patient. Certain drugs such as the eyedrops, pilocarpine, may have a duration of activity of only a few hours and may need to be used three to four times a day to yield satisfactory results. The terms relating to a drug should be understood.

A *solution* is a liquid vehicle for drug delivery to the eye. The problem with solutions is their short contact time (measured in minutes) with the eye and their absorption systemically, particularly when they drop through the lacrimal punctum and travel down the nasolacrimal duct and empty into the nose where they are absorbed into the general circulation.

The *pH* of a drug refers to its acid-base balance. Most ophthalmic solutions with a range of 3.5 to 10.5 are acceptable to the eye.

Tonicity refers to the amount of sodium chloride in solution. Initially, ophthalmic solutions were prepared to make them *isotonic* with tears having a 0.9% sodium chloride equivalent. To achieve this, many *buffers* were used, the phosphate buffer being the most commonly used at present. The range of tolerance of sodium chloride equivalents is quite broad, ranging from 0.7% to 2%.

Solutions that are below normal saline concentrations are referred to as *hypotonic.* Those that are stronger than normal saline are referred to as *hypertonic.*

Some solutions are affected by exposure to air as they *oxidize*. Epinephrine and phenylephrine hydrochloride oxidize in the presence of air, and when this occurs they turn brown and alter their chemistry. Physostigmine partially oxidizes and changes to a pink color. Some solutions alter or *hydrolyze* on exposure to water.

Sterility means that the solution is free from all vegetable organisms such as bacteria, viruses, or fungi or their spores. Some bacteria grow well in fluid media, so the active pharmaceutical is prescribed dry and reconstituted in solution when dispensed. Fluorescein is frequently prepared dry on strips to avoid contamination by the bacterium *Bacillus pyocyaneus (Pseudomonas aeruginosa)*.

Most drugs are sterilized by autoclaving. Once a drug container has been opened, it can easily be contaminated. This happens by touching the orifice of the bottle or dropper to the eye. So for surgical cases when the eye is opened, single-dose solutions are used.

To keep a solution sterile, a *preservative* is needed. Preservatives inhibit the multiplication of organisms. This is important for any drug that is going to be used more than once. Preservatives can be irritating. The more commonly used preservatives include *benzalkonium chloride, chlorobutanol,* quaternary ammonium compounds, phenols, and organic mercurials.

Administration of drugs

Iontophoresis is a method of achieving better drug penetration. The drug is applied to the eye with an eyecup that has an electrode. The charged eyecup creates a difference in potential that aids the passage of the drug across the corneal barrier. It is not used too often in modern therapeutics.

Subconjunctival injection refers to the injection of a drug under the conjunctiva or Tenon's capsule. This approach is used to treat severe intraocular infections and to dilate a pupil bound down by adhesions.

A *retrobulbar injection* is an injection behind the eye with a long needle. It is used to anesthetize and immobilize the eye before cataract surgery and also for chorioretinal infections.

A *peribulbar injection* is an injection that is given around the eye rather than in the muscle cone behind the eye.

Drug therapy

Alkaloids are solutions with a pH greater than 7. Ophthalmic solutions are more stable if the pH is reduced artificially to 5. As the pH is lowered, the stability of the drug increases. Frequently a 2% boric acid solution is used to reduce the pH to 5.

An *alkaloid* is a solution in dissociated or undissociated form. In dissociated form it is water soluble, and in the undissociated form it is fat soluble. Alkaloids are ideal for passing through the cornea, since both types of solubility are present to enable penetration through corneal epithelium and stroma. Solutions are often used for daytime delivery of drugs.

Ophthalmic ointments are more stable, and a petrolatum base is most commonly used. In such a matrix there is no worry about tonicity, pH, oxidization, or ionization. Ointments are usually not sterilized with autoclaving or preservatives. They are used at bedtime for a longer duration of effect.

Chelating agents such as ethylenediaminetetraacetic acid (EDTA) are used to remove calcium deposits in the cornea. The epithelium of the cornea is removed, and the EDTA is kept in contact with the eye with an eyecup. The calcium ions become incorporated into the molecule of EDTA.

A *staining agent* is a dye used to demonstrate epithelial defects of the cornea. Fluorescein is the most commonly used.

Tattooing is a method of injecting mineral pigments into the cornea to change the color of an ugly white corneal scar. *Gold and platinum salts* are introduced into the stroma of the cornea. When they oxidize (by exposure to the air), they produce a black color, the same as the pupil of the eye, and thus tattoo the cornea by obliterating the unsightly white color of a corneal scar.

Drugs given in the form of eyedrops are called *topical drugs.* Many topical drugs such as antibiotics do not enter the eye. The epithelium of the cornea is a barrier to any drug that is not fat soluble. Penicillin has a low lipid solubility, and therefore it does not enter the anterior chamber of the eye. Chloramphenicol has sufficient lipid solubility to enter the eye. Corticosteroids penetrate the eye but only as far as the anterior chamber.

Systemic drugs are those taken by mouth or given intramuscularly or intravenously. Such drugs are used for inflammations of the lids, orbits, retina, and optic nerve. For these areas it is the only way to reach the site of the problem. A drug must be lipid or fat soluble to pass the blood-aqueous barrier.

Parasympathomimetic agents stimulate structures innervated by the postganglionic parasympathetic nerves. These agents enhance the release of acetylcholine, which activates smooth muscle, skeletal muscles, sweat glands, and all autonomic ganglia. They are called *cholinergic* drugs. They cause secretion by salivary, gastric, lacrimal, and bronchial glands. They also stimulate involuntary muscles such as in the bladder, bronchi, and gastrointestinal tract. These agents also activate the ciliary muscle and the sphincter muscle of the iris. Because of this action, they are used to constrict the pupil. Pilocarpine falls into this category of drugs.

Sympathomimetic agents stimulate structures innervated by the sympathetic nerves, that is, heart, blood vessels, and the dilator muscle of the iris. Because of this action, they are used to dilate the pupil. In ophthalmic practice, they are used to dilate the pupil before ophthalmic examination. Phenylephrine hydrochloride

(Neo-Synephrine) is such a drug. These drugs are called *adrenergic* agents because their action is similar to that of epinephrine (Adrenalin).

Drugs that block the action of acetylcholine are called cholinergic blocking agents. Included in this group are atropine, scopolamine, cyclopentolate (Cyclogyl), and homatropine.

Anticholinesterase drugs permit the accumulation of acetylcholine by inactivating the eyzyme cholinesterase. The most commonly used drugs in this category are physostigmine or eserine and neostigmine. These agents cause constriction of gastrointestinal, urinary, and bronchioli muscles. They also cause increased salivation, sweating, and lacrimation. In the eye, they cause pupillary constriction and stimulate the ciliary muscle.

Complications of drug therapy

The major complications of drug therapy are *hypersensitivity* and *toxic reaction.*

Hypersensitivity reaction is an inflammatory response to a drug that previously had sensitized the tissues. For example, the drug neomycin is quite sensitizing to ocular tissues. When neomycin is given locally for infection, the condition may seem to become worse if a local hypersensitivity inflammatory response is initiated. The most common type of allergic reactions are skin eruptions. Other areas of sensitivity include asthma, drug fever, hepatitis, and anaphylactic reactions.

An *idiosyncrasy* is a peculiarity in which an individual reacts in a bizarre fashion to a drug.

A *toxic reaction* is predictable and is an exaggerated response to the medication. Sometimes a toxic effect can occur with small doses, whereas in other instances the tissues are so devitalized that the response to the drug is toxic and not beneficial.

Toxic substances

A *toxic* substance is defined as any substance that can cause damage to the eye. A reaction may be dependent on dose, having a largely beneficial effect within a given range and a harmful effect when this range is exceeded.

Acid burns to the eye depend on the type of acid and its pH. If the pH is 2.5 or lower, the degree of acid burn may be devastating. Yet between a pH of 7 to a pH of 2.5, such acid solutions induce a strong stinging sensation but no real destruction of the affected tissues. The worst acids as far as tissue destruction is concerned are rather common and include sulfuric acid, hydrochloric acid, and phosphoric acid. Weak acids such as boric acid are so safe that they are used as eyewashes (Murine).

Alkali burns generally cause a more toxic reaction to the eye than acid burns,

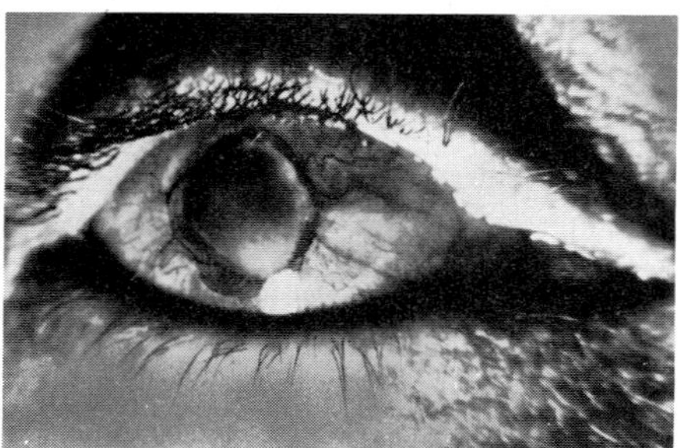

Fig. 4-1. End result of lime burn of cornea.

the severity of which is largely related to the pH of the eye. The higher the pH is above 7, the more severe the tissue destruction. Alkali burns are very common simply because these chemicals are found in many households. Frequently offending alkalis include *lime* (calcium hydroxide) (Fig. 4-1), *lye* (sodium hydroxide), and *ammonia* (ammonium hydroxide). But the pH is not the sole factor in tissue reaction. The severity of alkali burns also depends on the length of exposure, the area of the eye struck, the concentration of the alkali, and the pH. Over 11.5 pH values usually mean that the eye will be severely damaged. Some chemicals penetrate the eye easily, whereas others do their damage superficially. For instance, ammonia, which is most dangerous as liquid ammonia, can cause opacification of the cornea, iritis, and lens damage. The internal damage is related to ammonia's ability to penetrate the tissues, especially the cornea, and to cause destruction of the walls forming the anterior chamber, including the lens. So hypopyon, hemorrhage, and glaucoma frequently result from ammonia burns.

On the other hand, calcium hydroxide penetrates the cornea more slowly. It is one of the most common toxic substances—it is better known as lime, which is the basic ingredient of mortar, plaster, cement, and whitewash. The grayish white pasty lime becomes very adherent to the cornea, which makes irrigation very difficult. It can cause the cornea to become white with extensive tissue destruction but does not usually go deeper than the cornea. Lime burns are dreaded because they do not lend themselves to immediate correction by simple irrigation of water. They form an adherent complex with the cornea which causes damage for hours and even days after the event. First-aid treatment of lime burns still involves washing the eyes with running water, the removal of solid particles, and irrigation with sodium EDTA.

Some of the most commonly used ophthalmic drugs can cause toxic damage. Local anesthetics that are routinely used for glaucoma testing frequently cause stinging of the eyes and can cause irregularity of the cornea. Since local anesthetics create depression of wound healing, it is important to use local anesthetics in the office only and not as a pain reliever. It is easy to comtemplate the cycle of events that can result from the wanton use of local anesthetics. The eye is injured, which causes pain. The local anesthetics depress the pain but enlarge the injury or retard its healing, which makes the need for pain relievers even greater. In cases where a local anesthetic agent has been used to control discomfort, the corneal epithelium appears as a heaped-up gray ridge surrounding a crater of bare stroma.

Common household items can be toxic to the eyes. *Hair sprays* and *lacquers* are largely composed of polyvinyl pyrrolidone or shellac dissolved in alcohol. Hair spray can cause erosion of the corneal epithelium, which can vary from a mild stinging sensation to a severe punctate keratitis that needs a day or two to recover. If the person also happens to be wearing contact lenses, the lens may be spoiled, and the corneal reaction more severe because the congestion of the tissues with swelling causes the lens to form an airtight bond with the cornea.

Even ordinary *talc* has been incriminated as a toxic agent. Talc is powdered magnesium or steatite and is used as a dusting powder for surgeon's gloves. The talc can cause the formation of granulomas in the eye. It is for this reason that surgeons attempt to remove the talc powder from their gloves before commencing surgery. In the anterior chamber talc can cause an iritis with secondary glaucoma.

Some agents are erroneously implicated as being toxic. *Selenium sulfide,* which is the basic ingredient of many antidandruff solutions sold on the commerical market, does not cause any permanent eye damage whatsoever. Occasionally it can cause a chemical conjunctivitis that is brief and mild or a transient keratitis that is self-limiting. Yet the warnings on the bottles of these solutions create such anxiety that the thought of allowing some of this shampoo to enter the eyes fills many people with dread of imminent blindness.

A germicidal soap, *pHisoHex,* also can create minor irritation to the eyes. It contains hexachlorophene and a detergent. It is the detergent, known as Triton, that can cause conjunctival congestion and corneal edema. In rare cases, the corneal edema has been severe with a marked reduction of vision.

Smog is one of the commonest toxins to the eye and is endemic in many cities. The eye irritation is believed to be caused by unsaturated hydrocarbons in the atmosphere which come mainly from automobile exhaust systems. The effects of smog are irritating to the eyes but do not cause permanent injury. The features of smog irritation include redness and tearing of the eyes with variable degrees of irritation. It is worse when the sun is highest, and its effects diminish as the sun goes down. Los Angeles has one of the worst smog conditions because of its climate and the prevalence of automobiles.

The more common toxic substances found in industry, home, or recreational areas are listed in the following glossary.

A

acetaldehyde: a volatile liquid that can cause superficial injury to the cornea.

acetazolamide (Diamox): a drug available in tablet or syrup form and used to reduce intraocular pressure. Side effects include pins-and-needles sensation in the hands, loss of appetite, myopia, urinary stones, skin rashes, and dizziness.

acetic acid (vinegar): a solution that causes corneal irritation and swelling or permanent corneal damage with scarring.

acetone (solvent): a liquid that if splashed in the cornea causes superficial injury with no permanent side effects.

acetylsalicylic acid (aspirin): a drug used as an antipyretic (reduction of fever), an antiinflammatory (for arthritis), an anticoagulant (after coronary occlusions), and an analgesic (relief of common headaches). Mild chemical irritant to the eyes.

acid-resistant penicillins (propicillin, phenbenicillin): forms that can be used orally because of their resistance to gastric acid inactivation.

acids: solutions with a pH less than 7. Acids with a pH of 2.5 or lower can cause permanent ocular damage. Severe burns can cause loss of corneal tissue up to Descemet's membrane.

ACTH: adrenocorticotropic hormone of the anterior pituitary gland. The output of ACTH depends on the blood level of adrenal steroids.

Adrenalin: see *epinephrine.*

alkalis: solutions with a pH greater than 7. At pH 12 or greater, the ocular damage is profound. Calcium hydroxide (lime) has the slowest penetration into the eye, whereas ammonium hydroxide (ammonia) is the worst. Alkali binds to the corneal stroma with tenacity. There is a tendency for damage to the cornea to occur 1 to 3 weeks after injury.

aluminum chloride: a compound used in a 10% to 25% solution as a deodorant and antiperspirant. It can cause corneal irritation.

aluminum metal: metal particles that are well tolerated in the eye.

ammonia: a colorless gas used as refrigerant or fertilizer. Household ammonia is a 7% solution and is the most toxic to the eye. It can cause edema of the cornea, iritis, and lens damage.

amphetamine ("speed"): a stimulant that can cause dilation of the pupils and blurring of near vision. It also causes loss of appetite, restlessness, and insomnia.

amphotericin B (Fungizone): an antibiotic agent used intravenously for the treatment of fungus infections—histoplasma, blastomyces, cryptococcus. Side effects include renal toxicity, gastrointestinal upset, chills, and fever.

analgesic: a pain reliever.

androgens: a hormone of the adrenal gland that governs the development of sexual features.

Anectine: see *succinylcholine.*

anesthetics, local: anesthesia by injection in which only the area infiltrated is locally treated. Agents used in ophthalmology include procaine and lidocaine (Xylocaine).

anesthetics, topical: anesthetics applied to the surface, the most popular being tetracaine (Pontocaine), cocaine, and proparacaine (Ophthaine). They provide surface anesthesia of conjunctiva and cornea. Topical anesthetics such as Pontocaine or cocaine can depress corneal healing and can cause irregularity of the surface of the cornea.

antibiotics: antibacterial drugs originally derived from bacteria and fungus molds. Synthetic antibiotics are common.

Drug	Comment
bacitracin	used topically and systemically. Can cause kidney damage.
chloramphenicol	wide-spectrum antibiotic fallen into disfavor because of connection with aplastic anemia, especially in children.
erythromycin	an antibiotic that can cause nausea and vomitting and is mainly effective against gram-positive bacilli.
methicillin (Staphcillin)	a synthetic penicillin.
neomycin	a wide-spectrum antibiotic with a high incidence of allergic reactions. Used topically only.
penicillin	a bactericidal drug effective against gram-positive cocci. Hypersensitivity in allergic people. Results in urticaria, asthma, fever, rash, and at times death from anaphylactic reaction. Not used locally because of high incidence of allergic reaction.
streptomycin	given intramuscularly. Can cause hypersensitivity reactions and deafness. Rarely used in ophthalmology.
synthetic penicillin	used for penicillin-resistant bacteria. Includes methicillin and ampicillin. The penicillin-resistant bacteria produce penicillinase, which does not interfere with the activity of the synthetic group.
tetracycline (Aureomycin, Achromycin, Terramycin)	broad-spectrum antibiotics. Cause gastrointestinal upset and superinfections of the bowel.

antihistamines: drugs used in treatment of allergies; occasionally cause dilation of the pupils and impairment of accommodation.

Apresoline: see *hydralazine.*

Aralen: see *chloroquine.*

Atrabrine: see *quinacrine.*

atropine: a drug obtained from *Atropa belladonna* to block parasympathetic nerves. In the eye it causes pupillary dilation and can last 2 to 3 weeks. If this drug is absorbed, it can cause fever, dryness of the skin, skin rash, and acceleration of the heart. Available as a drop, ointment, injection, or tablet.

B

bacteriocidal agents: antibacterial agents that include penicillin, polymyxin B, bacitracin, neomycin, kanamycin, colistin, vancomycin, ristocetin, and streptomycin.

bacteriocidal antibiotic: a drug that destroys bacteria, such as penicillin.

bacteriostatic agents: bacteria-inhibiting agents that include tetracycline, the sulfonamides, erythromycin, novobiocin, amphotericin B, and chloramphenicol.

bacteriostatic antibiotic: a drug that inhibits bacterial replication; such as tetracycline and sulfa drugs.

barbiturates: a group of drugs used as sleeping pills and in ophthalmology as preanesthetic sedatives. Phenobarbital and Seconal are common barbiturates. The shorter acting drugs are usually prescribed (Nembutal and Seconal).

bee stings: iritis, hypopyon, congestion of the eye, and corneal edema can result if a bee sting penetrates the cornea. If Descemet's membrane is not perforated, the lens remains normal.

belladonna: a leaf or root from the plant *Atropa belladonna.* It yields several alkaloids including atropine, hyoscyamine, and scopolamine.

Benadryl: see *diphenhydramine hydrochloride.*

benzalkonium: a quaternary ammonium wetting agent used as an antiseptic. At dilutions of 1:1000 it can cause mild keratitis.

benzalkonium chloride (Zephiran): a quaternary ammonium antiseptic and preservative.

benzoquinone: see *quinones.*

bishydroxycoumarin (dicumarol): a synthetic anticoagulant that acts by inhibiting prothrombin formation. It must be monitored with prothrombin time tests to avoid bleeding.

boric acid: an antiseptic with germicidal powers. Used mainly as an eyewash (Murine).

botulismotoxin: a toxin produced by *Clostridium botulinum.* It can cause severe food poisoning, leading to death. In less severe cases it can cause ophthalmoplegia and pupillary dilation.

brake fluid: product composed of alcohol, glycols, and a lubricant; causes superficial injury to the cornea if splashed into the eye.

broad-spectrum antibiotic: an antibiotic effective against bacteria that consist of rods and cocci, for example, chloramphenicol. *Bacteriocidal agents* effective against cocci include penicillin, bacitracin, and vancomycin. *Bacteriostatic agents* effective against rods include streptomycin and colistin.

burdock burs: prickly bracts from the plant *Happa algaris.* If caught in the eye, the bristles can cause severe conjunctival and corneal reactions.

Butazolidin: see *phenylbutazone.*

C

caffeine: an alkaloid in tea or coffee that has no effect on vision.

calcium carbonate chalk: an agent that has no toxic effect in contact with the eye.

calcium hydroxide (lime): product used for mortar, cement, and whitewash; one of the most common causes of alkali burns to the eye.

calcium hypochlorite (bleaching powder): chemical that causes superficial injury to the epithelium of the cornea.

Candrase: see *ethoxzolamide.*

cannabis (marijuana, hemp, hashish): drug with ocular effects that include dilation of the pupil, impairment of accommodation, and visual hallucinations. Impairment of color vision may also ensue.

carbachol: a cholinergic drug that causes miosis, spasm of accommodation, and a fall in intraocular pressure from improved aqueous flow. Used mainly as a drop for control of glaucoma; it is contraindicated in people with asthma, cardiac problems, or peptic ulcer.

carbon: element that has no toxic effect in the eye. As part of graphite or soot, the carbon complex may cause inflammation of the lid and cornea.

carbon monoxide: a nonirritant gas that results from the incomplete combustion of gasoline, coal, or wood; found in the exhausts from automobiles and furnaces. It can cause loss of vision, convulsions, and death.

carbon tetrachloride: a solvent used for dry cleaning. General absorption can cause optic neuritis and death.

caterpillars: larvae of butterflies or moths. Their sharp hairs are very irritating to conjunctiva and cornea and can cause severe keratitis and iritis.

cephalothin: a derivative of cephalosporin C; active against gram-positive bacteria, including penicillinase-producing staphylococci and many gram-negative bacilli. Allergic reactions are absent.

chloramphenicol (Chloromycetin): a broad-spectrum antibiotic that when taken systemically can cause optic neuritis or fatal aplastic anemia.

chlordiazepoxide (Librium): a drug that is used as a sedative and muscle relaxant. It can cause skin rashes, mental problems, constipation, and blurring of near vision.

chlorine: a gas, liquid, or solid used for water purification, which can cause self-limiting ocular irritation when used in pools. No serious or permanent damage occurs.

chloroacetophenone (tear gas): substance that causes blepharospasm and tearing. The effects are usually transitory, although occasionally corneal scarring has occurred.

Chloromycetin: see *chloramphenicol.*

chloroquine (Aralen, Resochin): a synthetic quinoline used for the treatment of malaria, arthritis, and lupus erythematosus. It can cause a bull's-eye maculopathy, pigment degeneration of the retina, whorls of corneal deposits, and skin rashes.

chlorpheniramine (Chlor-Trimeton): a histamine antagonist used in allergic-based disorders such as asthma and hay fever. Can be given orally, intramuscularly, or intravenously. It also has mild sedating effects. Used to treat allergic eye conditions.

chlorpromazine (Thorazine, Largactil): a tranquilizer without ocular complications; may reduce intraocular pressure.

Chlor-Trimeton: see *chlorpheniramine.*

cocaine: a potent topical anesthetic agent that causes mydriasis and partial cycloplegia. An addictive drug that also can cause rapid heartbeat, delirium, chills, fever, and convulsions.

codeine: a mild analgesic that is a derivative of morphine. Available by tablet, solution for injection, or syrup.

corticosteroids (cortisone, hydrocortisone, triamcinolone, prednisone, dexamethasone): steroids that are used locally for the treatment of nonspecific ocular inflammation including iritis, keratitis, and blepharitis. Postsubcapsular cataracts can occur with use of steroids for 1 year. Local steroids can cause a rise in intraocular pressure.

corticotropin: a hormone derived from the anterior lobe of pituitary glands from farm animals; stimulates the secretions of the adrenal cortex to produce all the steroid hormones with the exception of aldosterone. It is used intramuscularly and intravenously and is effective only if normal adrenal cortical tissue is present.

Cyclogyl: see *cyclopentolate.*

cyclopentolate (Cyclogyl): a rapid-onset, short-acting synthetic drug that causes mydriasis and cycloplegia after being dropped into the eye. Used before refraction, especially in children.

Coumadin: see *warfarin sodium.*

D

Daranide: see *dichlorphenamide.*

Daraprim: see *pyrimethamine.*

demecarium bromide (Humorsol): a cholinesterase inhibitor that causes miosis and improved facility of outflow of aqueous. Used to treat glaucoma (open-angle) and esotropia.

Demerol: see *meperidine hydrochloride.*

detamide (M-delphine): a liquid insect repellent (Off). Can cause a temporary mild keratitis.

DFP: see *isoflurophate.*

Diamox: see *acetazolamide.*

dichlorphenamide (Daranide): a potent carbon anhydrase inhibitor used to lower intraocular pressure in glaucoma. Side effects include paresthesias, depression, loss of appetite, and tremor. Should not be used in people with respiratory depression and kidney disease.

digitalis: drug derived from the dried leaves of *Digitalis purpurea;* contains digitoxin, used in the treatment of heart failure. Side effects to vision include flickering of light and yellow, orange, or green coloration.

dicumarol: see *bishydroxycoumarin.*

dimethyl sulfate: a gas that causes burns to the skin and eyes. When absorbed by the skin, it can cause convulsions, kidney damage, liver and heart toxicity, and death.

2,4-dinitrophenol: a drug formerly used to treat obesity until the complication of cataracts was discovered and it was banned.

diphenhydramine hydrochloride (Benadryl): antihistamine used for nasal allergies and hay fever. Side effects include dryness of the mouth, tremors, nervousness, and loss of appetite. It has a mild sedative effect.

E

echothiophate iodide (Phospholine Iodide): a long-acting inhibitor of cholinesterase that is used in open-angle glaucoma; a potent drug that can cause severe spasm of accommodation and miosis. Iris cysts and cataracts are other side effects that limit its use.

edrophonium chloride (Tensilon): a curare antagonist that is given to myasthenic patients and causes a brief increase in muscle power. Its main use is as a diagnostic agent for myasthenia gravis when given intravenously.

EDTA: see *ethelenediaminetetraacetic acid.*

epinephrine (Adrenalin): drug used to treat glaucoma; tends to stain the conjunctiva with brown spots when oxidized and to sting when applied locally.

ethanol: see *ethyl alcohol.*

ethelenediaminetetraacetic acid (EDTA): a solution that absorbs calcium into its molecular structure and is used to remove calcium deposits from the cornea. Used as a preservative in ophthalmic solutions.

ether: a general anesthetic whose vapor can cause a transient irritation to the eye.

ethoxzolamide (Cardrase): a diuretic used in the treatment of glaucoma.

ethyl alcohol (ethanol): a liquid used as an antiseptic and a solvent. As a drink it is the basis of the alcohol industry. It is available commercially with toxic additives that make it unfit to drink. If splashed into the eye, it causes a transitory irritation. Whisky, brandy, gin, or vodka in the eye causes a temporary blurring of vision and stinging sensation. Some shampoos with high alcohol content can do the same. Systemic effects from alcohol ingestion include nystagmus, esophoria, and pupillary dilation. Chronic alcoholism can cause ocular muscle palsies. Optic neuritis and blindness can follow the ingestion of toxic ethyl alcohol.

ethylene glycol (antifreeze): water-soluble liquid that can cause death from cerebral edema if ingested.

eucatropine hydrochloride (Euphthalmine): a weak cholinergic blocking agent used to dilate pupils or to provoke angle-closure glaucoma in suspect patients.

euphthalmine: see *eucatropine hydrochloride.*

F

fire extinguisher fluid: a fluid that may be carbon tetrachloride, tetrachloroethylene, or methyl bromide. Water-filled extinguishers may contain sulfuric acid. A dry type may contain powdered sodium or potassium bicarbonate.

Floropryl: see *isoflurophate.*

fluorescein: a phthalein dye used to outline abrasions or defects in the corneal epithelial surface, to assess the fit of contact lenses, to outline lacrimal patency, and in retinal angiography. The solution form is easily contaminated by *Pseudomonas* bacteria so it is used either in its dry form, in impregnated filter strips, or in freshly prepared solution. It produces an intense green fluorescent color in alkaline solution.

fuel for model airplanes: fuel that may be a mixture of methyl alcohol, nitropropane, and castor oil. It can cause swelling and loss of the corneal epithelium if splashed into the eye.

Fungizone: see *amphotericin B.*

G

galactose: an enzyme that if not present in a child can cause cataracts. If diagnosed before 3 months of age and galactose is eliminated from the diet, the cataracts may disappear.

Garamycin: see *gentamicin.*

gentamicin (Garamycin): an antibiotic with a broad range of activity against gram-positive and gram-negative bacteria. It is unique in that it can also work against *Pseudomonas, Proteus,* and *Staphylococcus* bacteria.

glucocorticoids: a hormone of the adrenal gland that has its effect on the metabolism of fat, protein, and carbohydrate. Cortisone is the prime example of this hormone. It is used basically for its nonspecific inflammatory effect. Systemic side effects are frequent and serious. These include acne, diabetes, hypertension, bone fractures, psychoses, cushingoid facies, hirsutism, cataracts, and amenorrhea. Local side effects include glaucoma, depression of wound healing, and potentiation of growth of viruses, especially important for herpes simplex keratitis.

Therapeutic uses of glucocorticoids in ophthalmology include iritis; nonspecific keratitis; phlyctenular conjunctivitis; alkali burns of the cornea; superficial punctate keratitis; allergic blepharitis, keratitis, and conjunctivitis; temporary arteritis; optic neuritis; episcleritis; traumatic iritis; postoperative traumatic iritis; sympathetic ophthalmia; marginal corneal ulcers; and toxic keratitis from soft lens cleaners.

Drugs used as systemic glucocorticoids

cortisone acetate (cortisone)
hydrocortisone (Cortone, Hydrocortone)
prednisone (Deltasone, prednisolone)
triamcinolone (Aristocort, Kenacort)
methylprednisolone (Medrol)
dexamethasone (Decadron)

Drugs used as topical glucocorticoids

dexamethasone phosphate (Decadron)
prednisolone acetate (Predneferin forte)
hydrocortisone suspension (hydrocortisone acetate)
dexamethasone solution (Maxidex)

glycerol: a clear, colorless, syrupy liquid with a sweet taste; often combined with lemon juice to reduce the sickly, sweet taste. At full strength it is used to clear the haze of corneal edema. It is absorbed in the intestine and causes a rise in the osmotic pressure and withdrawal of fluid from the eye. It should not be used if diabetes is present. Usual amount used is 1 to 1.4 ml/kg.

golf-ball paste: the sodium hydroxide in the core of the ball that squirts out when the ball is cut. There have been many ocular injuries reported from the playful misuse of golf balls.

H

hair sprays or lacquers: products that contain polyvinyl or shellac dissolved in alcohol. Cause mild keratitis in the eye.

hair tonics: liquids consisting largely of alcohol with perfumes. Cause transient stinging and redness of the eye.

henna: a natural reddish dye used for tinting the hair. It has no ocular side effects or toxicity.

Herplex: see *idoxuridine.*

homatropine (1% to 5%): a synthetic alkaloid with the same effects and complications of atropine but much weaker. Mydriasis and cycloplegia last only 72 hours.

Humorsol: see *demecarium bromide.*

hydralazine (Apresoline): a drug used in the treatment of high blood pressure; can cause swelling of the lids, flushing of the face, headache, stuffy nose, and blurred vision.

hydrochloric acid: a common acid that can cause mild irritation to total opacification of the cornea, depending on its dose.

hydrochlorothiazide (Hydrodiuril): a diuretic and an antihypertensive agent. It may relieve some lid edema, conjunctival chemosis, and orbital swelling.

Hydrodiuril: see *hydrochlorothiazide.*

hydrogen peroxide: a liquid that can cause damage to the eye in high concentrations. Pharmaceutical concentration is 3%, whereas in industrial use the concentration is 30%, and for use in rockets, it is 90%. It is used as a cleaning and disinfecting agent for soft contact lenses.

hydrogen sulfide: a poisonous gas with an odor of rotten eggs, it can cause a superficial punctate keratitis. Deeper penetration is rare.

hydroquinone: see *quinones.*

hydroxyamphetamine hydrobromide (Paredrine): a synthetic sympathomimetic drug that produces mydriasis and no cycloplegia. It is used for ophthalmoscopy.

hydroxyzine pamoate (Vistaril): an antihistamine used as a preanesthetic agent for its calming and tranquilizing effects.

hyoscyamine: an alkaloid occurring in the plant *Hyoscyamus niger,* it causes temporary dilation of the pupil and paralysis of accommodation for near vision.

I

IDU: see *idoxuridine.*

insulin: pancreatic secretion that allows the proper metabolism of blood sugar. Without it a diabetic mellitus occurs.

interferon: a substance used to prevent the multiplication of viruses. Not available commercially, it has been shown that it will increase host resistance to herpes simplex and vaccinia. It has also been used as an anticancer agent.

iodine: a solution that is irritating to the eye but causes no permanent damage. It is used to chemically cauterize the epithelium of the cornea infected by herpes simplex virus.

idoxuridine (IDU, Stoxil, Herplex): a metabolic antagonist of the synthesis of DNA. It inhibits the use of thymidic acid. It is used to treat herpes simplex keratitis and vaccinia keratitis.

ipecac: a plant material used to induce vomiting. In a powdered form, it can be irritating to the eyes.

iron: a toxic mineral when it becomes an intraocular foreign body; it stains rust brown any tissue with which it is in contact and destroys it. The retina, lens, and iris are most prone to suffer the toxic effects of iron.

isoflurophate (DFP, floropryl): a potent parasympathomimetic drug that causes an intense miosis and spasm of accommodation and an increase in aqueous outflow. It is used primarily to treat refractory glaucoma. Iris cysts and headaches are common side effects.

isoniazid: a drug used to treat tuberculosis. Optic neuritis may be a complication of continued use of this drug.

K

kerosene: a petroleum hydrocarbon used as a fuel or a solvent that causes no permanent injury to the eyes after contact.

L

lanolin: wool fat, consisting largely of cholesterol esters and cholesterol and used as a base for cosmetics. Lanolin applied to the eye is not toxic.

Largactyl: see *chlorpromazine.*

lead poisoning: a condition that can cause headache, convulsions, and coma. Ocular involvement can occur with toxic effects found in the optic nerves, cranial nerve palsy to the external muscles of the eye causing facial palsy, ptosis, or strabismus. A lead line in the gums or lead in the urine is usually found in these severe cases.

lewisite: a war gas. Both the vapor and liquid cause a severe keratitis with profuse tearing and blepharospasm.

Librium: see *chlordiazepoxide.*

lidocaine hydrochloride (Xylocaine): a rapidly acting, common local anesthetic agent used for infiltrative, nerve block, or topical purposes. Serious side effects are not common.

lime (calcium hydroxide): product composed of sand, cement, and water; causes severe alkali burn to the eye that may lead to marked corneal scarring.

lincomycin: an antibiotic effective against most gram-positive bacteria, including pencillin-resistant strains of *Staphylococci.*

LSD-25: see *lysergic acid.*

lysergic acid (LSD-25): an alkaloid derived from ergot that causes mental aberrations and visual hallucinations.

M

manganese: metallic particles that can be absorbed by fumes or inhaled as dust; toxic effects include fatigue, ataxia, and decreased movement of the lids and eyes.

mannitol: a hydroxy alcohol used to lower the intraocular pressure in glaucoma (narrow-angle) and before cataract surgery. It does this by osmotic effect. It is an aldehyde sugar that resembles dextrose in its properties.

mascara: a cosmetic for the eyelashes that is largely lampblack kaolin and sulfonated castor oil. The pigments can accumulate in the tarsus and cause a slight folliculosis. No serious side effects are known.

Mellaril: see *thioridazine.*

meperidine hydrocloride (Demerol): a potent synthetic analgesic drug that is highly addictive for the euphoria it induces. It is used as a preoperative analgesic but it can cause vomiting and hypotension.

mercury oxide (yellow): a heavy powder that can cause lens opacities and staining of the conjunctiva. Corneal staining consists of a graying ring just anterior to the endothelium.

mescaline: alkaloid obtained from the mescal buttons (flowering heads) of a cactus; when taken internally, it can cause wild visual hallucinations.

methazolamide (Neptazane): a diuretic similar in action to Diamox, it is a carbonic anhydrase inhibitor and a sulfonamide-type drug. It is used to lower intraocular pressure.

methyl alcohol: a liquid known as methanol or wood alcohol and used as a commercial solvent, antifreeze, and fuel. It resembles ethyl alcohol in taste and has been used as a substitute. Toxic reactions occur within 1 to 2 days and include nausea, vomiting, headaches, loss of vision from mild loss to total blindness, and respiratory failure and death. Severely toxic patients also show features of acidosis.

methyl salicylate (wintergreen oil): an oily liquid used for flavoring and liniments; taken internally, it is quite toxic causing loss of vision, convulsions, and stupor.

methylene blue: a dye used as a stain in bacteriology; if splashed into the eye, it causes no serious ocular effects. It may be used for skin markings and for dyeing sutures.

mineralocorticoids: hormones of the adrenal gland concerned with the regulation of fluid and electrolyte metabolism. Aldosterone and desoxycorticosterone are examples.

miotics: agents used in the treatment of glaucoma, including pilocarpine, carbachol, physostigmine, demecarium, phospholine iodide, and diisopropyl fluorophosphate (DFP). These drugs may cause lid twitching, conjunctival hyperemia, iris cysts, ciliary muscle spasm, myopia, and cataracts.

morphine: an addictive drug that is a powerful analgesic and produces a tremendous euphoria. It causes miosis of the pupil, respiratory depression, vomiting, and constipation.

mustard gas: a war gas that causes corneal ulceration, vascularization, and scarring. In severe cases keratoplasty is required.

Mycostatin: see *nystatin.*

Mydriacyl: see *tropicamide.*

N

nail polishes: enamels and lacquers that can cause swelling and blisters of the lids. Itching is also common.

nail polish remover: product largely consisting of acetone, alcohol, and benzene that removes polish from the nail. If splashed in the eye, it causes a mild keratitis that lasts a day.

Nembutal: see *pentobarbitol sodium.*

neostigmine (Prostigmin): a potent inhibitor of acetylcholinesterase. Used for the diagnosis and treatment of myasthenia gravis.

Neo-Synephrine: see *phenylephrine hydrochloride.*

Neptazane: see *methazolamide.*

nickel: metal that causes contact dermatitis.

nitrous oxide: a general anesthetic; called laughing gas. Toxic if not accompanied by adequate oxygen.

Novocain: see *procaine hydrochloride.*

nystatin (Mycostatin): an antifungal agent primarily effective against *Candida albicans* (moniliasis and thrush). Used topically as a cream for skin infections or in the eye with a dosage of 100,000 units per milliliter.

O

oil of cloves: a flavoring agent, topical anesthetic, and aseptic in dentistry. Can cause a severe keratoconjunctivitis if splashed into the eye.

Ophtaine: see *proparacaine hydrochloride.*

Ophthetic: see *proparacaine hydrochloride.*

opium: a drug that contains several alkaloids including morphine, codeine, and papaverine. It has few toxic effects, but miosis is a telltale sign of drug usage.

ozone: an oxidizing gas produced by action of the ultraviolet in sunlight on the oxygen of the air. At concentrations greater than 1 ppm in air, ozone is an ocular irritant.

P

Paredrine: see *hydroxyamphetamine hydrobromide.*

parasympatholytic agents: agents that relax accommodation and dilate the pupil. Systemically they may cause dryness of the mouth, increased pulse rate, disorientation, and visual hallucinations. In predisposed patients they may cause angle-closure glaucoma.

pathogens: organisms that cause disease.

penicillinase (methicillin, oxacillin, cloxacillin, nafcillin, ampicillin): an agent that inactivates regular penicillin. Penicillin resistant, the drugs listed are resistant to hydrolysis or inactivation by penicillinase. For ocular use, methicillin and ampicillin are the most useful. NOTE: Hospital-resistant *Staphylococcus aureus* is the major producer of penicillinase.

pentobarbital sodium (Nembutal): a hypnotic (sleeping agent) and sedative; effective sedation occurs 30 minutes after ingestion.

Pentothal: see *thiopental.*

pepper: the dried unripe fruit of the plant *Piper nigrum,* it causes a mild inflammatory reaction including swelling of the lids and redness of the eyes.

perphenazine (Trilafon): drug used as a tranquilizer and antiemetic. Can cause blurring of vision and a parkinsonian-like condition.

Phenergan: see *promethazine.*

phenobarbital sodium: a barbiturate drug that is a strong, long-acting hypnotic, sedative, and anticonvulsant. It causes a hangover-like condition resulting from its prolonged effect.

phenol (carbolic acid): liquid that in a dilute solution is used as an antiseptic. Concentrated solutions can burn the skin and eyes. A 2.5% solution of phenol will give a serious burn to the cornea.

phenothiazine derivatives: drugs used in the treatment of major psychoses and as tranquilizers and antiemetics. Complications include pigmentary retinopathy and parkinsonian-like movements of the eyes.

phenothiazines: drugs used as antiemetics. The most popular ones are promethazine (Phenergan), triflupromazine (Vesprin), and chlorpromazine (Thorazine). These drugs also are the mainstay of antipsychotic therapy. They are used to potentiate the effects of barbiturates and opiates. Complications of this group of drugs include parkinsonian-like symptoms, motor restlessness, chorioretinopathy (Mellaril), skin eye, purple-gray skin, as well as purple-gray pigmentation of the cornea and conjunctiva (Thorazine).

phenylbutazone (Butazolidin): an antiinflammatory agent used for arthritis, gout, and traumatic bursitis. It appears to help in uveitis. Also used as an analgesic and antipyretic. Side effects are common, including skin rashes, gastrointestinal disorders, vertigo, anemia, and cardiac problems.

phenylephrine hydrochloride (Neo-Synephrine): a synthetic sympathomimetic compound that on local application to the eye produces mydriasis without cycloplegia. It is used for dilating pupils for examination in a 2.5% solution and as a decongestant (Visine) in a 0.125% solution. A 10% solution of the drug has caused death from systemic absorption. It should not be used in patients with heart disease or hypertension nor should it be used routinely in the 2.5% solution.

pHisoHex: germicidal soap used before surgery, it contains hexachlorophene and a detergent. It can cause a transient irritation to the conjunctiva and cornea.

Phospholine Iodide: see *echothiophate iodide.*

picric acid: strong acid that in 0.3% to 0.5% solution is used as an antiseptic. It can be sensitizing and cause allergies.

pilocarpine: a drug that is used as a parasympathomimetic agent. In the eye it causes increased facility of outflow, miosis (pupillary contraction), and ciliary spasm. It is primarily used to treat open-angle glaucoma. It has a duration of activity of 4 to 6 hours.

pitch: a black residue from distilling tar. Exposure over years can cause staining of the exposed eye, the cornea, and conjunctiva.

plastics: substances that are generally inert and do not injure the eye. They are used for artificial eyes, contact lenses, spectacle lenses, and intraocular lenses. Damage to the eye from hard or soft plastic contact lenses is related to fit, the solutions used, or improper care, but not to the plastics used.

poison ivy (Rhus radicans) and poison oak (Rhus toxicodendron): species that on contact cause a delayed skin and ocular inflammation.

Pontocaine: see *tetracaine hydrochloride.*

potassium hydroxide (potash): a fertilizer, it is one of the potent alkalies.

potassium permanganate: chemical that in dilute solutions is used as an antiseptic. It can cause a severe keratoconjunctivitis.

procaine hydrochloride (Novocain): an effective local anesthetic, it cannot be given in drop form.

promethazine (Phenergan): a potent antihistamine drug used to treat allergic states and to control motion sickness. Preoperatively it is used as a sedative.

proparacaine hydrochloride (Ophthaine, Ophthetic): an excellent local ocular anesthetic agent that offers fast action but a short duration of activity. Toxic side effects are rare, although on rare occasions a diffuse temporary clouding of the corneal epithelium may occur.

Prostigmin: see *neostigmine.*

Prussian blue (ferric ferrocyanide): a blue inert pigment used to tattoo the cornea.

pyrimethamine (Daraprim): a synthetic antimalarial drug that is a folic acid antagonist. It is used to treat malaria and toxoplasmosis. It can be toxic and cause bone marrow depression of platelets, red blood cells, and white blood cells.

Q

quinacrine (Atabrine): a drug used to treat malaria, rheumatoid arthritis, and lupus erythematosis, it can cause blue-gray staining of the conjunctiva and corneal deposits. Cessation of the drug stops the corneal deposits, but the retinal changes may be permanent. A related drug, chloroquine, also causes a bull's-eye maculopathy with subsequent permanent visual loss.

quinine: a natural drug derived from cinchona bark and used as an antimalarial drug; can be very toxic, causing mild blurring of vision to blindness, and can cause extreme narrowing of retinal vessels and optic atrophy.

quinones (benzoquinone, hydroquinone): drugs that cause staining of the outer eye in workers exposed to the vapors of aniline dyes, but the inner eye is not affected by these drugs.

R

reserpine (Serpasil): an alkaloid derived from *Rauwolfia serpentina,* it is a popular drug for the treatment of hypertension. It can cause conjunctival vascular congestion and slight miosis.

Resochin: see *chloroquine.*

rose bengal: a dye that in a 5% solution is used to stain devitalized tissue, such as filamentary keratitis in keratoconjunctivitis sicca. It has no toxic effect to the eye.

S

salicylic acid: see *acetylsalicylic acid.*

scopolamine hyoscine: an atropine-like drug that is antiparasympathetic. In the eye its effect is shorter than that of atropine, but it is seldom used because of its hypnotic effect (induces sleep). As with atropine, it causes mydriasis, cycloplegia, dryness of the mouth, central nervous system excitement, tachycardia, and skin flush.

secobarbital sodium (Seconal): a short-acting barbiturate, it is used as a sedative and to induce sleep. Skin eruptions, excitement, and vertigo can occur with use.

Seconal: see *secobarbital sodium.*

selenium sulfide: a topical antiseborrheic in combination with a detergent; used to treat dandruff, it can cause a low-grade keratitis but never do severe damage to the eyes.

Serpasil: see *reserpine.*

silica (quartz): a substance that is nontoxic to the ocular tissue.

silver compounds: agents that on local contact can stain the eye gray, particularly the cornea at the level of Descemet's membrane and the conjunctiva. A 1% silver nitrate solution was used for years to prevent ophthalmia neonatorum. The silver stain is harmless in dilute solutions. In 5% to 50% solutions silver nitrate can cause gross corneal scarring.

smog: a mixture of fog and smoke that causes ocular irritation. The chemicals in the air, which include oxides of nitrogen and unsaturated hydrocarbons, are promoted by sunlight. The hydrocarbons are a product of automobile exhausts. By-products of these reactions are ozone and aldehydes. Although the smog reaction to the eye is unpleasant, no permanent injury has been reported.

sodium carbonate (washing soda): product that is mildly toxic to the cornea and should be diluted with water on contact with the eye.

sodium chloride (table salt): a salt that is harmless to the eye in solution.

sodium hexametaphosphate: a chemical that is the principal component of water softeners; not harmful to the eye.

sodium hypochlorite: agent used as a bleach (Chlorox) and in Javelle water; can cause transient corneal edema.

Stelazine: see *trifluoperazine*.

Stoxil: see *idoxuridine*.

streptomycin: an antibiotic that causes vestibular damage but is not harmful to the eye. It is rarely used for ocular disturbances.

strychnine: a poisonous alkaloid. Poisoning is accompanied by painful convulsions, deviations of the eye, and dilation of the pupils.

succinylcholine (Anectine): a drug used with general anesthesia as a muscle relaxant; it may cause a transient rise in ocular pressure and a temporary contraction of the extraocular muscles. The effect of succinylcholine is potentiated by previous use of phospholine iodide eye drops.

sulfa drugs: drugs used in the treatment of bacterial infections, they are the major component of carbonic anhydrase inhibitors. Ocular side effects include myopia, conjunctivitis, pemphigoid lesions, and retinal hemorrhages.

sulfonamides: a group of drugs that are effective against gram-positive organisms and some gram-negative bacilli. These drugs are bacteriostatic in that they prevent the replication of bacteria. Against bacteria these drugs prevent the formation of folic acid, an essential growth ingredient, and also stop bacteria from using *p*-amino benzoic acid. Toxic effects include skin rashes, gastrointestinal upsets, fever, renal lesions, and peripheral neuritis. Some sulfonamides in use systemically are sulfadiazine, sulfisoxazole (Gantrisin), sulfamethoxypyridazine (Kynex), succinylsulfathiazole (Sulfasuxidine), and sulfadimethoxine (Madribon). Sulfa drops are commonly used locally. They have a broad spectrum of activity and rarely cause serious side effects except for a tendency to irritate.

sulfur dioxide: a chemical used for preserving fruit and as a bleaching agent. As a gas, it is irritating to the eyes and to the respiratory tract. Serious injury to the eye is rare, although severe burns of the cornea by liquid dioxide have been reported. Oddly enough, discomfort is not acute because the chemical damages the corneal nerves and renders an anesthetic effect to the eye. The most injurious form of sulfur dioxide is liquid sulfurous acid. In this form the acid penetrates rapidly through the corneal epithelium.

sulfuric acid: drug also used as battery acid; can chemically burn the eye.

surfactants: agents that are surface active. Three types are (1) ionic, the most toxic (benzalkonium chloride); (2) anionic, the middle range (soap, Triton); and (3) nonionic, the least harmful (Span, Tween).

synergism: the use of agents that work together for a more beneficial effect than can be expected with the use of one agent alone. For example, the antibiotics neomycin, bacitracin, and polymyxin B are often used together to treat conjunctivitis.

T

tear gas: see *chloroacetophenone.*

TEM: see *triethylenemelamine.*

Tensilon: see *edrophonium chloride.*

tetracaine hydrochloride (Pontocaine): a long-acting surface anesthetic agent applied in drop form. It can also be injected. Topical use can cause mild but transient corneal edema.

thallium: a heavy metal used to kill insects and rodents. In the past it was used as a depilatory. It is very toxic. Systemic disturbances include paralysis of a limb, mental derangements, and even death. Optic neuritis can occur with chronic poisoning.

thioglycolates: sodium and ammonium varieties used as a cold wave for hair. Optic neuritis has been reported with its use. Local splashing into the eye can cause corneal damage and scarring.

thiopental (Pentothal): a short-acting barbiturate given before general anesthesia.

thioridazine (Mellaril): a drug used in psychotherapy that can cause pigmentary retinopathy.

Thorazine: see *chlorpromazine.*

thyroid: a natural hormone in humans that can be obtained from farm animals and used as a replacement in hypothyroid states.

timolol (Timoptic): a beta blocker used for glaucoma. Very few ocular side effects.

Timoptic: see *timolol.*

toad poisons: toxins secreted by the glands of the skin of the toad. Corneal damage has been reported.

trichloroacetic acid: a strong acid used in 10% to 25% solutions to cauterize the surface of the cornea in bullous keratopathy. It has been used to chemically remove xanthoma about the eye.

triethylenemelamine (TEM): a cytotoxic drug used in ophthalmology to treat retinoblastoma.

trifluoperazine (Stelazine): a phenothiazide used to treat psychotic people. It can cause Parkinson's disease.

triflupromazine (Vesprin): a phenothiazine derivative used to treat psychotic disorders and vomiting. The worst side effect is an induced parkinsonian condition.

Trilafon: see *perphenazine.*

tropicamide (Mydriacyl): a short-acting (up to 4 hours) mydriatic and cycloplegic agent used in refraction, in retinal photography, and to dilate pupils in which the iris is bound down by inflammation.

turpentine: a volatile distillate from pine trees, it can cause a superficial epithelial keratitis if in contact with the eye.

U

urea: an osmotic agent, it creates a hypertonic solution in the blood that draws tissue fluids into it. It is used to lower intracranial pressure, brain volume, and intraocular pressure.

urethane: a drug used in pesticides, cosmetics, and in the treatment of leukemia and multiple myeloma. Crystals in the cornea may occur from its use.

V

Vesprin: see *triflupromazine.*

Vistaril: see *hydroxyzine pamoate.*

vitamin A: vitamin present in cod liver oil; overdosage can cause skin rashes, enlarged spleen and liver, loss of hair, sores at the angles of the mouth, and raised intracranial pressure with papilledema.

vitamin D: vitamin that when used to excess can cause kidney stones, headaches, stomach upsets, and band keratopathy of the cornea.

vitamin K: a fat-soluble vitamin needed to form prothrombin in the liver. Given orally, intramuscularly, or intravenously. Its absence results in bleeding.

W

warfarin sodium (Coumadin): an anticoagulant that works by depression of prothrombin formation in the liver. It is given orally or intravenously.

wasp sting: sting that causes a greater and more powerful eruption than the sting of a bee. If the eye is hit, it can cause iritis and corneal opacity.

X

Xylocaine: see *lidocaine hydrochloride.*

Z

Zephiran: see *benzalkonium chloride.*

CHAPTER 5

GENETICS

Genetics (Greek *gennan* "to produce") is the study of heredity and human variation. *Chromosomes* (Greek *chroma* "color" + *soma* "body") are darkly staining bodies of genetic material that are passed from parent to offspring. Each human cell has 46 chromosomes, constituting 23 matched or homologous pairs. One member of each chromosome pair is inherited from the father and the other from the mother. Each normal *sperm* (Greek *sperma* "seed") or *ovum* (Latin *ovum* "egg") contain 23 chromosomes, one representative from each pair; thus each parent transmits half of the genetic information to each child. Of the 46 chromosomes, 44 are *autosomes* or non–sex-determining chromosomes, and two are sex-determining chromosomes. Males can pass either an X or Y chromosome to their offspring. Females have 2 X chromosomes and no Y chromosomes and therefore can pass only an X chromosome to their offspring. If the offspring inherits an X and a Y chromosome, a male child will be born. If the offspring inherits 2 X chromosomes, a female will be born.

Genes are located on the chromosomes and are responsible for determining specific traits of individuals. *Genotype* refers to the total genetic pool of information of an individual. *Phenotype* refers to the total observable physical, physiologic, or biochemical characteristics of an individual that are determined by the genotype but often modified by the environment.

Genes at a specific location (locus) on each pair of chromosomes can have a variety of forms referred to as *alleles* (Greek meaning reciprocals). If both members of a pair of alleles are identical, the individual is *homozygous.* If the allelic genes are distinct from each other, the individual is *heterozygous.*

Disease entities that are dependent on an abnormal gene can be classified as being: *autosomal dominant, autosomal recessive, sex linked, or multifactorial.* When an autosomes allele leads to an abnormality in the heterozygote, the gene is termed *dominant.* With dominant genes, the term *penetrance* is used and refers to the presence or absence of a phenotypic effect of the gene. If a dominant gene has any evidence of its phenotypic effect, the gene is termed *penetrant;* if it is not expressed to any level of detection, it is *nonpenetrant.* An autosomal dominant trait is transmitted by an affected person *(heterozygote)* to an average of 50% of the offspring. Neurofibromatosis and Marfan's disease are examples of autosomally dominant inherited diseases.

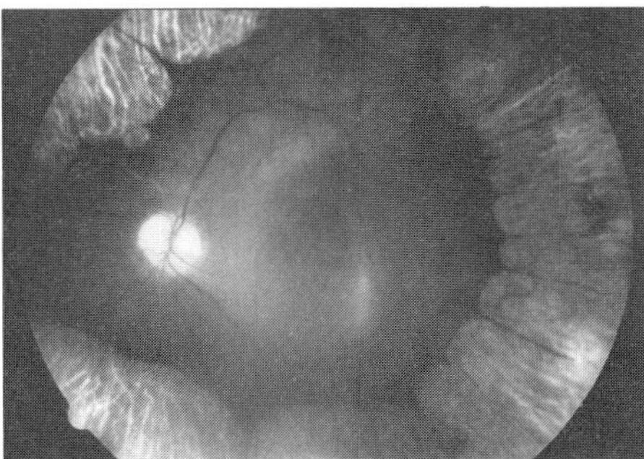

Fig. 5-1. Gyrate atrophy, an autosomal recessive disease, characterized by patchy areas of chorioretinal atrophy. The macula is usually preserved until late in the disease as is demonstrated here. (Courtesy Department of Ophthalmology, Mayo Clinic.)

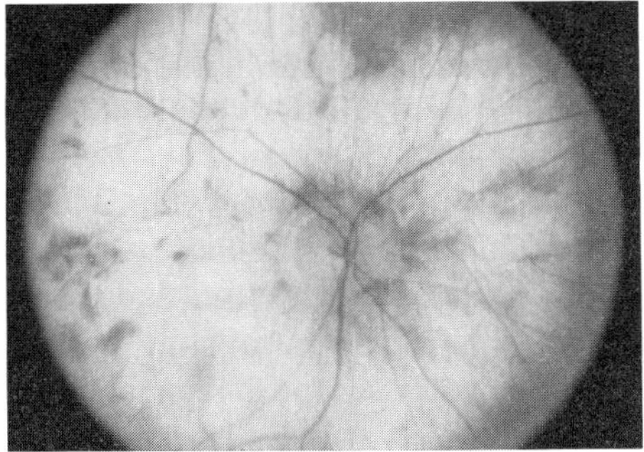

Fig. 5-2. Choroideremia, an X-linked recessive condition, characterized by diffuse chorioretinal atrophy. (Courtesy Department of Ophthalmology, Mayo Clinic.)

An autosomal recessive disease is expressed fully only in the presence of a double dose of the mutant gene. Therefore for offspring to be affected both parents must pass the mutant gene. An average of 25% of the siblings will be affected. Tay Sachs disease, oculocutaneous albinism, and gyrate atrophy (Fig. 5-1) are examples of the diseases that are inherited by autosomal recessive genes.

A trait determined by genes carried on either of the sex chromosomes is properly termed *sex linked.* X-linked genes can be X-linked dominant or X-linked recessive. In X-linked dominant disorders, females are affected more often than males, and all daughters (no sons) of affected males are affected. In X-linked recessive diseases, the females are carriers (heterozygotes), and only males are affected. All daughters of affected males are carriers. Choroideremia (Fig. 5-2), juvenile retinoschisis, and ocular albinism are examples of X-linked recessive disorders.

A condition that exhibits multifactorial inheritance means that it is determined by multiple factors, genetic and nongenetic, each with only a minor affect.

Genetic disease may also occur with chromosomal abnormalities that may be either structural or numerical and may affect either autosomes or sex chromosomes. Down's syndrome (after John L. H. Down, an English physician 1828-1896, who first described it) is the most common chromosomal syndrome in humans. It is usually the result of an extra number 21 chromosome and therefore is referred to as *trisomy 21.* Characteristic eye findings include: slanted lid folds *(epicanthal folds),* white spots of the iris *(brushfield spots),* progressive thinning of the central cornea *(keratoconus),* cataracts, and myopia. Edwards' syndrome *(trisomy 18)* is the second most common multiple malformation syndrome. Affected persons usually die in the nursery before 4 months of age, although some live as long as 15 years. Ocular findings include a small eye *(microphthalmos),* corneal opacities, congenital glaucoma, and lid droop *(ptosis).* Partial chromosome deletions can occur that are associated with a variety of disease entities. A deletion of the long arm (q) of chromosome 13 can be associated with *retinoblastoma,* a potentially lethal eye tumor in children. Deletion of the short arm (p) of chromosome 11 can be associated with aniridia and a kidney tumor that is referred to as a Wilms' tumor.

Genetic counseling imparts knowledge of human disease to the patient and his or her family, including a genetic diagnosis and its ocular and systemic implications, and information about the risk of occurrence or recurrence of the disorder within the family. *Genetic screening* is a method of testing of persons designed to detect potential genetic handicaps in them or their progeny. *Amniocentesis* (Greek *amnion,* "bowl," + kertesis, "to prick") is a technique performed in certain genetic settings on the pregnant woman. This procedure involves making a needle puncture of the uterus through the abdominal wall to allow amniotic fluid and fetal cells to be withdrawn; these then can be subjected to tests for various genetic diseases. One such test involves chromosomal analysis by the technique of banding, in which cells are stained with quinacrine (Q-banding) or modified Giemsa (G-banding) techniques. This produces a characteristic pattern of cross-bands that allows for individual identification of each chromosome pair. *Karyotype* is the name given to a photograph of a set of chromosomes that are usually arranged in pairs by size, shape, and banding pattern. At the present time amniocentesis has not been applicable to detect any eye disorders. Recently researchers have been searching for DNA markers that may be linked to some genetic eye diseases in the hope of providing accurate prenatal and genetic counseling.

A

alleles: different forms of a gene that may occur at the same locus on homologous chromosomes.

aneuploidy: an abnormal number of chromosomes, i.e., when the chromosomes number other than 46.

B

biochemical genetics: the science concerned with the chemical and physical nature of genes and the means by which they control the development of man.

C

carrier: an individual who has a gene pair consisting of one "normal" and one "abnormal" (or mutant) gene. The abnormal gene is usually recessive; therefore, the carrier does not express the disease.

centomere: the center portion of the chromosome.

clinical genetics: the study of the possible genetic factors influencing the occurrence of a pathological condition.

codominance: the state in which two different alleles of a pair of chromosomes are expressed to produce specific physical or metabolic traits.

congenital: present at birth, with no implications about the origin or heritability of the trait.

consanguinity: a genetic relationship by descent from a common ancestor.

E

expressivity: describes the variation in clinical manifestations between patients with a particular medical disorder; the variability may be either a difference in age of onset or in severity.

F

first-degree relatives: individuals who share one-half of their genetic material with the proband (parents, siblings, offspring).

forme fruste: an expression of a genetic trait so mild as to be of no clinical significance.

G

geneticist: a specialist in genetics.

H

haploid: the chromosomal number in the normal gamete, designated IN, N = 23.

hemizygous: a term that applies to the genes on the X chromosomes in a male;

since males have only one X, they are hemizygous (not homozygous or heterozygous) with respect to X-linked genes.

hereditary: genetically transmitted or capable of being genetically transmitted from parent to offspring.

heterogeneity: describes disorders that were once thought to be identical, which are found on further scrutiny to be two or more distinct entities.

I

inborn error: a genetically determined biochemical disorder in which a specific enzyme defect produces a metabolic disturbance that may have pathological consequences.

isolated: a trait occurring in a single member of a family, whether or not the trait is heritable.

L

linkage: genes that are tightly located so that the combination between the two loci does not occur and is therefore not transmitted together; e.g., retinoblastoma is tightly linked to esterase D on the q-arm of chromosome 13.

locus: the unique physical location on a chromosome occupied by a specific gene.

M

mendelian disorder: a trait or medical disorder that follows patterns of inheritance suggesting that the entity is determined by a gene at a single locus.

molecular genetics: that branch of genetics concerned with the molecular structure and activities of the genetic material.

mutation: any alteration in the genetic material regardless of whether the change has a positive, indifferent, or negative effect.

P

p-arm: the short arm of a chromosome, with relationship to the centromere.

pedigree chart: a shorthand method of visually recording genetic family data.

pleiotropism: multiple phenotypic abnormalities produced by a single mutant gene.

polymorphism: the occurrence together in a population of two or more genetically determined phenotypes, each with an appreciable frequency.

polygenic inheritance: the interaction of a number of genes that act additively to determine a given trait.

proband: the affected family member who first draws attention to a pedigree of a given trait; also called propositus or index case.

Q

q-arm: the long arm of a chromosome with relationship to the centromere; as apposed to the p-arm.

R

recombinant DNA: artificially synthesized DNA in which a gene or part of a gene from one organism is inserted into the genome of another.

S

second-degree relatives: individuals who share one fourth of their genetic material with the proband (grandparents, aunts, uncles, grandchildren).

CHAPTER 6

EMBRYOLOGY

Embryology is the science that deals with the origin, structure, and development of the embryo. It is derived from the Greek *"em"* meaning in and *"bryein"* meaning swelling. The fascinating world of embryology leads us to understand some of the congenital defects that arise. A *coloboma* is a defect of ocular tissue such as the lid, iris, retina, and choroid that usually results because of failure of the fetal fissure to close in embryonic life. *Microophthalmus* is a small disorganized eye that often has a *microcornea* or a small cornea of less than 9 mm in horizontal diameter. A multiple number of eye defects can occur and are listed below.

A

agenesis: absence of an organ resulting from failure of the developmental tissue to form.

aniridia: absence of the iris.

anisocoria: unequal size of the pupils in diameter.

anlage: primitive tissue from which an organ or part develops; the term primordium has a similar meaning.

anophthalmos: absence of the eye caused by a developmental defect (Fig. 6-1).

aplasia: lack of development of an organ or tissue.

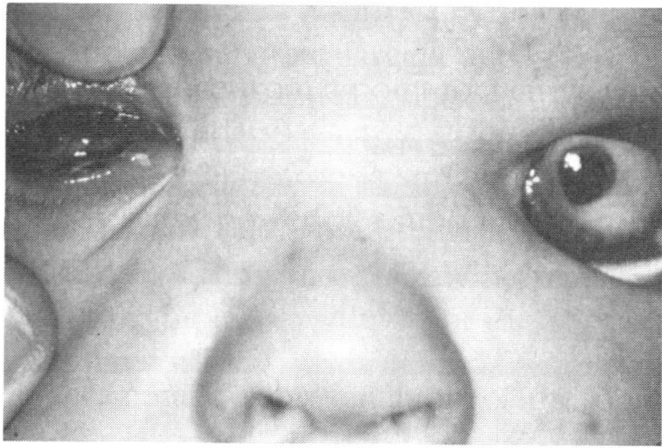

Fig. 6-1. Anophthalmos, a rare developmental condition, is manifested by the absence of an eye. (Courtesy Department of Ophthalmology, Mayo Clinic.)

C

Chievitz layer: an embryologic term that refers to a layer of the retina that disappears by the eleventh week of embryonic life.

choristoma: a mass of tissue histologically normal for an organ or part of an organ other than the site at which it is located.

coloboma: a defect of some ocular tissue; e.g., lid, iris, retina, and choroid, which usually results from failure of the fetal fissure to close in embryonic life (Fig. 6-2).

corectopia: deformed pupil.

cryptophthalmos: a developmental anomaly in which the skin is continuous over the eyeballs without any indication of the formation of eyelids.

cyclopia: a lethal developmental anomaly characterized by a single orbit, within which the globe may be absent, rudimentary, or single.

D

dysgenesis: defective development.

dysplasia: abnormal development of tissues or cells with retention of some features resembling normal structures.

E

ectoderm: one of the primary tissues of the embryo that goes on to form three cell lines: (1) neuroectoderm—which forms the retina, retinal pigment epithelium, ciliary epithelium, iris epithelium, optic nerve, and sphincter and dilator muscles of the iris; (2) surface ectoderm—which forms the lens and the epithelium of the cornea, conjunctiva, lacrimal gland, lacrimal excretory apparatus, and the lids; and (3) neural crest cells—which form the corneal

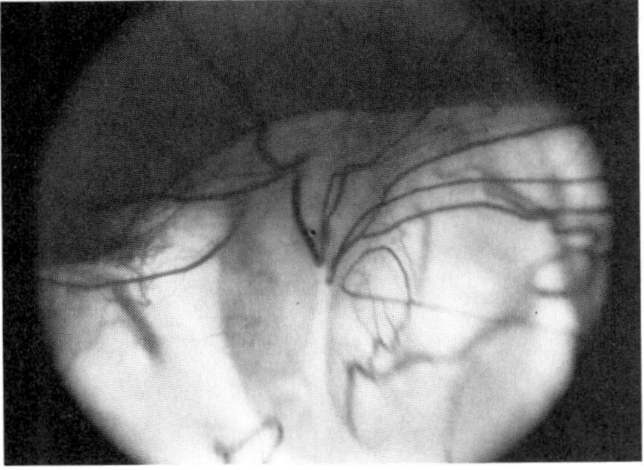

Fig. 6-2. Coloboma of the retina and choroid is present inferior to the disc. (Courtesy Department of Ophthalmology, Mayo Clinic.)

stroma and endothelium, iris stroma, trabecular meshwork, ciliary body, choroidal stroma, sclera, and orbital bones.

ectopia: displaced pupil.

embryogenesis: the earliest stages of development of a new individual from a fertilized ovum.

L

lens placode: a thickened area of ectoderm in the early embryo from which the lens develops.

leukoma: a congenital corneal disorder characterized by discrete, white, opacified areas in the central or peripheral cornea.

M

megalocornea: a large cornea, greater than 12 mm in horizontal diameter.

mesenchyme: the meshwork of embryonic connective tissue from which are formed the connective tissues, blood vessels, and lymphatic vessels of the body.

mesoderm: one of the primary tissues of the embryo that gives rise to the endothelium of the blood vessels and the extraocular muscles.

microcornea: a small cornea, less than 9 mm in horizontal diameter; frequently found in microphthalmia.

microphthalmos: a small, disorganized eye.

N

nanophthalmus: a rare developmental anomaly in which the eyeballs are abnormally small but are without other deformities.

neural tube: a tubular structure of the embryo that goes on to form the central nervous system.

O

optic cup: a cup-shaped part or structure of the primitive eye formed from the optic vesicle.

optic pits: a stage of ocular development that follows the formation of the optic primordia.

optic primordia: the first identifiable structure destined to become the eye.

optic vesicle: a structure of the embryonic eye formed from the optic pit.

orbital encephalocele: herniation of cranial contents, e.g., meninges, brain, into the orbit through a bony defect.

organogenesis: the development or growth of organs; period of development after embryogenesis, begins about the fourth week in ocular development.

P

polycoria: presence of many openings in the iris.

posterior embryotoxin: a congenital opacity of the margin of the cornea; also called arcus juvenilis.

primordium: the earliest discernible indication during embryonic development of an organ or part; called also anlage or rudiment.

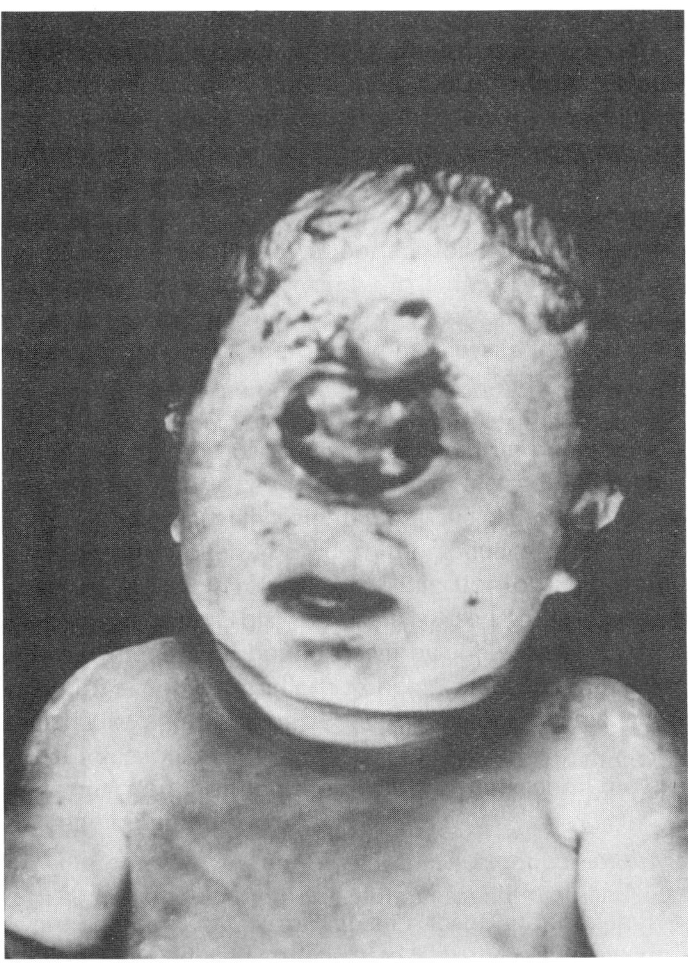

Fig. 6-3. Synophthalmos, a developmental anomaly, is characterized by the eyes being partly joined in the midline. (Courtesy Department of Ophthalmology, Mayo Clinic.)

S

sclerocornea: the scleral rim extends anteriorly, replacing the peripheral cornea and leaving 2 to 3 mm of clear cornea centrally.

spherophakia: a spherical lens that has a tendency to dislocate; often associated with various joint diseases; e.g., Marfan's syndrome and Weill-Marchesani syndrome.

synophthalmia: a lethal condition in which parts of the two eyes are joined in the midline (Fig. 6-3).

T

teratogen: an agent or factor that causes physical defects in the developing embryo.

teratoma: a true neoplasm made up of a number of different types of tissue, some of which is native to the area in which it occurs.

tunica vasculosa lentis: the vascular envelope that encloses and nourishes the developing lens of the fetus.

CHAPTER 7

RESEARCH TERMS

Statistics is the field of study concerned with (1) the organization and tabulation of data, and (2) the drawing of inferences about a body of data when only a part of the data is observed. There are a number of ways that studies can be designed so as to collect important information. A *retrospective* (case-control) study is one in which a group is identified with some specific disease (case group) and another group is identified without the disease (control group). The two groups are then compared as to the presence or absence of an antecedent factor to determine its association with the risk of developing a disease (Fig. 7-1). A *prospective* (cohort) study is one in which a group of subjects is identified that is exposed to some specific factor (exposed group) and another is identified that is not exposed to that factor (nonexposed group). Both groups are then followed to determine the association of the factor with the frequency of occurrence of some subsequent event; e.g., the risk of developing a disease (Fig. 7-2). A *clinical trial* is a controlled experiment on human beings designed to investigate the efficacy of some form of medical treatment. This experiment may be done in a *double-blind* fashion such that neither the physician nor the patient is aware of which treatment the patient has received (Fig. 7-3).

Commonly used statistical terms and their definitions are presented below.

The *mean* is the arithmetic average i.e., the total of values of a set of observations divided by the number of values. The mean age of five patients are obtained as follows:

$$\text{mean age} = \frac{35 + 71 + 65 + 65 + 44 \text{ years of age}}{5} = 56 \text{ years of age}$$

The *median* is the middle value of data, ordered from lowest to highest. If the number of values is odd, the median will be the middle value when all values have been arranged in order of magnitude. When the number of observations is even, there is no single middle observation, but two middle observations. In this case the median is taken to be the average of these two middle observations. To obtain the median value of the ages in the sample above, we would arrange the values in order of magnitude; e.g., 35, 44, 65, 65, and 71. Since this is an odd number of values the median is the middle value, or 65.

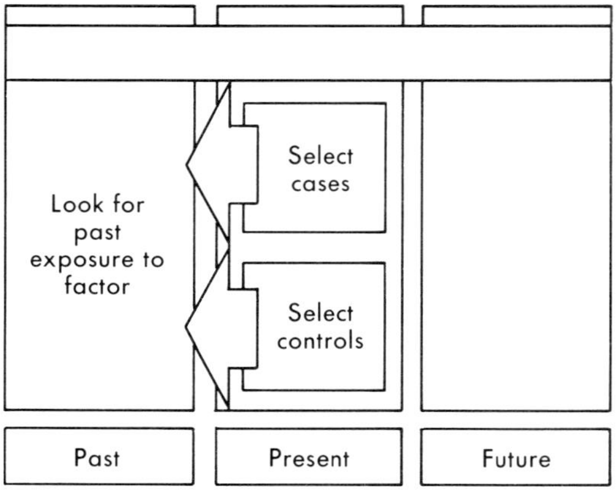

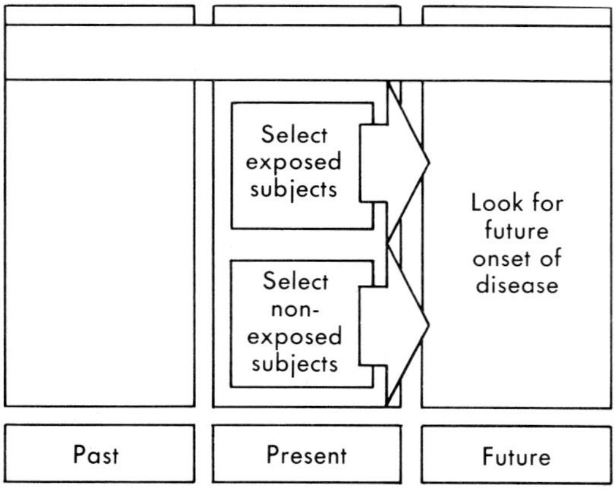

Look for
past
exposure to
factor
Select
cases
Select
controls
Past
Present
Future

Fig. 7-1. Retrospective study.

Select
exposed
subjects
Select
non-
exposed
subjects
Look for
future
onset of
disease
Past
Present
Future

Fig. 7-2. Prospective study.

Subjects
randomized
Exposed
group
Non-
exposed
group
Look for
future
onset of
disease
Present
Future

Fig. 7-3. Clinical trial.

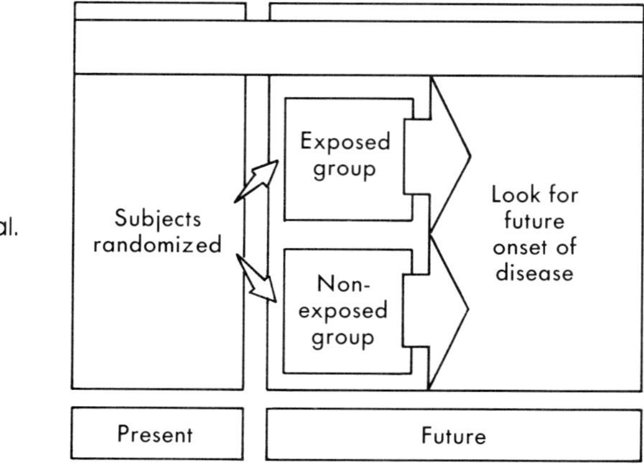

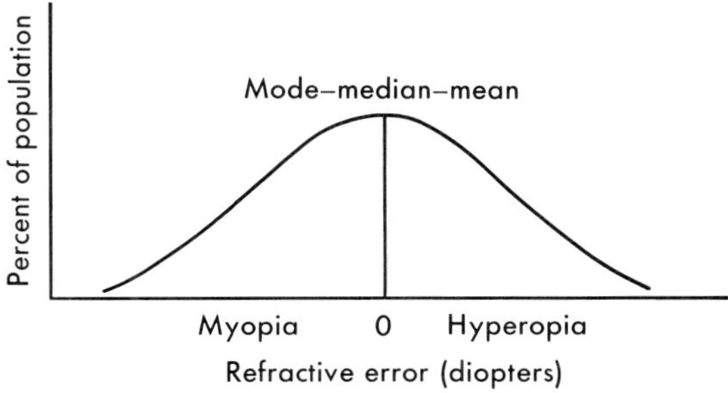

Fig. 7-4. The normal (Gaussian) distribution of refractive errors in the general population.

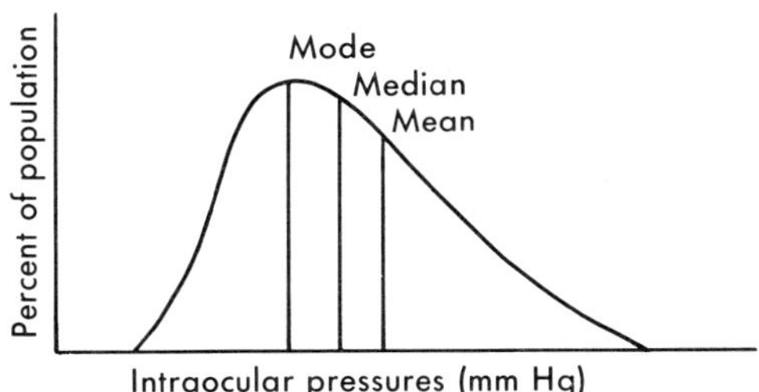

Fig. 7-5. The median value of data is the middle value when all values are arranged in order of magnitude. The mode is the most frequent value. The mean is the arithmetic average of all values.

The *mode* is the most frequent value of a set of observations. If all the values are different there is no mode; on the other hand, a set of values may have more than one mode. In the example above, the mode value would be 65 years of age since it occurs more frequently than the other values.

A *normal distribution* is a bell-shaped (Gaussian) distribution in which the mean, median, and mode are the same (Fig. 7-4). For example, let us consider the ages for cataract surgery of nine patients: 65, 67, 68, 70, 70, 70, 72, 73, and 75. In this sample, the mean, median, and mode are all equal to 70 years of age. If the mean, median, and mode differ at all from each other, as in our initial example, than a skewed distribution results in contrast to the normal bell-shaped distribution (Fig. 7-5).

Variance is a measure of variability. When the values of a set of observations lie close to their mean, the variance is less than when they are scattered over a wide range. To compute the variance, subtract the mean from each of the values, square the differences, and then add them up. This sum is then divided by the sample size, minus one, to obtain the variance.

Standard deviation is a measure of dispersion obtained by taking the square root of the variance. The standard deviation of a normal frequency distribution (a bell-shaped curve) may be used with the mean to indicate the percentage of items that fall within specified ranges. Thus if a population of observations is in the form of a normal distribution, the following relationships apply:

mean + 1 SD includes 68.3% of all items
mean + 2 SD includes 95.5% of all items
mean + 3 SD includes 99.7% of all items

In interpreting data it is important to question the reliability or significance of the information. For example, suppose a study found that 33% of patients who had intraocular pressures greater than 30 mm Hg developed visual loss. It is apparent that if the study involved a large sample of patients it would be more reliable than if only a small group was investigated. The χ^2 (*Chi squared*) test and the *t* test allow one to measure the statistical significance that is determined by the *"p" value*. In theory, a p value of less than 0.01 means that, if the same experiment were repeated 100 times, 99 times the same results would be obtained because of the experiment itself and one time as a result of chance alone. Thus p value less than 0.05 means that in less than 5 of 100 times the results would be the result of chance.

C

chance: the happening of events; the way in which things occur.

coefficient of variation: used to compare the variability of two groups with different units of measure, such as blood sugar level (mg/100 ml) with respiration (breaths/minute; it is the size of the standard deviation relative to the size of the mean (in percentage).

control group: comparison group for evaluating the effect of an experimental procedure.

correlation coefficient: a number that indicates the strength of association between two variables.

D

dispersion: refers to the variety that the values of the observation exhibit; if all the values are the same, there is no dispersion; if they are not all the same, dispersion is present in the data.

F

false-negative result: an error in a diagnostic test indicating a disease-free state when the disease really exists.

false-positive result: an error in a diagnostic test indicating a disease state when there is no disease.

finite population: a finite collection of individuals.

frequency: the number of occurrences of a given type of event, or the number of members of a population falling into a specified class.

H

histogram: a bar graph in which the values of the variable under consideration make up the horizontal axis, whereas the vertical axis has as its scale the frequency of occurrence.

I

incidence rate: the total number of new cases of a specific disease during a year, divided by the total population and multiplied by 100.

independent events: two events are independent if the probability of one is the same whether or not the other is given.

inference: estimation of population values (parameters) from sample data.

interpolation: the process of obtaining intermediate terms when other data are available.

O

ordered array: a listing of the values of a collection (either population or sample) in order of magnitude from the smallest value to the largest value.

P

parameter: a fixed figure (quantity) that characterizes a given population.

percentiles: values that divide a distribution of ordered data into 100 equal parts.

placebo: an inactive substance or preparation given to satisfy the patient's symbolic need for drug therapy and used in controlled studies to determine the efficacy of medicinal substances.

population: the entire group about which information is desired.

prevalence rate: defined as the total number of cases, new or old, existing at a point in time divided by the total population at that point in time, multiplied by 100.

R

range: differences between the highest and lowest values.

rate: the number of events (cases) in a period of time divided by the population exposed to the risk of this event.

S

sample: that portion of a population about which information is actually obtained.

sampling error: error resulting from chance in the sampling process resulting in some difference between the sample outcome and the complete count carried out in the same manner.

sensitivity: the probability that the diagnostic test will yield a positive result when given to a person who has the disease.

specificity: the probability that the diagnostic test will yield a negative result when given to a person who does not have the disease.

V

validity (accuracy): closeness with which a measured value agrees with the "true" value.

CHAPTER 8

BASIC COMPUTER TERMS

Computer terms have become buzz words in everyday use. New vocabulary is added regularly. Some basic terms should become part of each individual's vocabulary. Many readers may already be familiar with them; for others, this may be an entirely new area.

A *microcomputer* is a desk-top or portable computer for a single user. It is often called a personal computer or PC. *Memory* refers to the internal data storage capacity of the computer. A *memory chip* is a chip whose component forms thousands of cells, each holding a single bit of information. A *bit* is the smallest unit of information in a computer. The word "bit" is a contraction of the words *binary digit.* The *binary cord* is a system of representing things by combination of two symbols.

Hardware refers to the physical devices and components of a computer system. *Software* refers to programs that permit the computer hardware to do specific functions. The programs may be "stored" either as a *"hard" disk* that is part of the computer or as a *"floppy" disk* or "tape back-up". A *word processing* program is one that is able to handle textual material. *ROM* stands for "read only memory," where data are stored permanently and can be read by the user but not altered. *RAM* stands for "random access memory," in which the memory may be retrieved, altered, or erased by the user. *Networking* refers to a system in which two or more computers are interlinked.

A

ASCII: acronym for American Standard Code for Information Interchange.

B

back up: the process of creating a duplicate of the information stored in the computer.

binary number system: a numbering system with two symbols, 1 and 0, that has 2 as its base.

bit: the smallest unit of information, represented mathematically as a single digit consisting of a "one" or a "zero," sometimes considered an abbreviation for binary unit or binary digit.

bug: an error in a program caused, usually accidentally, by the programmer.

byte: a piece of computer memory representing a letter, digit, or punctuation mark. They are eight bits in length. A bit is the smallest unit of the computer information represented by a choice between two alternatives such as on-off, yes-no. A combination of bits makes up the codes for different characters.

C

cathode ray tube (CRT): viewing screen of the computer.

central processing unit (CPU): computer hardware that carries out data manipulation and controls the sequence of operations the computer performs.

chip: an integrated circuit on a small patch of silicon made up of thousands of transistors and other electronic components.

D

data: numeric or similarly coded information that is or may be converted into a suitable form for some computer storage medium.

data base: a file of data so structured that appropriate applications draw from the file and update it but do not themselves constrain the file design or its content.

data entry: the activity of putting information into a computer.

debugging: the technique of detecting, diagnosing, and correcting errors (also known as bugs) that occur in programs or systems (both hardware and software).

diagnostics: also known as diagnostic programs—programs written for the explicit purpose of testing certain devices or conditions; there are printer diagnostics, disk diagnostics, and even processor diagnostic programs.

digitizer: device for converting lines, circles, and other forms into numbers for storage on computer media. NOTE: A plotter takes digitized information and generates a drawing of lines, circles, and so on.

disk: rigid, circular platter, coated with magnetizable material, used to store information.

diskette: flexible plastic magnetic storage medium; often referred to as floppy disk.

disk controller: controls the flow of data between the disk and the internal memory.

display unit: the television-like display used for computer output; also called video display unit (VDU) and cathode ray tube (CRT).

do-it-yourself: mode of system development in which the user writes his or her own program.

dot matrix: a printing method or mechanism that forms images, such as the letters of the alphabet, from individual dots on the paper; the arrangement of dots is by rows and columns, hence the term matrix.

drive: also called a disk unit—the physical mechanism that reads information from and writes information onto a disk.

driver: the logical program or program module that controls the reading and writing of a device such as a disk or tape.

E

external memory: where data are stored, such as on disk and tape.

F

files: collections of data or program instructions recorded on a computer medium such as magnetic disk or diskette.

floppy disk: a thin disk with one or two magnetic recording surfaces (see *diskette*).

G

graphics: a specialized area of computer usage dealing with the generation, enhancement, or analysis of images.

H

hard copy: printed copies of information generated by a computer.

hardware: the physical devices and components of a computer system.

I

integrated circuit: an electronic circuit on a chip (e.g., a microprocessor) in which the circuit components themselves, the wires, and the insulators are all formed together in a single block of silicon as part of a single manufacturing process. The word "integrated" is used to distinguish this type of circuit from the older type in which components (such as transistors) were first made individually and then later formed into a circuit using wires and solder.

interface: a physical component designed to interconnect two devices; a format by which two program modules can be interconnected; in both cases a set of rules is associated with the interface.

internal memory: storage area in which programs are run and manipulated. There are two types of internal memory: RAM and ROM.

I/O: input/output.

J

joystick: a device for converting smooth movements of the arm and wrist into numbers for storage on computer media.

K

K: 1024 bytes of computer memory capacity; 2K represents 2 × 1204, or 2048 bytes.

keyboard: the principal data entry device for most computers; consists of keys most commonly arranged in the same fashion as the keys of a typewriter.

L

language: a set of symbols and a set of rules for expressing procedures and relationships with those symbols.

letter quality: of the same appearance as the print image produced by a top-quality typewriter.

line printer: a printing device that produces an entire print line at one time or in one movement; all the characters in the same line are generated at the same time.

M

machine code: the coding system adopted in the design of a computer to represent the instruction repertoire of the computer. The various operations that can be performed are represented by numeric function codes, and all store locations are allocated numbers to enable the data stored in such locations to be addressed. Also known as computer code, instruction code, instruction set, order code.

magnetic tape: this type of memory, which stores information in exactly the same way as an ordinary tape cassette, has the advantage of not needing an electrical power supply to keep the information stored. It has the disadvantage, for some applications, of taking seconds (or in the case of long tapes, minutes) to get at a particular item of information.

mainframe computer: originally implied the main framework of a central processing unit on which the arithmetic unit and associated logic circuits were mounted, but now used colloquially to refer to the central processor itself.

megabyte: one million binary digits.

memory: the part of a computer that holds instructions and data.

menu: a display format in which the computer user's options are presented as a series of entries in a list, as in a restaurant's menu.

microcomputer: a computer whose central processor is a microprocessor.

microprocessor: a computer processor usually characterized by small physical silicon chip and functions as the computer's central processing unit.

minicomputer: a computer whose central processor is faster, compared with micros, and whose instruction repertoire is quite large.

monitor: television-like viewing screen, usually higher resolution than a color television; may be monochromatic (black and white) or color, but usually monochromatic. This is comprised of a cathode ray tube that permits the visualization of the characters that are fed into the computer.

motherboard: a chassis or cabinet designed so that several electronic circuit boards can be connected into it.

mouse: a pointing device used to introduce a command.

MSDOS: disc operating system created by Microsoft.

multiuser: a system that has more than one visual display unit and more than one keyboard.

N

network: an arrangement of several computers interlinked over telecommunications lines.

O

operating system: a program that allows the computer to accept commands from the user, retrieve or record data on disk and/or tape, and send it to the printer and monitor.

P

parallel interface: a method of transmitting data from device to device in which an entire byte or word at a time has its component bits moved simultaneously along parallel wires to achieve a high rate of data transfer.

plotter: an output device for making images, usually through juxtaposition of tiny dots; the opposite of digitizer.

printer: output device that produces copy on paper.

programmer: one who writes or codes programs.

programs: collection or packages of instructions organized in a logical fashion so as to perform anything from a simple function to a complex application.

publication quality: suitable for reproduction in books or other printed forms.

punched card: a card containing data represented in the form of punched holes that can be sensed by a variety of machines in order to carry out various logical functions (such as addition, subtracting, comparing, collating, and printing).

R

random access memory (RAM): an internal memory of a program that may be altered or erased.

read: retrieve data from a storage medium.

ROM (read only memory): internal memory where data are stored permanently and will not be lost in the absence of power. Commonly used programs such as the operating system are in ROM so they may be run without first being loaded into RAM from disk or tape; also called firmware.

record: within a data file, the smallest logical entity that may contain a complete set of each type of data element in the file.

S

sequential access storage: a storage device in which data can be accessed only in the sequence in which they are stored in the device; i.e., an item can be processed only after all the preceding items have been accessed. An example of sequential access storage is magnetic tape.

simulation: using a computer to pretend to be, or setting up a correspondence between computer operations and, a physical mechanism such as a wind tunnel or a phenomenon such as the flow of people through an outpatient clinic.

slot: a position in the microprocessor chassis that is designed for connection to another device.

software: programs that allow the computer to perform specific functions.

storage: memory capacity or requirements of a system or application—either memory, or disk, or both.

T

terminal: an input/output device at which data leave or enter a computer system.

time sharing: a method for permitting several users or programs to have access to the same machine at the same time.

U

user: the person who is operating the computer or the person for whom the computer is programmed or operated.

W

word: unit of information processed by the CPU at one time, usually a multiple of a byte.

word processing: using a computer or other sophisticated device to handle textual material, usually for producing a typed end product.

write: to record data on a memory device.

PART TWO

REFRACTION, SPECTACLES, AND CONTACT LENSES

CHAPTER 9

REFRACTION

The term *refraction* refers to the sum total of *refractometry* (measuring the refractive error of an eye), assessing the visual needs of an individual and arriving at a clinical judgment as to which prescription to provide.

When light passes from one medium to another, it changes its direction or is *refracted* or bent back because light travels at different speeds in different media.

Emmetropia (Greek *em,* "within," *metro,* "measure," and *opia,* "the eye") is the measurement of a normal eye (Fig. 9-1, *A*). *Ametropia* is the measurement of an abnormal eye. *Hyperopia* (*hyper,* "beyond," *opia,* "eye") refers to a farsighted eye (Fig. 9-1, *B*). *Myopia* (Greek *my,* "close" and *opia,* "eye") refers to the nearsighted eye. Persons with myopia half close the eyelid to gain advantage of the slit to see better.

Hyperopia may be *latent* (hidden), in which case it is completely compensated by the eye's ability to *accommodate* or adjust. *Absolute* hyperopia cannot be compensated by the eye and requires a convex lens to correct the hyperopia (Fig. 9-1, *C* and *D*).

Myopia and *hyperopia* may be *axial,* meaning the eyeball is either too long *(axial myopia)* or too short *(axial hyperopia).* It may be *curvature myopia* or *hyperopia* caused by changes in the curvature of the cornea and lens, which bend the rays of light an improper amount; or it may be *index myopia* or *hyperopia* caused by changes in the index of refraction of the lens, as may occur in the presence of cataracts and diabetes.

Astigmatism is a refractive error in which the rays of light do not come to a point focus on the retina. It may be *regular astigmatism,* in which the rays of light come to two focal points on the retina and is correctable by cylinders, or *irregular astigmatism,* in which the cornea is damaged and irregular so that rays of light come to many focal points on the retina and which is not correctable by cylinders.

Astigmatism is said to be "with the rule" if the plus axis and the steepest meridian is in the vertical or 90-degree plane (Fig. 9-2, *A*). It is said to be "against the rule" if the plus axis and the steepest meridian is in the horizontal or 180-degree plane (Fig. 9-2, *B*).

Astigmatism may be *corneal astigmatism* if caused by different radii of cur-

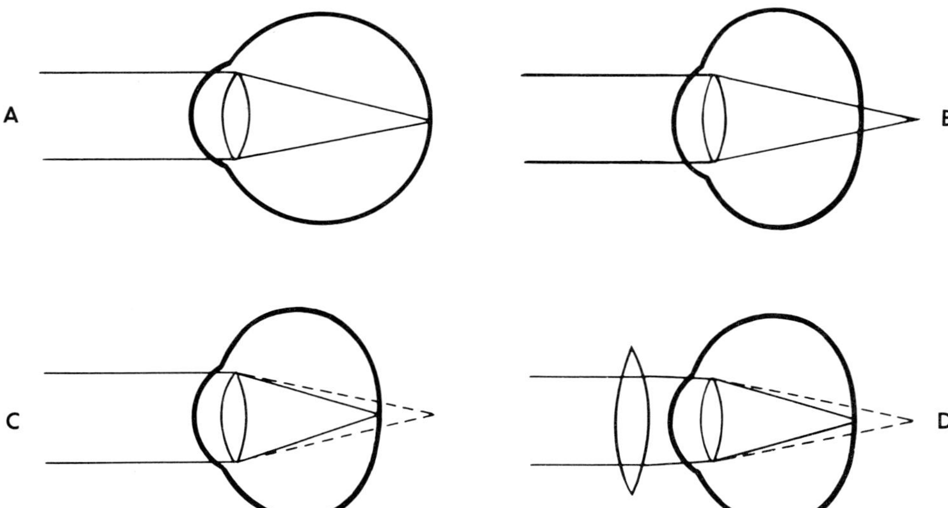

Fig. 9-1. **A,** Emmetropic eye. Parallel rays of light come to a focus on the retina. **B,** Hyperopic eye. Parallel rays of light come to a focus behind the retina in the unaccommodative eye. **C,** Latent hyperopia. Accommodation by the lens of the eye brings parallel rays of light to focus on the retina. **D,** Absolute hyperopia. A convex lens is required to bring rays of light to focus on the retina.

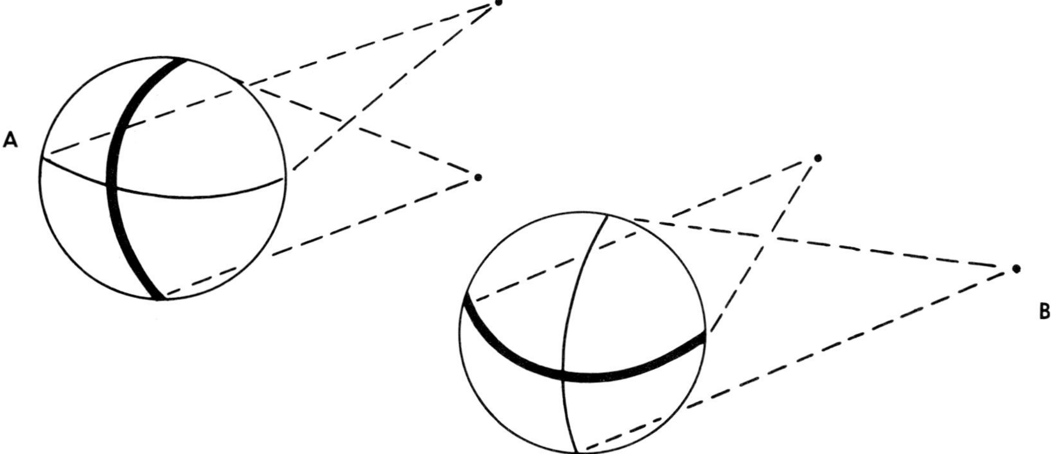

Fig. 9-2. **A,** Astigmatism with the rule. The vertical corneal meridian has the steepest curvature. **B,** Astigmatism against the rule. The horizontal meridian has the steepest curvature.

vature of the cornea, may be *residual astigmatism* if it remains after the corneal astigmatism has been neutralized, and is sometimes also called *lenticular astigmatism* because it is caused by the crystalline lens of the eye.

Anisometropia is a condition in which there is a difference in the refractive error of the two eyes. If the difference is very large, *aniseikonia* (Greek *an,* "not," *iso,* "equal," and *eikon,* "images") exists, and images of unequal size will appear on the retina and be transferred to the brain.

Aphakia (Greek *a,* "absent," *phako,* "lens") is the condition in which the crystalline lens is absent from the eye. *Presbyopia* (Greek *presbyo,* "old," and *opia,* "eye") or "old eye" is a condition in which the ability to accommodate for near vision falls off because of loss of elasticity of the crystalline lens of the eye and weakness of the ciliary muscle. The individual is no longer able to read clearly.

Photopic vision is that vision occurring in daylight when the eye is light adapted. Cones mediate daylight vision, precise vision, and color vision. *Scotopic* vision is that vision occurring at night when the eye is dark adapted. Rods are the active light receptors with scotopic vision.

Some other words relating to optics and refraction have been arranged in alphabetical order.

A

ac/a ratio: accommodative convergence/accommodation ratio; the ratio between the convergence caused by accommodation (in prism diopters) and the accommodation (measured in diopters).

addition or add: the total dioptric power added to a distance prescription to supplement accommodation for reading.

afterimage: image of an object that persists when the lids are closed.

amblyopia: loss of vision without any apparent disease of the eye.

amplitude of accommodation: the total amount of increase in the dioptric power of the eye made by maximum effort of the ciliary muscle.

angle kappa: the difference between the direction of gaze and the apparent direction in which the eye points; this normal structural feature may cause a false interpretation of strabismus.

anisometropia: a difference in the refractive power of the two eyes.

aperture: the opening that permits light to pass through an optical system.

asthenopia: eye fatigue caused by errors of refraction, driving, prolonged close work, dryness of the eyes, and so on. A wastebasket term that embraces a number of causes and situations.

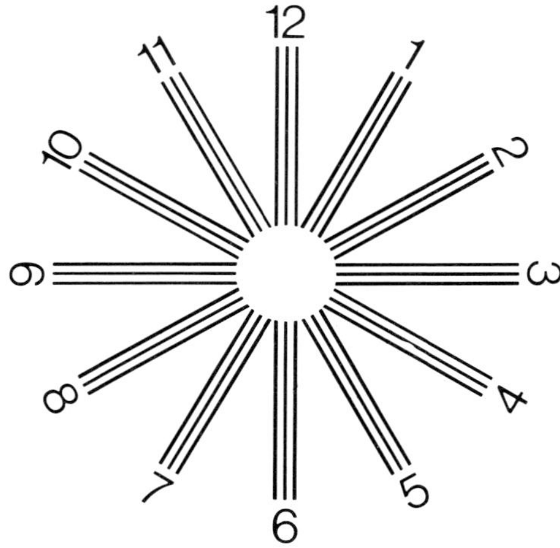

Fig. 9-3. Astigmatic clock.

astigmatic clock: clocklike pattern of lines used to determine the presence of astigmatism and to determine the orientation of astigmatism (Fig. 9-3).

C

convergence: the process of directing the visual axis of the two eyes inward to a new point.

convergence excess: a convergent deviation, greater at near points than at distance.

convergent insufficiency: inability to turn the eyes in at near.

cross cylinder: a lens consisting of two cylinders of equal power, one being plus, the other being minus, set 90 degrees apart. Frequently referred to as the Jackson cross cylinder.

cycloplegic: a drug often used in refraction, which temporarily places the ciliary muscle at rest and dilates the pupil. Used in refraction of children and young adults.

D

depth perception: ability to perceive the solidity of objects and their relative positions in space; also called stereoscopic vision.

distometer: a caliper used to measure the vertex distance, which is the distance from the cornea of the patient's eye to the back surface of the lens. It is inserted in the trial frame, phoropter, or glasses. The distometer consists of a scale in millimeters, an indicator, a movable arm, and a fixed arm (Fig. 9-4).

divergence: the outward rotations of the two eyes to see in the distance.

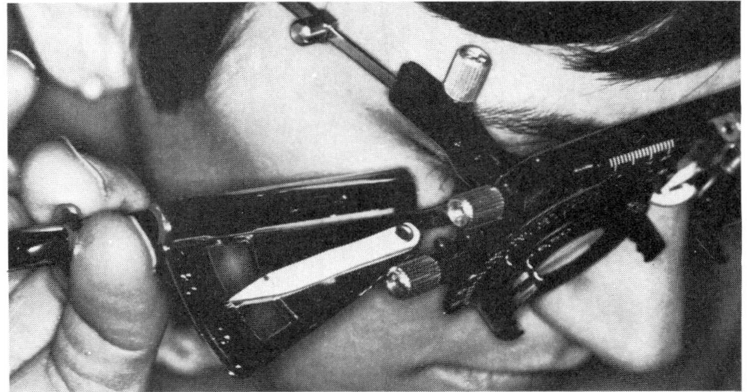

Fig. 9-4. Measuring vertex distance with a distometer.

E

eikonometer: an instrument that was designed to measure the relative size of images seen by the two eyes. No longer manufactured.

F

Farnsworth-Munsell color test: a color test containing 84 colors arranged in order of increasing hue.

fixation disparity: a condition in which the object of fixation does not fall on exactly corresponding retinal points, but in which the images still fall within Panum's fusional area, so that an object is seen singly.

Fresnel press-on prism: a series of small plastic prisms lying adjacent to each other on a thin platform of plastic. It has the same deviating power of the conventional prism but is only 1 mm thick. It is used as a temporary lens because it can peel off, become soiled, and generally has poorer optics than a glass prism.

fusional reserves: the range of convergence, divergence, and vertical vergence through which binocular single vision can be maintained. This may be measured in degrees or prism diopters.

G

glare: irregularly scattered light that interferes with the focused retinal picture and reduces visual acuity.

H

Halberg trial clip: a clip attached to spectacles to insert ophthalmic lenses to over-refract. See also *Janelli clip* (Fig. 9-5).

Hardy-Rand Ritter (HRR): a series of color plates to detect abnormalities of color vision.

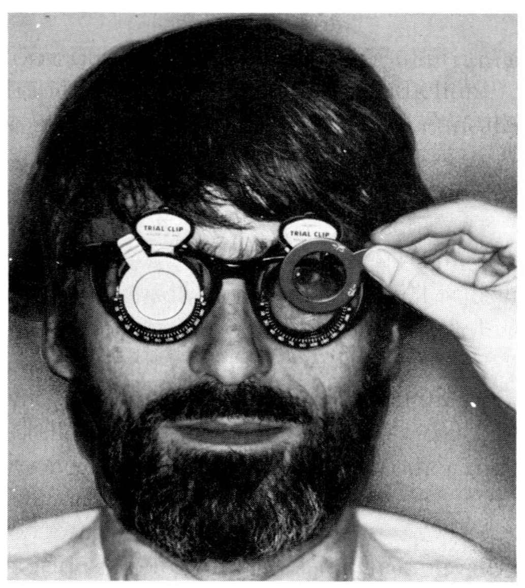

Fig. 9-5. Halberg trial clip used to refract over spectacles.

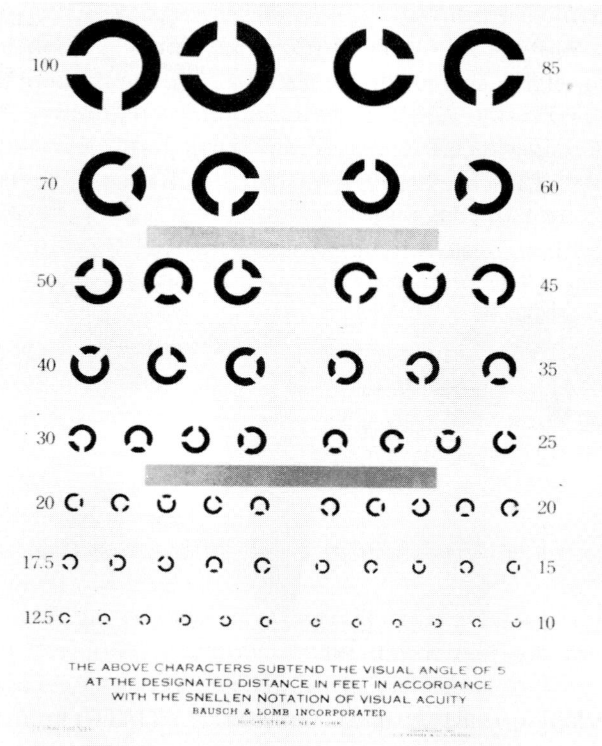

Fig. 9-6. Landolt's broken-ring test.

HRR: see *Hardy-Rand Ritter.*
hyperphoria: a latent tendency for an eye to deviate upward.

J

Jaeger: a numerical grading system for near vision devised by Jaeger in the latter part of the nineteenth century.
Janelli clip: a variation of the Halberg clip, having a bubble level, an extra trial lens cell, and a cylinder lock to keep the cylinder on axis.

K

keratometer: an instrument used to measure the radius of the interior surface of the cornea and the power and axis of the corneal cylinder if present. Based on the principle of utilizing the mirror effect of the front surface of the cornea.

L

Landolt broken-ring test: a test for the measurement of visual acuity consisting of a circle subtending 5 minutes of arc with the thickness of the ring and the gap subtending a 1-minute angle (Fig. 9-6).
lensometer: an instrument designed to measure the prescription of an optical lens (trade names include Lensmeter, Focimeter, Vertometer, Vertexmeter).
light perception (LP): ability to distinguish only light from dark.
light projection: ability to determine the quadrantal direction of light.
LP: see *light perception.*

M

Maddox rod: a lens composed of a parallel series of very strong cylinders. When viewed through a Maddox rod, a point of light appears as a red line. Used to measure the latent muscle imbalance or phoria of the eye.
magnification: increase in size achieved by a lens system (Fig. 9-7).

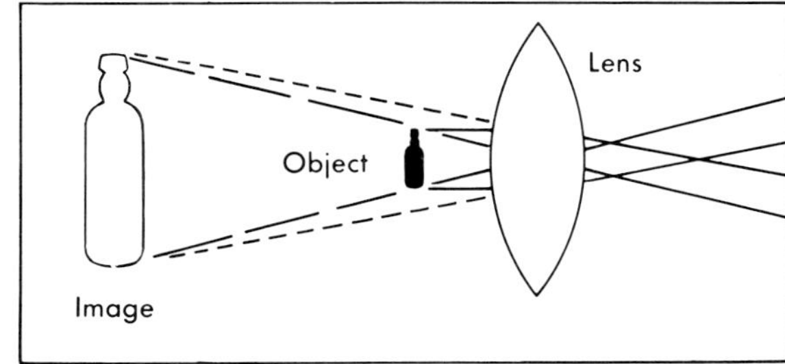

Fig. 9-7. Magnification by a convex lens is obtained by bringing the object within the focal distance of the convex lens. An erect magnified image is obtained.

minify: to reduce the apparent dimensions. The opposite of magnify.

monocular: pertaining to or affecting one eye.

multifocal: a spectacle or contact lens with more than one focusing power area.

N

near point of accommodation (NPA): the nearest point measured in centimeters that each eye can maintain clarity of small print when it is brought close to the eye.

near point of convergence (NPC): the nearest point measured in centimeters that a person can maintain binocular vision when an object is brought close in the midline. The nearest point an individual can hold fusion before seeing double.

night myopia: an increase in myopia that occurs after dark; caused by dilation of the pupil.

NPA: see *near point of accommodation.*

NPC: see *near point of convergence.*

O

orthophoria: a condition in which the eyes are straight; a condition in which the visual axes are parallel even when the eyes are dissociated.

P

Panum's fusional area: an area around corresponding retinal points, including slightly disparate retinal elements, whose stimulation will result in binocular fusion with stereopsis rather than diplopia.

Phoropter: trade name for a refractor. An instrument for determining the refractive state of the eye, phorias, and so on, consisting of a housing containing a rotating disc with lenses, occluders, prisms, and pinholes.

pinhole disc: a disc with one or more holes to eliminate peripheral rays of light and improve contrast. Used to determine the visual acuity by eliminating the refractive error of the eye.

progressive myopia: refers to myopia over 6 D that is increasing in dioptric power.

R

refractive error: a defect in the eye that prevents light rays from being brought to a single focus exactly on the retina.

retinal correspondence: corresponding retinal areas in both eyes that perceive the same point in space simultaneously.

retinoscopy: objective method of determining the refractive error of the eye by observing the movements of light reflected from the back of the eye.

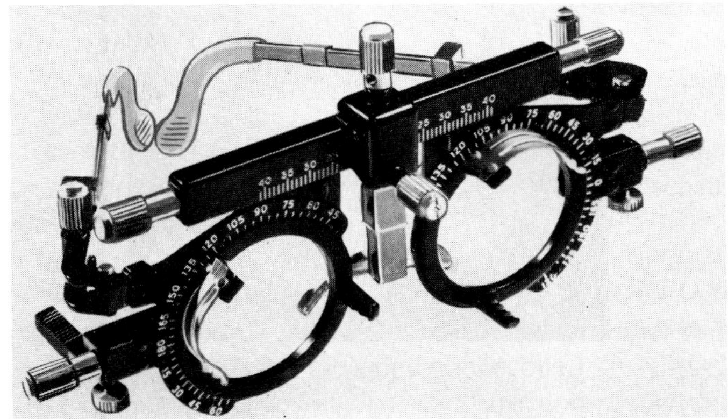

Fig. 9-8. Trial frame.

S

spherical equivalent: the equivalent of spectacle refraction expressed only as a sphere. To obtain it, take half of the cylinder and algebraically add it to the sphere.

spherocylinder: a lens with one spherical surface and one cylindrical (or toric) surface.

T

telescopic lenses: special lenses for persons with advanced degrees of sight impairment; two lenses, properly ground, and mounted in a spectacle frame with a short distance between them to form a Galilean telescope.

transposition: the process of changing a spectacle prescription from a plus to minus cylinder or vice versa without changing its refractive value.

trial case and lenses: a tray of ophthalmic lenses and accessories to determine the refractive error of the eye.

trial frame: an adjustable spectacle frame into which trial lenses are placed during the refraction procedure (Fig. 9-8).

trifocal: a lens with three focusing points such as distance, intermediate, and reading.

W

Wirt stereo test: a test to grade stereopsis or depth perception.

Worth four-dot test: an illuminated red, green, and white dot test to detect the presence of binocular vision or suppression.

CHAPTER 10

SPECTACLES

The use of lenses in optics was first mentioned by Roger Bacon in 1268. Thirteen years later spectacles were invented by either Alendresso della Spina or Salvino degli Armanti of Pisa. Over Armanti's tomb is the inscription "Here lies Salvino degli Armanti, inventor of spectacles; may God pardon his sins." Marco Polo recorded that the Chinese were using spectacles in 1270, but some sources claim that they served an ornamental rather than functional purpose in this period.

Spectacles, originating from the Latin *spectaculum* meaning a "spectacle" or "show," are optical appliances consisting of lenses and a *frame,* the latter with "earpieces," loosely called *temples,* extending over the ears. The *bridge* is the part of a spectacle frame that either joins the two lenses together in the rimless type or joins the eyewire of the front with lenses inserted in rigid frames. The lenses are held in the frame by means of screws or clamps as in a *rimless* frame or by means of an *eyewire* in a full frame. The eyewire may be composed of metal, plastic, a thread of nylon, or any combination of the three.

Frames

Frames are now most commonly made of *cellulose acetate,* a thermoplastic that is poorly flammable. They were formerly made (now banned in North America) from *cellulose nitrate,* a highly flammable material sometimes known as *celluloid, xylonite, zylonite,* or *zyl.* Frames may be made from *polymethylmethacrylate,* sometimes called *Plexiglass, Lucite,* or *Perspex,* which is the same material used to make hard lenses. This plastic is strong, retains its shape, and is available in solid colors. Frames may be made from nylon, which is flexible but becomes brittle with age, or from *Optyl,* a lightweight flexible material available in a variety of colors and popular because of its semitransparent appearance. *Molded frames* are injection-molded plastic frames, identified by plastic hinges and a seam and found in inexpensive sunglasses.

The bridges of frames are of two basic types, the *saddle* type and the *keyhole* type, designated by a shape resembling that of a saddle or keyhole. The saddle bridge with a wide nasal cut creates the illusion of shortening a long nose, whereas the keyhole bridge, with an elongated nasal opening, is used for round, short noses. *Pads* are the portions of the frame that rest on the sides of the nose. A

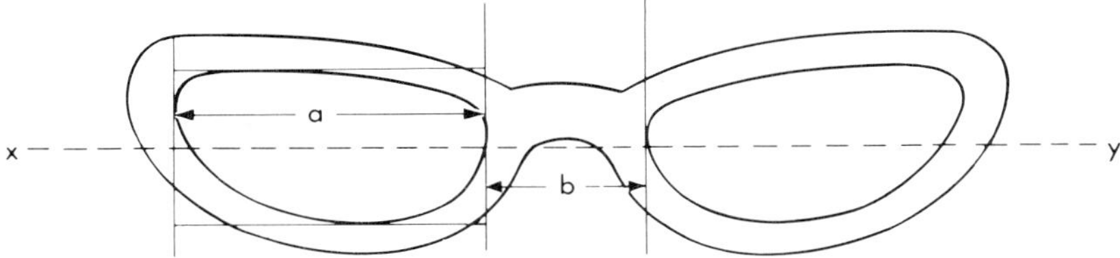

Fig. 10-1. Frame measurements; *a* represents the eye size; *b* represents the bridge size. The dotted line *xy* is the box system.

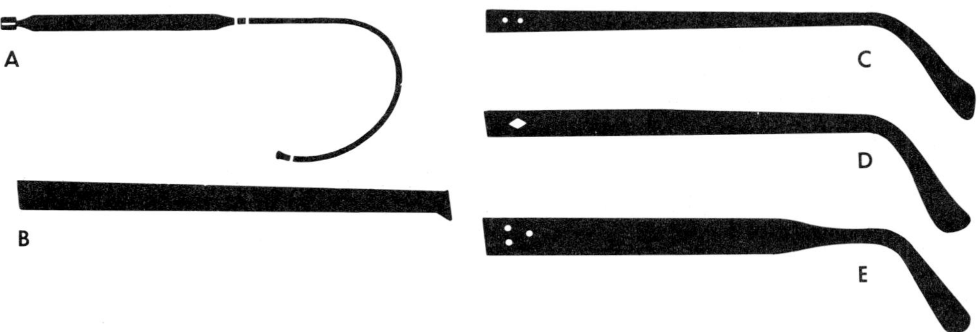

Fig. 10-2. **A,** Cable, riding bow, or curl side temples. **B,** Straight, loafer, or library temples. **C** to **E,** Paddle, skull, or hockey-end temples.

comfort bridge is a plastic insert, usually a saddle design, which inserts into the bridge of a metal frame. This displaces the weight over a greater area by resting equally on the bridge and the sides of the nose.

On the back of each frame are noted the millimeter measurements of the *eye size,* or the inside distance of the lens aperture measured horizontally, and the *bridge size,* the measurement of the width of the bridge. The *datum* line represents an imaginary line running through the center of the lenses (Fig. 10-1).

Cable temples, sometimes called *riding bow* or *curl temples,* have a flexible portion that can be shaped to contour and curve behind the ear. They are used for children, athletes, and active people. *Straight* temples, sometimes called *loafer, spatule,* or *library* temples, fit around the side of the head and are used for people who constantly remove their spectacles. *Spring hinge temples* maintain lateral tension for a longer period of time. The spring hinge may be used for any of the temple designs. *Paddle temples,* shaped like a paddle, are sometimes called *skull* or *hockey-end temples* and are the most popular (Fig. 10-2).

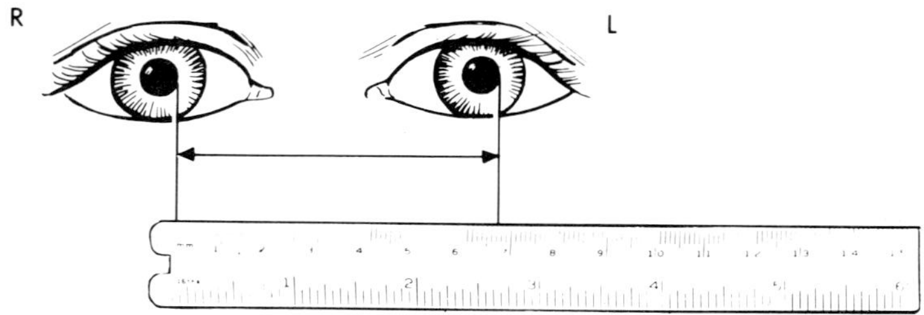

Fig. 10-3. Measurement of interpupillary distance. Measurements are commonly made from the nasal edge of one pupil to the temporal edge of the other pupil. Near ray measurements are several millimeters less than measurements at distance.

Measurements

The *interpupillary distance* or pupillary distance (PD) is the distance in millimeters between the center of the two pupils of the two eyes (Fig. 10-3). It is conveniently measured from the nasal edge of the pupil of one eye to the temporal edge of the pupil of the other eye. The *optical center* of a lens is the point on a lens in which light rays are not bent and corresponds to the thinnest portion of a minus lens and the thickest portion of a plus lens. Under normal circumstances the optical center of a lens is aligned with the corresponding pupil of the eye. The optical center of a lens does not necessarily coincide with the geometric center of a lens (Fig. 10-4) or the major reference point.

Lenses

Ophthalmic lenses are made of glass, the most popular being *crown glass,* which is primarily sodium silicate with a low refractive index (1.523), and *flint glass,* made of lead oxide with a high refractive index (1.62). *Hidex glass* is a high-index glass (1.86) used for myopia or hyperopia. Every lens has an anterior curve and a posterior base curve that is measured in diopters. The anterior is a frontal curve, whereas the base curve is the concave or posterior curve of the lens. The mathematical difference between the two curvatures produces the power of the lens measured in diopters. The base curve may be deliberately altered, minimally to allow for eyelash clearance.

Lenses may also have a secondary curve adjacent to, but 90 degrees away from, the base curve. These curves lie in different meridians of power, and their purpose is to correct astigmatism. When the cylinder correction is on the anterior plane of the lens, the lens has been made in "plus cylinder form"; and conversely lenses

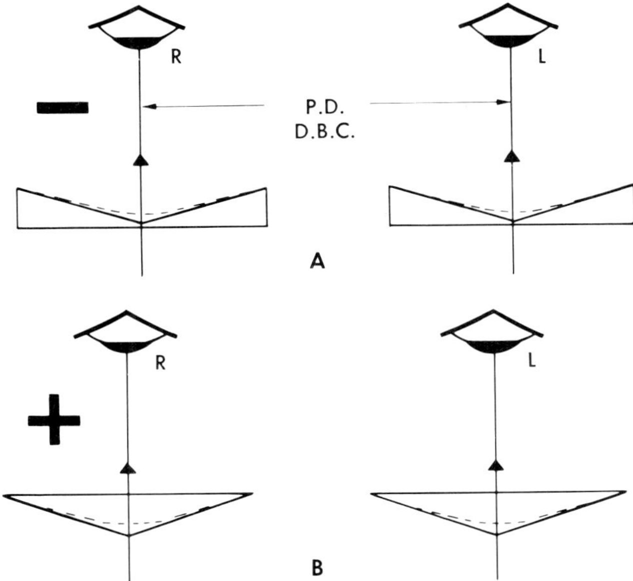

Fig. 10-4. **A,** Minus, or concave, lens. Optical center is at its thinnest part. **B,** Plus, or convex, lens. Optical center is at its thickest part. *P.D.,* Pupillary distance; *D.B.C.,* distance between centers of lenses.

designed in "minus cylinder form" would have the cylinder correction on the concave plane of the lens.

Lenses may also be made of hard resin plastics and polycarbonate. These lenses have superior impact resistance to glass lenses and are preferred for sports glasses and goggles. The scratch resistance capabilities are lower than those of glass, and therefore special coatings are available to reduce scratching.

Glass lenses may be treated by heat and are said to be toughened or incorrectly *hardened* to resist breakage. *Laminated lenses* are safety lenses made by sandwiching a sheet of plastic between two pieces of glass. *Chemically treated* lenses result in a thinner lens with superior impact-resistant qualities. *Lexan* is a soft polycarbonate semiflexible plastic that surpasses other materials for impact-resistant properties. *Blooming* a lens refers to coating a glass lens with magnesium flouride as an antireflection coating to minimize reflection. The name is derived from its purplish sheen similar to the bloom on a ripe plum. *Photochromatic lenses* are photosensitive plastic or glass lenses that darken when exposed to the ultraviolet light at the short end of the spectrum such as is found in natural sunshine.

Aberrations

Lenses may produce aberrations or distortions of light from normal (from Latin *ab,* "from," and *errare,* "to wander"). In *chromatic aberration* white light is broken up by a lens into its spectral color components and observed as color fringes. *Spherical aberration* occurs when a lens fails to focus a broad beam into a single point (Fig. 10-5). *Distortion* from an optical lens occurs when objects appear other than their true form. *Barrel distortion* occurs when lines of a square are bowed outward like a barrel. Such distortion appears when viewing an object through highly myopic lenses. *Pincushion distortion* occurs when the lines of a square are bowed inward similar to a pincushion (Fig. 10-6). This is seen with high-plus lenses such as those used for aphakia. *Astigmatism* may occur when oblique rays of light strike a spherical surface and may thus occur when spectacles are angled to the light striking the lens.

Special types of lenses

Toric lenses are lenses designed to compensate for *astigmatism,* a condition in which the refractive error is greater in one meridian than in the opposite 90-degree meridian.

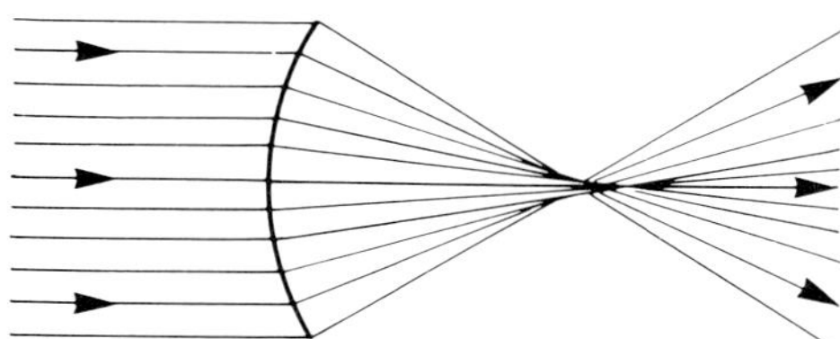

Fig. 10-5. Spherical aberration. The rays of light on refraction by the lens are converged to a meeting area rather than to a single focal point.

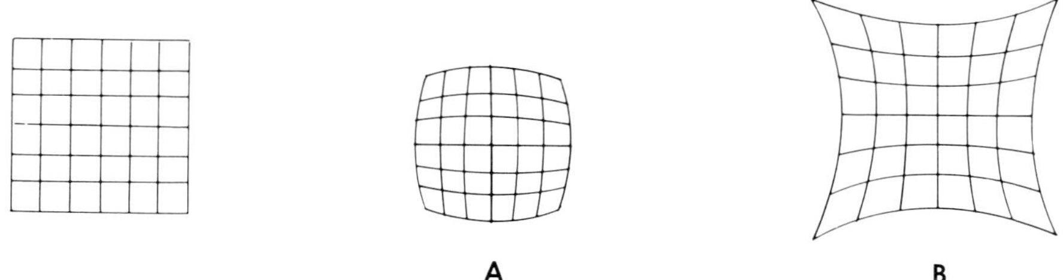

Fig. 10-6. Optical distortion produced by lenses. **A,** Strong concave lenses as in high myopic corrections distort a square to a barrel shape. **B,** Strong convex lenses as in high hyperopic or aphakic corrections distort a square to a pincushion shape.

Prismatic lenses are designed to compensate for or aid muscle imbalance in one or both eyes. A *prism* is any optical material shaped like a wedge. The apex of a prism is its thinnest portion. The base of the prism is the thickest edge. Light that passes through the prism will be deviated toward its base, although the image is seen toward the apex of the prism.

Lenticular lenses are designed to minimize distortion and reduce weight and are essentially smaller lenses mounted on a thin plano carrier lens that is edged to fit the frame. They appear as an inverted bowl or small lens placed on a flat surface (Fig. 10-7).

Aspheric lenses (from Greek *a,* "not," and *sphaira,* "a ball") are lenses that do not have uniform power. A high-plus lens has decreasing power toward the periphery (Fig. 10-8).

An *achromatic lens* is a lens that is corrected for chromatic (color) aberrations.

Multifocal lenses are lenses with more than one focal point, thus allowing a person with presbyopia to see at more than one near distance. A *slab-off* is a method of creating a *bicentric lens,* a lens with two centers, from a one-centered lens by grinding a prism-shaped slab from one surface of the lens so that the lens then has one center for distance and one for reading. Slab-off or bicentric grinding reduces vertical imbalance that results from vertical prismatic differences between two lenses of differing powers.

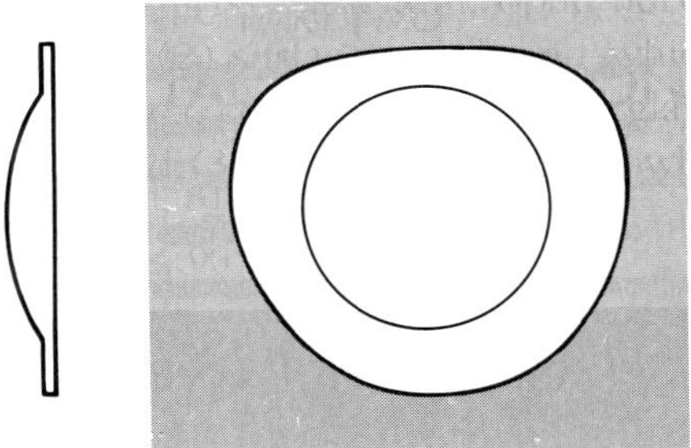

Fig. 10-7. Lenticular lens, single vision.

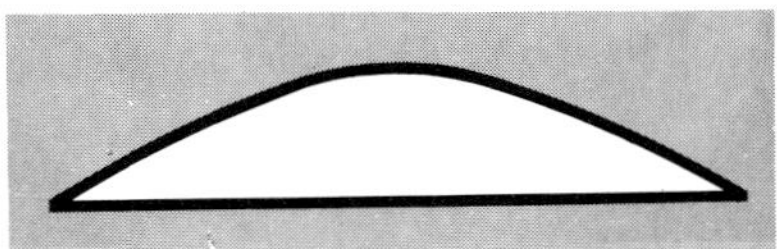

Fig. 10-8. Aspheric lens, side view. Note the flatter curve in the periphery of the lens. This eliminates many of the aberrations of the periphery of the lens and permits a greater field of vision.

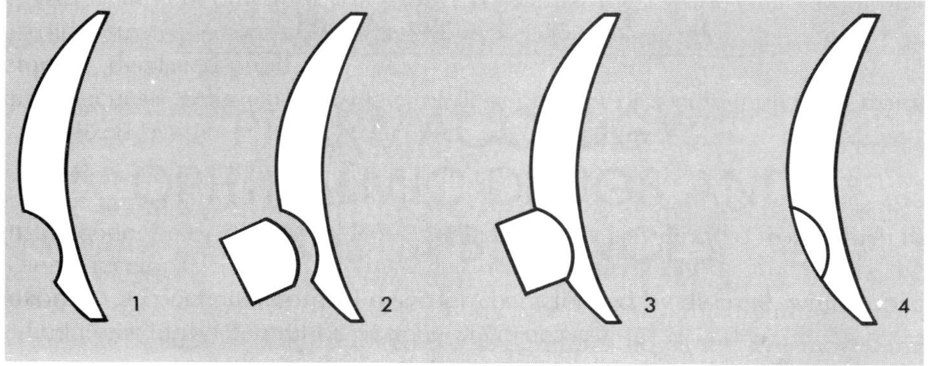

Fig. 10-9. Fused bifocal. *1,* Countersink is placed on the lens blank. *2,* Segment of a higher index of refraction is ground to fit into the countersink. *3,* Two lenses are fused together in an oven and cooled slowly. *4,* Excess lens is ground off and polished.

The *one-piece multifocal* lens is made from the same type of material (glass or plastic) throughout, whereas a *fused multifocal* lens uses glass with two or more indices of refraction in which one material is countersunk and fused into the other (Fig. 10-9).

Bifocal segments may be referred to as *flat top* or *round top* depending on the shape of the upper part of the bifocal segments (Fig. 10-10). *Cement bifocals* are two lenses that are fastened together with cement such as Canada balsam. *Invisible* or seamless bifocals are one-piece bifocals in which the reading sector is blended into the distance lens so that the reading segment cannot be seen. An *addition* or *add* is the additional lens power that is added to the distance prescription to supplement accommodation for reading.

Progressive multifocal lenses are lenses in which the top half is for distance and the bottom section for reading with a corridor joining the two in which the power gradually increases from distance to reading so that the lenses have a focus for all distances.

Spectacle manufacture

The first spectacles were made out of naturally occurring transparent quartz or beryl in the thirteenth century. Increased demand called for the use of glass, and this in turn led Venice (already a center of glassmaking) and later Nuremburg to become spectacle manufacturing centers. The late eighteenth and nineteenth centuries saw a rapid expansion in all technologies, including lens manufacture. In 1784 Benjamin Franklin invented the bifocal lens by fitting two lenses in each

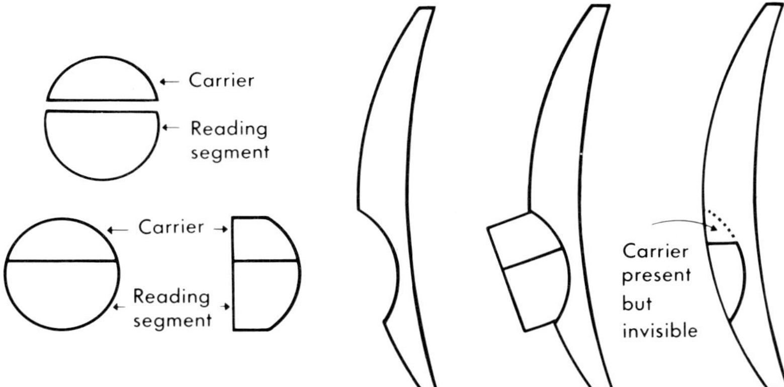

Fig. 10-10. Flattop bifocal. The reading segment is combined with a carrier of similar properties as the main lens. This button is then inserted into the countersink of the main lens, fused, and ground off to produce a flattop bifocal. The carrier is invisible, but the segment, being of a different type of glass, can be seen.

spectacle frame. This invention was improved in 1884 by cementing the lenses together, in 1908 by fusing them, and finally in 1910 by making a one-piece bifocal. As in the case of Franklin who made bifocals to correct his presbyopia, in 1827 Sir George Airy made the first cylindrical lens to correct his own visual defect, astigmatism. At first this was thought to be a rare disorder until F. C. Donders showed in 1864 how prevalent astigmatism was in the general populace.

Several terms are used in the manufacture of spectacles. A *blank* is a piece of glass or plastic molded to the rough shape of a spectacle lens. The lens blank is *blocked* by affixing a handle to the glass or plastic lens by a low-melting-point metal or adhesive pad so that the lens may be held firmly during the process of *generating, fining,* and *polishing,* the three steps involved in the manufacture of a spectacle lens. The term *deblocking* is the removal of the lens from the block.

In the manufacture of a lens, *generating* is the process in which the correct dioptric curve is ground into the lens blank. This results in a *frosted glass* appearance to the blank. *Fining* is a process in which an appropriate abrasive material polishes the frosted surface to a satinlike finish. In *polishing* the satin finish is changed to a highly polished surface by way of a *felt pad* for plastic lenses combined with the use of an earth compound as polishing material. This process results in an *uncut* lens, which is the term used for a lens with a prescription ground in but not cut to fit a spectacle frame.

A lens is *edged* when it is cut to fit a particular frame. It is considered *knife edged* if the edge is extremely thin. The edging may be a *flat edge* for rimless frames, a *beveled edge* for other frames, or a *microbevel* edge. *Chamfer* refers to putting a slight bevel on the edge of a lens to prevent chipping.

Mounting, or *glazing,* is the term used for inserting the lens in the frame.

Tinting is the term used for the process in which hot dye solutions are added to produce a color or tint on plastic lenses. In glass lenses, the color may be a surface coated or a solid tint produced by adding oxides to distribute the color through and through. Specific metal oxides are used to create a specific color and/or absorption.

Coating is a term used for the vacuum treatment of glass lenses to add *antireflection coating, color coating,* or *mirror coating.* Coating may be single- or multilayered. Multilayered coating reduces residual reflectance to a greater degree, thereby increasing light transmission. This is accomplished as each and every layer is applied for a specific wavelength of the visual spectrum.

Edge coating is a process used to darken the edge of a high-minus lens, which eliminates the "myopic ring" and thus improves the appearance of the lens cosmetically.

Box measurement of a lens or frame is the standard now in use by spectacle manufacturers. The shape of the lens or front is "boxed" by horizontal and vertical lines.

Other terms used in conjunction with spectacles are given in the following glossary.

A

acetone: a liquid ketone that serves as a solvent for many organic compounds used for repairing plastic spectacle frames and as a cleaning agent for plastic lenses before tinting.

achromatic: corrected for chromatic aberration (color aberration).

anneal: a regulated process of heating materials (glass and metals) and the subsequent slow, controlled cooling to eliminate internal strains.

B

back vertex power: the reciprocal of the back focal length in meters. The power of the lens or optical system in diopters as measured from the back surface of the lens.

bevel edge: The V-shaped edge ground on the periphery of a lens (about 135 degrees) to hold the lens in a spectacle frame.

C

Canada balsam: a liquid resin from balsam fir tree, which grows in Canada and is used to glue lenses.

carbolite: a graphite-based material produced in Japan and used for making plastic frames.

cataract glasses: usually a high-plus lens to compensate for the removal of the lens in the human eye (cataract operation).

Chavasse glass: a lens with a crinkled surface on the back side to serve as a partial occluder. According to the planned irregularity of the surface, visual acuity is reduced to 20/200 or less.

compound lens: a generic spherocylinder lens (plus on plus or minus on minus) as distinct from a cross cylinder lens (minus on plus or equals on minus).

coquille: blown-glass plano lenses usually used for goggles, approximately 12.00 D curve; mi-coquille lenses have a curve of about 6.00 D. Today lenses of this class are made by "drooping" (sagging) a flat lens with heat.

corrected lenses: a curving of the lens to correspond approximately with the movement of the visual axis while rotating the eyeball.

CR39 (allyl diglycol carbonate): a thermal-setting optical plastic used for the majority of plastic ophthalmic lenses. It is the standard for all plastic lenses and was named after the thirty-ninth trial by the first manufacturer, Columbia Resin Co.

cylinder lens: a lens ground to give one power measured in diopters at one axis and a different power (also in diopters) at right angles to the first axis, e.g., a cylinder lens of + 2.00 + 1.00 × 90 has two focal points: one at 50 cm (+2.00 sphere) and one at 33 cm (the spherocylinder combination).

D

DBC: distance between centers (the frame PD, pupillary distance).

DBL: distance between the nasal lines of a frame.

decenter: to displace. In the fabrication or the design of an ophthalmic lens, the optical center is displaced with respect to the geometric center depending on the size or power and fitting of the lens plus whether it is used for distance or near vision.

decentration: eccentric positioning of a lens to produce a prism effect.

densitometer: instrument to measure the amount of light transmission through a lens.

detachment: see Chapters 16 and 22.

Diamond Dye: a trade name of BPI Company coating system to eliminate ultraviolet light.

diopter: the unit of measurement of the refractive power of a lens. The reciprocal of its focal length in meters. For example, a lens of 2.00 D has a focal point of 0.5 M.

dispersion: the spreading of light waves such as occurs when a prism breaks up light into its component colors or wavelengths.

distometer: a caliper used to measure the vertex distance, usually from the back surface of the lens to the closed lid.

distortion: an aberration through optical glass that causes objects to appear in other than their true form. Strong plus lenses (aphakic) produce pincushion distortion (straight lines appear concave), whereas high myopic lenses cause a barrel effect (a bowing outward of straight lines).

E

endpiece: the extension attached to rimless lenses, metal frame eyewires, or plastic frame rims that contains the joint or hinge to which the temples are attached.

executive: a type of one-piece bifocal or trifocal lens with the segment across the entire lower portion of the lens. A modern version of the original Franklin bifocal. The distance and near optical centers are vertically aligned as opposed to the near optical center being decentered nasally approximately 1½ to 2 mm, as occurs with standard bifocals.

F

fitting triangle: the imaginary triangle that has its apexes at the tops of the ears and the point of contact on the bridge of the nose.

focal length: the distance between the plane of a lens and the focal point of an object from infinity. The dioptric power is the reciprocal of this measurement in meters. All optical testing instruments and prescriptions use back focal lengths or back dioptric powers.

Focimeter: see *Lensmeter*.

folding spectacle: a term given to eyeglasses that can be folded to fit into a small pocket.

frame scotoma: a ring of blind area at the periphery of the visual field caused by the spectable frame.

Franklin bifocal: a split bifocal made of sections of two lenses held together in a frame. It was the first bifocal and invented by Benjamin Franklin.

Fresnel press-on prism: a series of small plastic prisms lying adjacent to each other on a thin platform of plastic. It has the same deviating power of the conventional prism but is only 1 mm thick.

Ful-vue: a glass with high refractive index (1.62), containing lead and sometimes used in spectacle glass and bifocal segments. Trade name of a spectacle frame or mounting in which the temples are attached 15 to 30 degrees above the datum line.

G

geometric center: a point midway between all edges of a spectacle lens.

glare: irregularly scattered light that interferes with the focused retinal picture and reduces visual acuity.

glasses: colloquial name for spectacles.

H

hemianopic glasses: a type of spectacle, incorporating a reflecting mirror or a beam-splitter plano filter lens as an aid to patients with complete blindness in one half of the visual field (Fig. 10-11). The purpose of the mirror is to perceive within the observed field of vision caused by the hemianopic field defect.

I

image jump: the sudden prismatic displacement created by the edge of the segment in a bifocal, especially one with a round segment. The amount of jump is dependent on the strength of the add and the distance the optical center of the reading segment is from the optical center of the main lens—the less its distance, the less the jump.

index of refraction: the ratio of the velocity (V) of light in one medium to the velocity of light in the next medium. Index equals V first medium divided by V second medium.

infinity: the far distance (20 feet or 6 meters or over).

injection molded: a method of injecting plastic into a mold to obtain a plastic cast of the mold. Used for making some frames such as nylon and some lenses.

K

Kryptok: the name of one of the earliest types of round-segment fused bifocal lenses.

L

lap: a cast-iron or aluminum tool used in the grinding and polishing of lens surfaces.

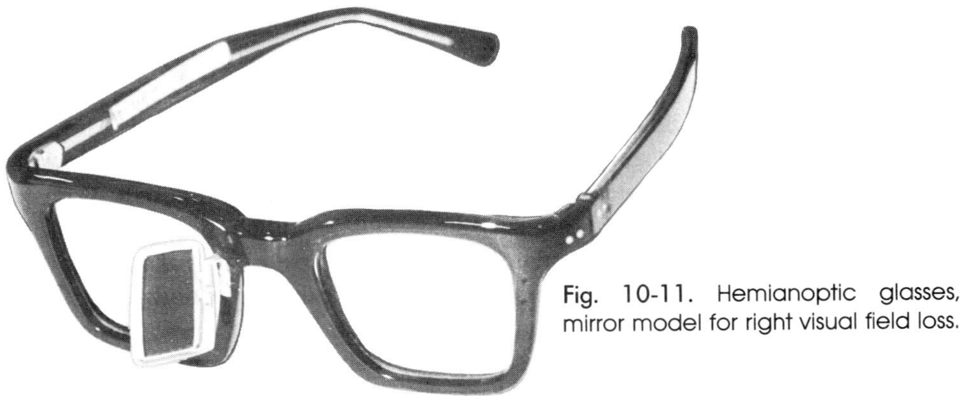

Fig. 10-11. Hemianoptic glasses, mirror model for right visual field loss.

Lensmeter: instrument designed to measure the back vertex power of an optical lens (see lensometer). Trade names include Lensmeter, Vertexmeter, and Vertometer.

light transmission: the percent of incident light that passes through a given lens.

line of sight: the line that connects a point in space with the center of the entrance pupil of the eye; the point does not have to be the point of fixation, i.e., visual axis.

lorgnette: spectacles that are attached to a handle, or a folding case that also serves as a handle, to hold the lenses before the eyes.

Lucite: see *polymethylmethacrylate;* trade name of E. I. du Pont Co.

M

magnification: approximate magnification of a device can be calculated by dividing dioptric power by 4. Alternately, 25 divided into the back focal distance in centimeters will give approximate magnification. (The measurement in meters divided into 10 will give the same answer.)

MED (minimal effective diameter): a system in which semifinished blanks are ground to the smallest diameter creating the thinnest lens.

meniscus lens: a lens with a profile similar to a crescent, having one surface convex and the other curved.

minify: to reduce the apparent dimensions. The opposite of magnify.

mirror sunglasses: a type of sunglass with coating to act as a one-way mirror.

Multilux: see *Varilux.*

N

n: usually the symbol for index of refraction, e.g., $n = 1.523$ for crown glass.

near visual point (NVP): the point in a lens that one looks through in the act of reading. Usually about 8 mm down and 2 mm nasalward from the distant optical center of a lens.

neutral filter: a light gray filter that dampens illumination by reducing the visible spectrum about equally and causing no color changes.

neutralization: the combining of two lenses of opposite powers to produce a resultant power of zero (one lens neutralizes the other).

P

Panoptik: the trade name of a series of fused multifocal lenses formerly made by Bausch & Lomb.

pantoscopic angle: the angle of spectacle lenses when rotated on the x-axis to set the lens normal to the fixation axis below the horizon. Commonly measured as the angle between spectacle temple and the plane of the eyewear as angulated back from the perpendicular.

Perspex: see *polymethylmethacrylate;* trade name of Imperial Chemical Industries, Ltd.

photochromatic lens: photosensitive glass that darkens on exposure to light.

photogray lens: lens that darkens in sunlight to 75% of its maximum in the first minute. It has maximum light transmission of 85% and at the darkest 45% to 50%.

photo sun lens: lens that darkens in sunlight more than do photogray lenses and in which transmission varies from 65% to 20% maximum. It is primarily used for sunglasses.

pince-nez: eyeglasses without temples and supported by tension pads that clip on the nose.

plano: a lens having no refractive strength.

Plexiglas: see *polymethylmethacrylate.* (Rohm & Haas trade name.)

polarized: a sheet of optical plastic containing crystals of an iodine compound that are all oriented in one direction. The plastic is sometimes laminated in glass. Light polarized by this material is used for stereoscopes, three-dimensional pictures and movies, and a test for strain in glass, including heat-treated impact-resistant lens. Lenses are made with the axis of the polarizing material placed so the glare coming off a flat horizontal surface is not transmitted. One of the major uses of polaroid lenses is for sunglasses, especially for protection from reflected light on water, snow, and highways. Polaroid is a corporate name.

polymethylmethacrylate: a strong rigid plastic sometimes used for frames. Also used for hard contact lenses and intraocular lenses. Trade names are Lucite, Plexiglas, and Perspex.

Prentice's rule: a 10 D lens decentered 1 mm creates 1 D of prism.

ptosis crutch spectacles: a spectacle frame in which a small spring wire has been attached nasally to lift a drooping upper eyelid.

R

reflex pupillometer: a device for measuring the distance between the visual axis of the eye.

refraction: deviation in the course of rays of light in passing from one transparent medium into another of different density.

refractometry: the sum of steps performed in arriving at a decision as to what lens or lenses (if any) will most benefit the patient.

riding bow: a spectacle bow or temple that extends to the lobe of the ear and is shaped to the crotch behind the ear.

rimless frames: frames with no fronts or eyewires, thus eliminating the frame scotoma.

ring scotoma: a ring of blind area in a high-plus lens created by the prismatic effect from the thick center to the thin edge.

RLX coating: trade name of 3M coating for plastic lenses that reduce scratching.

S

scotoma, frame: see *frame scotoma.*

soule: to cut off a portion of an optical lens, usually the lower nasal quadrant to give clearance for the side of the nose.

spherical equivalent: the arithmetically spherical dioptric power of a cylindrical or spherocylindrical lens. It is the spherical power of the lens plus half the power of the cylinder. For example, + 2.00 + 1.00 × 90 lens has the spherical equivalent of +2.50.

standard notation: the method of denoting cylinder axis or prism base-apex axis in which from the patient's side the horizontal axis 0 to 180 degrees is the origin for angles measured clockwise beginning from the left side.

strap: the lens holding part of a rimless mounting consisting of two plates between which a lens is secured by a screw or cement and two arms that are fitted to the periphery of the lens.

T

telescopic lenses: a compound lens system for persons with advanced stages of sight impairment; two lenses, properly ground, and mounted in a spectacle frame with a short distance between them to form a magnifying lens system.

transposition: the process of changing a spectacle prescription from a plus to a minus cylinder or vice versa without changing its refractive value. A + 2.00 + 1.00 × 90 lens is equivalent to a + 3.00 − 1.00 × 180 lens. The rule is to add the cylinder to the sphere, change the sign of the cylinder, and rotate the axis by 90 degrees.

trial frame: a spectacle frame into which lenses are placed during the refraction procedure.

trigeminal shield: a type of side shield affixed to spectacle frames and used to prevent exposure of the eye after a seventh or fifth nerve paralysis or both.

V

Varilux, Multilux: trade names for a type of invisible multifocal lens in which the power progresses from the distance area to the reading area through a channel, giving continuous focus at all distances from far to near.

vertex distance: distance from the posterior surface of the lens to the anterior surface of the eye (for measuring purposes, the closed lid). Important in aphakic prescriptions and high myopia.

Vertexmeter: see *Lensmeter.*

Vertometer: see *Lensmeter.*

X

x-axis: the imaginary line connecting the centers of rotation of the eyes. The line connecting the geometric centers of a pair of spectacle lenses.

Y

y-axis: an imaginary line perpendicular to the x-axis and fixation axis through the center of rotation. A line perpendicular to the x-axis of the spectacle lens and optical axis.

CHAPTER 11

CONTACT LENSES

Contact lens refers to any lens that is placed on the surface of the cornea and sclera, either for *optical* purposes (improvement of visual acuity) or for *therapeutic* purposes (treatment of eye disorders).

Types of lenses

Scleral contact lenses are contact lenses that cover not only the cornea but also the conjunctiva overlying the sclera (Fig. 11-1, *A*). *Corneal contact lenses* are those lenses confined to the cornea (Fig. 11-1, *B*). *Semiscleral lenses* are those that bridge the limbus and lie partially on the conjunctival tissues overlying the sclera adjacent to the limbus (Fig. 11-1, *C*).

Lenses may be *hard* or *soft,* depending on the nature of the material composition. Hard lenses are sometimes referred to as "rigid lenses." *Extended-wear* or *prolonged-wear lenses* are lenses that may be worn for 24 hours or more. *Gas-permeable lenses* are lenses that permit the passage of oxygen and carbon dioxide through the material. *Cosmetic lens* is the term for a colored lens used to cover an unsightly blind eye; this term is sometimes applied to lenses that are used to replace spectacles for nonpathological conditions, to enhance cosmetic appearance. The latter should be referred to as *refractive lenses.* "Tinted lenses" are colored lenses that change or enhance iris color. A *bandage lens* is used over the cornea to protect the cornea from external influences and permit healing of underlying pathology. Soft lenses may be also classified as to whether they are *hydrophobic* (hate water) or *hydrophilic* (love water).

Design of lenses

The *base curve* of a lens is the curvature of the central portion of the back surface of a lens and is measured in millimeters of radius of an arc. This is the *central posterior curve (CPC).* Most lenses are either *bicurve,* having one base curve and one secondary curve, or *multicurve,* having one base curve and two or more secondary curves. These latter lenses have an outer *peripheral posterior*

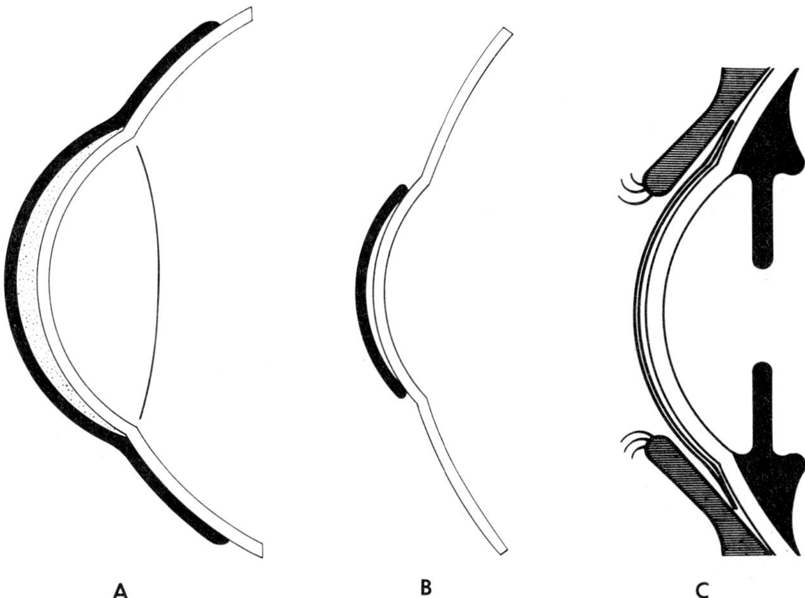

Fig. 11-1. **A,** Scleral contact lens. The contact lens fits over the cornea and sclera. **B,** Corneal contact lens. **C,** Semiscleral lens that bridges the limbus and lies partially on the conjunctival fissure.

curve (PPC) and one or more *intermediate posterior curves (IPC).* At each junction of these curves, there is a *junctional zone.* The smoothness of this junction can be obtained by *blending* the zone to remove the sharp junctional line between zones.

Not every lens has a smooth spherical back surface. Some lenses have an *aspherical* or nonspherical back surface that is not of uniform radius but shaped like a parabola. The radius of curvature of these aspheric lenses must be measured at the apex or center of the lens; this measurement is called the *posterior apical radius (PAR).*

Every contact lens has a diameter or *chord diameter,* which represents the width or measurement from one edge of the lens to the opposite edge. Each of the curves referred to previously, the CPC, the PPC, and the IPC, also has its own *curve widths.*

The *central thickness* of a lens is the separation between the anterior and posterior surfaces at the geometric center of the lens.

The *sagittal depth* or *height* of a lens is the distance between a flat surface and the back surface of the central portion of the lens (Fig. 11-2). The greater the

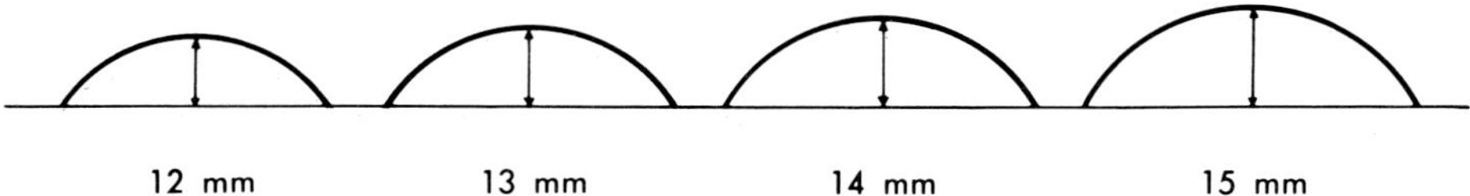

Fig. 11-2. Sagittal height. When the radius is kept constant and the diameter increased, the sagittal height of the lens is increased, and the lens becomes steeper.

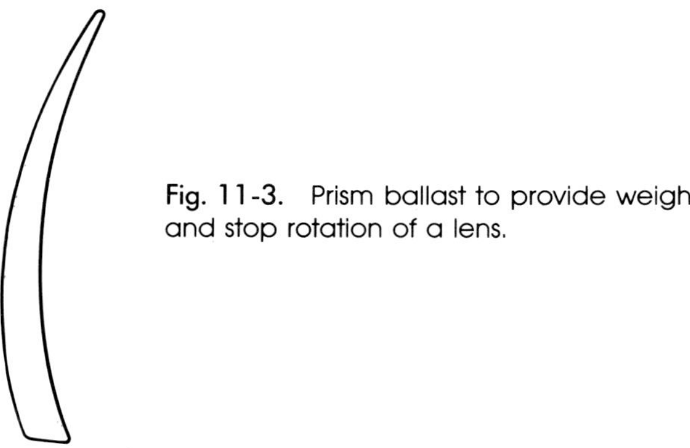

Fig. 11-3. Prism ballast to provide weight and stop rotation of a lens.

sagittal height, the greater the *vaulting* of the lens and thus the steeper the lens. This is often referred to as the *sagittal vault.*

A *ballasted lens* is one that has a cross-sectional shape with a heavier base so that it orients inferiorly when the lens is worn. It is usually *prism ballasted* because of the employment of a prism wedge to weight the lens (Fig. 11-3). A *truncated* lens is one that is cut off to form a horizontal base. The amputation of the lens is usually at the inferior pole of the lens, although superior and inferior truncations have been used. Truncation is frequently used to add stability to a soft toric lens by lying along the lower eyelid.

The *optical zone (OZ)* of a lens is the central zone that contains the refractive power of the lens. The *back vertex power* of a lens refers to the effective power of lens measured from the back surface. The *wetting angle* of a lens is the angle that the edge of a bead of water makes with the surface of the plastic. The smaller the angle, the greater the wetting ability (Fig. 11-4).

Toric lenses or *toroidal lenses,* derived from Latin *torus* meaning "swelling," are lenses with different radii of curvature in each meridian. These lenses are used to correct for astigmatism. A *front surface toric lens* has an anterior surface with two different radii but a posterior surface that is spherical. A *back surface*

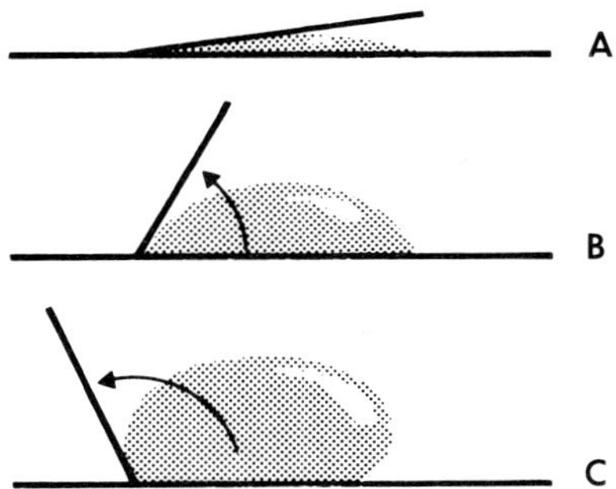

Fig. 11-4. Wetting angles. The smaller the angle of contact *(Θ),* the greater the spreading of a liquid over a solid. A hard lens is hydrophobic and has a 60-degree angle of contact with water. **A,** Low-wetting angle. **B,** Wetting angle of methylmethacrylate hard lens. **C,** Large wetting angle with droplet of mercury.

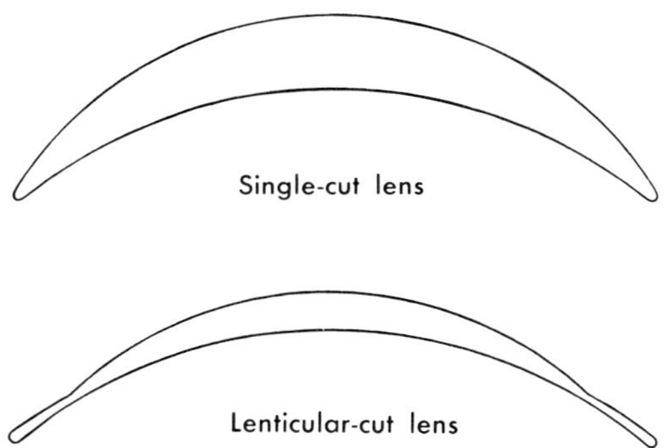

Fig. 11-5. Single-cut and lenticular-cut lenses.

toric lens has a posterior surface that has two different radii and an anterior spherical surface. In a *bitoric* lens both the anterior and posterior surfaces have different radii.

Higher power plus lenses are often designed with a *lenticular bowl* or central area that has the appearance of an upside-down bowl-like lens sitting on the underlying lens (Fig. 11-5).

Hard or rigid lenses

Hard lenses may have a *standard,* or *thin,* thickness. They may be composed of a material made of *polymethylmethacrylate,* sometimes referred to as *PMMA,* a hard transparent plastic with a long history of acceptance. They may also be composed of *cellulose acetate butyrate (CAB),* a combination of *silicone* and *PMMA* often called "silicone acrylate," or of a hard resin silicone. "Fluorocarbon" is a newer material that can be used either in its pure form or in combination with other polymers such as silicone and PMMA to provide more oxygen permeability to the lens. These latter groups of materials transmit sufficient oxygen to label these lenses as *gas-permeable lenses.*

Rigid lenses may be modified by *fenestration,* which is the drilling of one or more holes through the plastic. The lens may be *polished*, or the edges refinished by the *Con-Lish, rag-wheel method,* or use of a *felt disc polisher.*

Soft lenses

Soft lenses are composed either of *hydrogel* material, a watery gel-like material that contains more than 10% water, or of *silicone.* Soft lenses may be manufactured by the *spin cast process,* using liquid material revolving in a given mold at a controlled speed and temperature to produce the resultant curvature, design, and power. Silicone lenses are molded by placing liquid in a metal or glass mold of known design. Silicone lenses are more flexible than hard lenses, but still belong to the group of essentially hard lenses. Many soft lenses are *lathe cut* by a machine lathe used to grind lens design, size, and power. Most hydrogel soft lenses are made with HEMA, which stands for *hydroxyethylmethacrylate,* as their basic ingredient but are often copolymerized with other materials. Non-HEMA lenses are also available and are hydrogels.

Oxygen flow and contact lenses

The oxygen transmission through a given material as a laboratory measurement is often referred to as the "DK" value, where D is the diffusion coefficient of oxygen movement in a lens material and K is the solubility coefficient of oxygen in the material. DK or oxygen permeability is a characteristic of a given material obtained in a given condition at a given temperature in the laboratory only. *Oxygen flux* is the amount of oxygen that will pass through a given area of the material in a given amount of time driven by a given partial pressure difference of oxygen across material. The oxygen flux is the relationship of the DK of the material and the lens thickness so that the thinner the lens the more the oxygen flux there is. The term *oxygen transmissibility* is used to indicate the oxygen permeability (DK) divided by the thickness of the lens (L) so that DK/L = oxygen transmissibility. A more meaningful importance is the total oxygen passing through a lens. This measurement is called the *equivalent oxygen performance* (EOP).

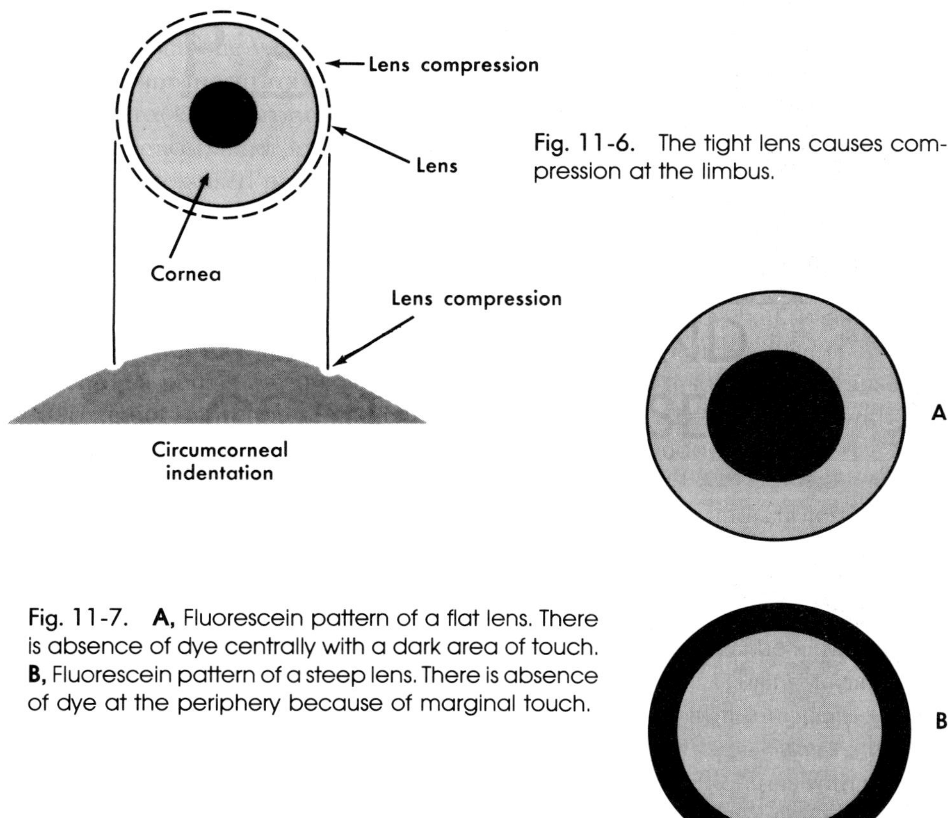

Fig. 11-6. The tight lens causes compression at the limbus.

Fig. 11-7. **A,** Fluorescein pattern of a flat lens. There is absence of dye centrally with a dark area of touch. **B,** Fluorescein pattern of a steep lens. There is absence of dye at the periphery because of marginal touch.

Contact lens problems

When a lens or base curve is said to be made *steeper,* it means that the posterior radius of curvature is decreased, or shortened. When a lens or base curve is said to be made *flatter,* it means the opposite, that the posterior radius of curvature is increased, or lengthened.

Decentration of a lens indicates that the lens is sliding off center and may give rise to poor vision or *arcuate staining* or both. Arcuate staining is arclike staining in the periphery of the cornea. *Vertical striae* are small vertical lines in the cornea caused by folds in Descemet's membrane and are an early sign of corneal hypoxia. *Limbal compression* occurs with soft lenses that are too tight and cause pressure at the periphery of the cornea (Fig. 11-6). *Fluorescein* is a dye used to analyze hard lens problems because it mixes with the tear film and glows in the presence of ultraviolet light or cobalt blue light (Fig. 11-7, *A* and *B*).

A

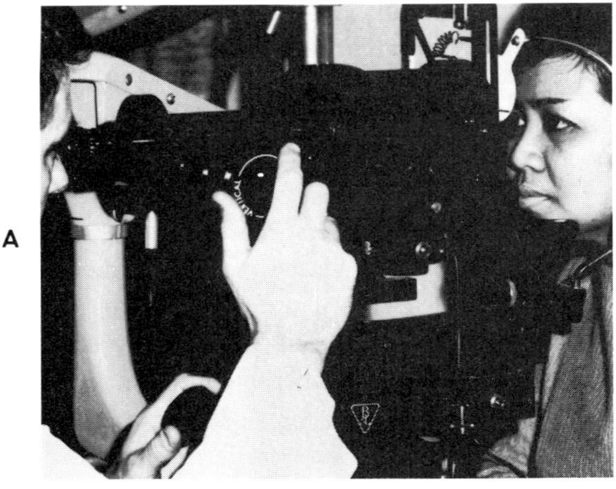

B

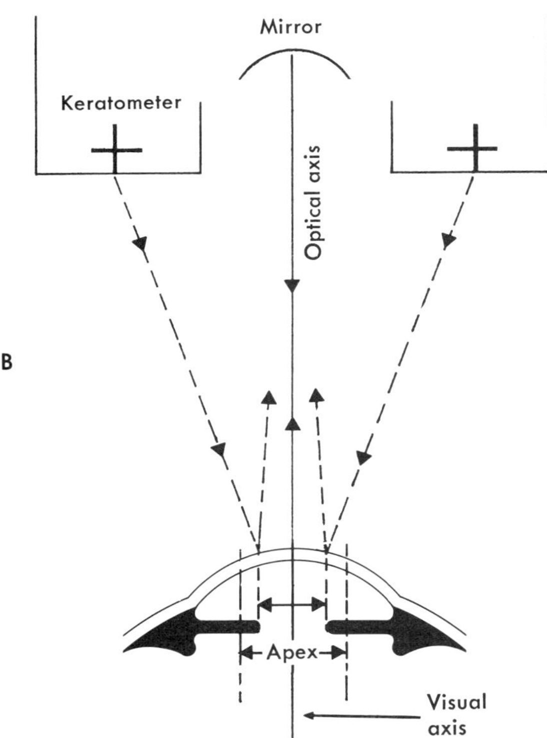

Fig. 11-8. **A,** Taking a K reading. **B,** The principle of the keratometer. The visual axis is aligned along the optical axis of the instrument so that the central front surface of the cornea, acting as a mirror, reflects the mires of the keratometer.

Instrumentation

An *ophthalmometer* is an instrument designed to measure the radius of curvature of the cornea, using the mirror effect of the cornea's front surface (Fig. 11-8). This instrument is most commonly referred to as a *keratometer,* the name originated by Bausch & Lomb from *kerato* meaning "horn" (cornea) and *meter,* "to measure." The instrument measures a small portion of the *corneal cap,* the central zone of the cornea, and the measurement is often called the *K reading.* The size of the corneal cap measured varies with the instrument used but is usually about 3.36 mm chord length. The *mires* of the ophthalmometer are the targets that are reflected back from the cornea (Fig. 11-9).

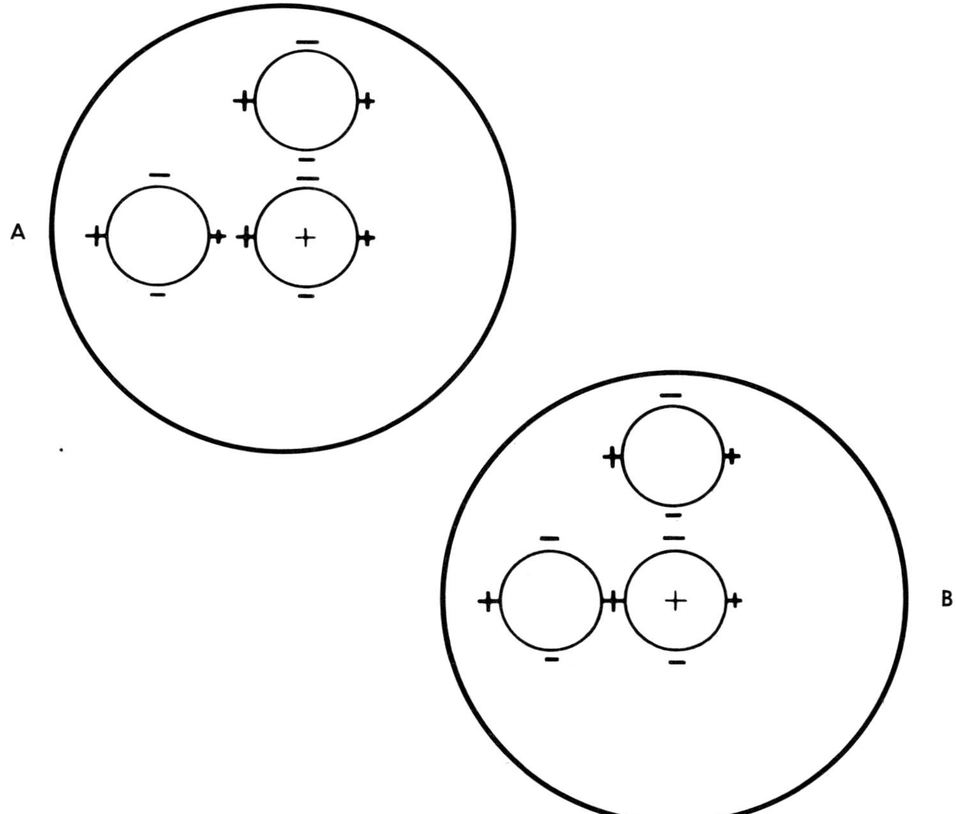

Fig. 11-9. Keratometer mires. **A,** Alignment of the mires for axis. **B,** Apposition of the plus-sign mire to measure one meridian of corneal curvature.

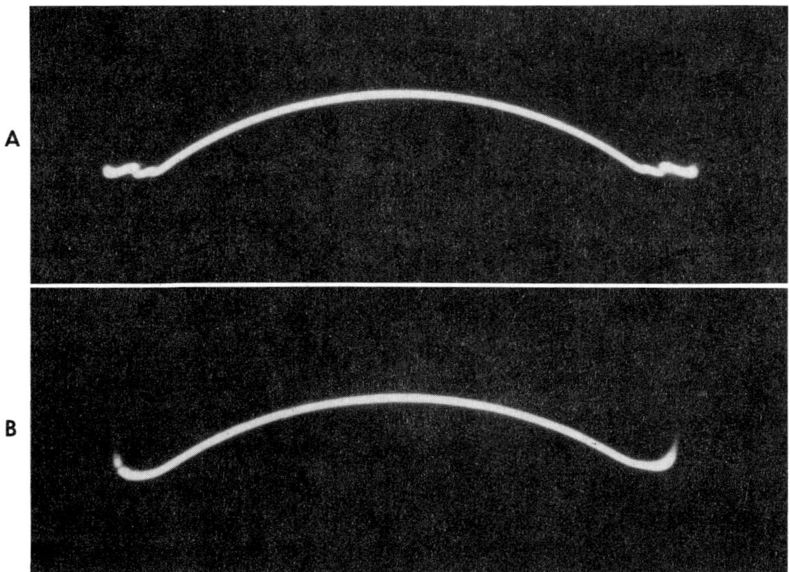

Fig. 11-10. **A,** Poorly finished transition zone as determined by the profile analyzer. **B,** Perfect transition zone with ski contour at its periphery.

The *topogometer* is a keratometer attachment with a movable light designed to localize the apical zone or corneal cap of the cornea to be measured by the keratometer. The limiting margin of the apical zone is determined by the points on the corneal surface where the radius of curvature of the cornea begins to flatten. The average diameter of the apical zone is about 6.0 mm.

The *radiuscope,* a term coined by American Optical Company and often referred to as a microspherometer, is an instrument that measures the radius of curvature of a hard contact lens. A *profile analyzer* is an instrument used to assess the junctional zone blending of a hard lens (Fig. 11-10). A *shadow graph* is an instrument that projects and magnifies a contact lens. It is used to examine defects in a lens and determine measurements.

A *wet cell* or *hydrometric chamber* is used to retain a soft lens for evaluation and measurements of power and edge configuration (Fig. 11-11). *Templates* are small elevated plastic domes of known radius of curvature for evaluating base curves of soft lenses in a number of existing soft lens analyzers.

The *photokeratoscope* is an instrument that photographs the front surface of the eye and provides a permanent record of a large corneal area.

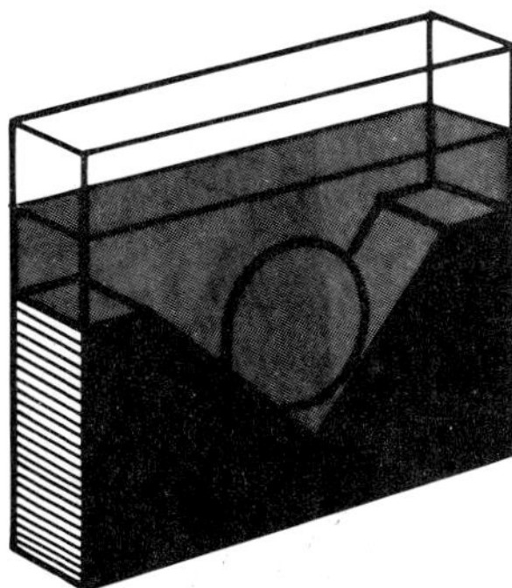

Fig. 11-11. Water cell used to measure power of a soft lens in the hydrated state. The soft lens is floated in normal saline solution and measured in a regular lensometer.

A

annular bifocal contact: a lens with distance portion ground into the center of the lens and near power ground into the periphery.

anoxia: a diminished supply of oxygen.

aphakic lenses: lenses designed for postcataract fitting.

apical zone of cornea: area of the central portion of the cornea with a constant radius of curvature. Sometimes called the corneal cap.

artificial tears: wetting agents for the cornea to supplement the loss of tear formation (Methylcellulose, Liquifilm, and so on).

aspheric lens: a continuous lens with an elliptical shape that has a flatter peripheral curvature.

B

bacteriocide: a chemical that disinfects and kills pathogenic organisms.

benzalkonium chloride: a preservative used in contact lens solutions because of its germicidal qualities.

biomicroscopy: microscopic examination of the cornea, anterior chamber lens, and posterior chamber contents with a slit lamp microscope. The magnification is approximately 10 to 50 times.

bullous keratopathy: total swelling of the cornea with painful blister formation at the epithelial level; treated frequently with therapeutic soft lens.

burton lamp: an ultraviolet light used to excite the fluorescein dye that is used to analyze the fit of a hard contact lens.

BUT: see *tear film break-up time (BUT).*

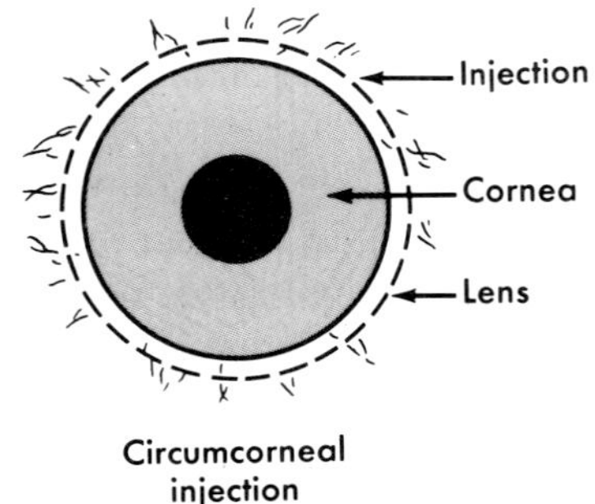

Fig. 11-12. Circumcorneal injection as noted by the considerable vascularity at the limbus.

C

chlorhexidine: a chemical used for disinfection.

chlorobutanol: an antimicrobial agent used in soaking solutions.

circumcorneal injection: redness around the limbus of the eyes surrounding the cornea (Fig. 11-12).

conjunctivitis, giant papillary: see *giant papillary hypertrophy (GPH).*

contact lens blank: a sheet or rod of plastic, which can be methylmethacrylate or hydroxyethylmethacrylate, used to make either hard or soft lenses.

contact lens wetting angle: the angle between the liquid and lens surface.

contour lens: a tricurve lens designed to conform to the curvature of the cornea that flattens as it extends in the periphery.

copolymer: two or more chemicals that are combined to form a new chemical compound.

corneal cap: the apical zone or central zone of the cornea that has a constant area of curvature.

corneal diameter: the diameter of the cornea, usually taken along the horizontal meridian.

corneal edema: swelling of the cornea caused by hypoxia or insufficient oxygen.

D

dehydration: the drying out of a soft lens.

deturgescence, corneal: the state of relative dehydration maintained by the normal intact cornea that enables it to remain transparent.

diagnostic fitting set: a limited set of trial lenses used to gain a dynamic overview of the fit of a contact lens.

discoloration: a change in color of a contact lens.

disinfection: physical or chemical procedures that kill common pathogenic organisms but may permit some nonpathogenic organisms to survive.

DK value: a measure of the oxygen permeability through a given material where D is the diffusion coefficient for oxygen movement in the lens material and K is the solubility of oxygen in this material.

double slab-off lenses: sometimes called thick-thin lenses; the upper and lower portions of the lens are reduced in thickness so that when the lens is placed on the eye, these portions lie under the upper and lower eyelid. The thin zones aid in stabilizing toric soft lenses.

dry spots: areas of drying as noted by absent areas of fluorescein-stained tear film on the cornea when the patient stares.

Dyer nomogram system of lens ordering: a simplified system of ordering hard lenses based on clinical experience, corneal topogometry, and charts of associated lens parameters.

E

EDTA: see *ethylenediaminetetraacetic acid.*

elasticity: the ability of a lens to stretch and return to the same configuration. Lens memory.

endophthalmitis: an inflammation of the entire eye including the outer coats.

enzyme cleaner: a cleaning agent that acts on a soft lens by a digestion of protein.

epithelial edema: edema of the superficial layer of the cornea.

esthesiometer (Cochet-Bonnet): a device used to evaluate corneal sensitivity, consisting essentially of a nylon thread mounted in a handle so that its length may be varied and calibrated in milligrams of weight necessary to bend a given length of the thread when pressed against the cornea.

ethylenediaminetetraacetic acid: a chemical used for disinfection.

eversion of the eyelid: the folding back of the eyelid on itself.

F

finished lens: a complete lens with anterior and posterior curves, a specified diameter, a designated peripheral curve, and edge design.

fitting set: a complete inventory of lenses of graduated powers and base curves.

flare: flutterings or fringing of lights, caused by a lens with an optical zone too small, a decentered lens, or an excessively loose lens.

flat cornea: a cornea with a K value less than 41 D.

fluid lens: power created by having a very convex or concave tear film; in most cases the power of the tear film is negligible, because this layer is too thin (less than 0.02 mm) to have an appreciable effect on the power of the lens.

fluorescein: an organic compound that is inert and used to stain the tear film for contact lens fitting and to assess the integrity of the cornea.

G

galilean telescope: telescope with a minus ocular lens combined with a plus objective lens.

germicide: a chemical used for disinfection, such as chlorhexidine.

giant papillary hypertrophy (GPH): large elevated papules on the tarsal conjunctiva. Usually associated with soft lens wear but can occur with any contact lens. It is regarded as an autoimmune response to the patient's own protein. Also referred to as giant papillary conjunctivitis (GPC).

GPH: see *giant papillary hypertrophy*.

H

haptic: the part of a contact or intraocular lens that supports the optical portion.

Harrison Stein nomogram: a series of lens specifications for prescribing a gas-permeable contact lens from silicone-PMMA material.

hydrogen peroxide: a bacteriocide used for soft lenses.

hypoxia: low in oxygen.

K

Korb lens: a PMMA lens that is fitted in a manner to position on the superior portion of the cornea regardless of weight or power and designed to move vertically over the cornea on blinking as if attached to the upper eyelid.

L

LD + 2: the longest diameter (LD) of the optical zone plus 2 mm (for the intermediate and peripheral curves) yields the diameter of a lens; determined by using the topogometer.

lenticular lenses: relatively large lens most suitable for large, flat eyes; consists of a central optical zone and a surrounding nonoptical flange.

limbal zone: junction between the periphery of the cornea with the sclera.

loose lens: a contact lens with excessive movement; it can be caused by a lens that is too small in diameter, too thick, or too flat.

M

magnification: the ratio of image size to object size.

methylcellulose: a wetting agent.

microthin lens: a lens less than 0.10 mm in thickness.

minus carrier: a lens designed with an edge configuration similar to that of a minus lens that is thicker at its periphery.

monovision: single vision contact lenses used for presbyopic people in which the power of the lenses is such that one eye is used for distance vision and the other is used for near vision.

Morgan's dots: small discrete subepithelial corneal opacities resulting from corneal hypoxia; sometimes called epithelial microcystic edema.

N

nomogram: a table of precalculated mathematical values used to arrive at a hard lens design.

O

orthokeratology: the technique of flattening the cornea and thus correcting refractive errors by the use of a series of progressively flatter contact lenses.

overwearing syndrome: a misnomer for acute corneal hypoxia characterized by a latent interval after removal of the lens; extreme pain and congestion of lids, cornea, and conjunctiva are experienced. Overwearing syndrome is more common with hard lenses.

oxygen flux: a measure of the amount of oxygen that will pass through a given area of material in a given unit of time.

oxygen permeability: the degree in which a lens permits the passage of oxygen across it. It depends on composition of the plastic (that is, silicone has excellent permeability, whereas PMMA has no permeability), the thickness of the lens, and its water content. It is often expressed as the DK value.

oxygen transmissability: the ability of a lens to permit oxygen to flow through to the cornea. It is the oxygen permeability divided by the thickness of the material.

P

pachometer: an instrument used to measure the thickness of the cornea and depth of the anterior chamber.

photokeratoscope: an instrument designed to photograph annular rings of the cornea and to aid in making a contact lens that will contour to the cornea. The data are often fed to a computer for a readout for a lens design.

photophobia: sensitivity to light.

Placido's disc: a disc with concentric rings to determine the regularity of the cornea when its reflection is revealed on the corneal surface.

plano lens: a lens with zero dioptric power.

polymer: a chain of linked molecular units of dimension greater than 5 monomer units.

polymerization: the union of molecules of a compound to form larger molecules and a new compound.

polyvinyl alcohol: a wetting agent.

polyvinylprolidone (PVP): a polymer often copolymerized with other plastics in hydrogel lenses.

prism ballast lens: contact lens with based-down prism added inferiorly to improve the stability of the lens. Usually 1 to 1.5 D of prism is added.

PVP: see *polyvinylprolidone.*

Q

quaternary ammonium chloride: known commonly as quat, it is a compound used for disinfecting contact lenses.

R

residual astigmatism: the astigmatism present after the corneal astigmatism has been nullified by a contact lens. It is the astigmatism usually created by the lens of the eye.

retroillumination: light is focused on deeper structures such as the iris, while the microscope is adjusted to study the cornea; best method of showing fine corneal edema.

S

Schirmer test: measures normal tear secretion; the ability of the eye to wet in 5 minutes 15 mm of a 5 × 35 mm strip of filter paper.

scratched lens: a defect in the lens surface consisting of a groove and ridge.

semifinished blank: a contact lens blank in which the posterior curve of the contact lens has been fabricated.

semifinished lens: a polished lens with an anterior and a posterior curvature.

soaking solution: a solution designed to keep a lens moist and free from contamination.

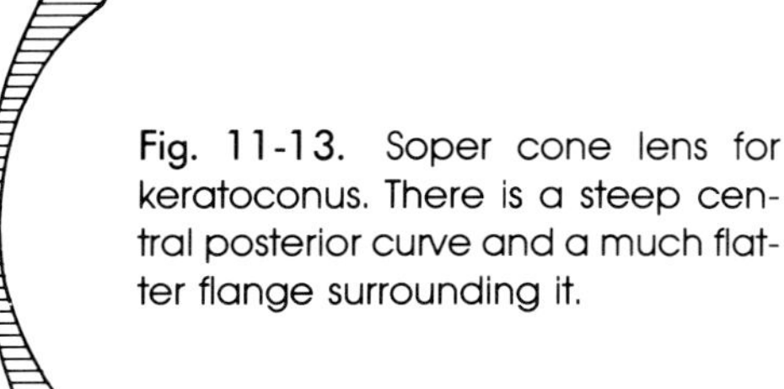

Fig. 11-13. Soper cone lens for keratoconus. There is a steep central posterior curve and a much flatter flange surrounding it.

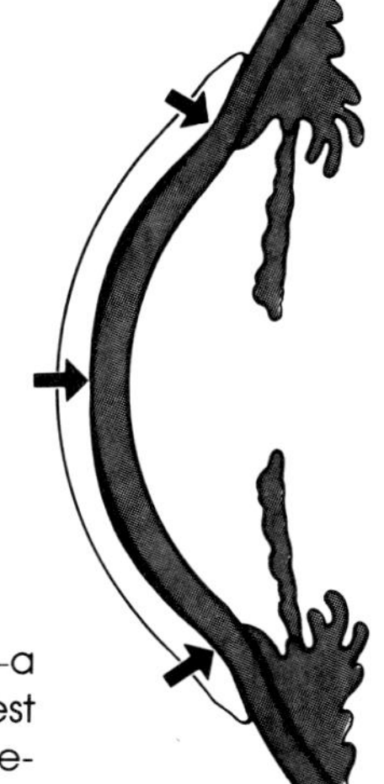

Fig. 11-14. Three-point touch—a normally fitting soft lens will rest lightly at the apex and at the periphery of the cornea.

Soper cone lens: a hard lens designed by Joseph Soper with a steep central posterior curve to accommodate large cones of keratoconus (Fig. 11-13).

spectacle blur: blurred vision that lasts for 15 minutes or longer after a contact lens is removed and spectacles are used.

specular reflection: a reflection from a mirror surface such as the back of the cornea.

spherical equivalent: It is the spherical power of the lens plus half the cylindrical power. It represents the dioptric power of a cylindrical or spherocylindrical lens from the vertex to the plane of the circle of least confusion (the midpoint of the interval of Sturm).

SPK: see *superficial punctate keratitis.*

stable vision: visual acuity that does not fluctuate.

sterilization: the complete death of all forms of bacteria, fungi, and spores.

stippling: dotlike staining of the cornea.

superficial punctate keratitis (SPK): diffuse stippling of the cornea.

surfactant: a cleaner that acts on the surface of a contact lens.

T

taco test: a test to determine that a soft contact lens is not inside out by grasping the lens near its apex and folding it so the edge will roll in like a Mexican taco if it is not everted.

tear film break-up time (BUT): an evaluation of tear quality; the tear film will normally break up in 10 to 30 seconds and show dry spots. Any dry spot that appears in less than 10 seconds is pathological.

tears: a composite of secretions from lacrimal glands, accessory glands of Kraus and Wolfring, mucin-secreting goblet cells of the conjunctiva, meibomian-secreting tarsal glands, and oil-secreting glands of Teis.

thermal disinfection: disinfection of a lens by heat.

thickness of a lens: the measurement of the center of a lens; a variable that depends on the posterior vertex power, the central base curve, the index of refraction of the lens material, and the lens diameter.

thimerosal (Merthiolate): a mercurial agent used for disinfection.

three and nine o'clock staining: erosion of the cornea at the three and nine o'clock position; seen commonly in rigid lenses.

three-point touch: a lens that rests on the sclera and on the center of the cornea (Fig. 11-14).

tight lens: a lens that has minimal or no movement.

transitional zone: that area of the cornea between the apical zone and the limbal zone.

Trantas' dots: small peripheral limbal infiltrations caused by delayed hypersensitivity, as seen in vernal conjunctivitis.

U

ulceration of the cornea: a large defect in the cornea that may be caused by hypoxia, trauma, or infection.

V

V-groove gauge: a ruler measure with a groove to measure the diameter of a hard lens (Fig. 11-15).

vascularization: increased blood vessels occurring in a cornea.

VID: see *visible iris diameter*.

viscosity agent: sticky or gummy substance used for lubrication and cushioning in certain contact lens solutions.

visible iris diameter (VID): a term that represents the iris diameter and aids in selecting the initial lens; often used in place of the corneal diameter.

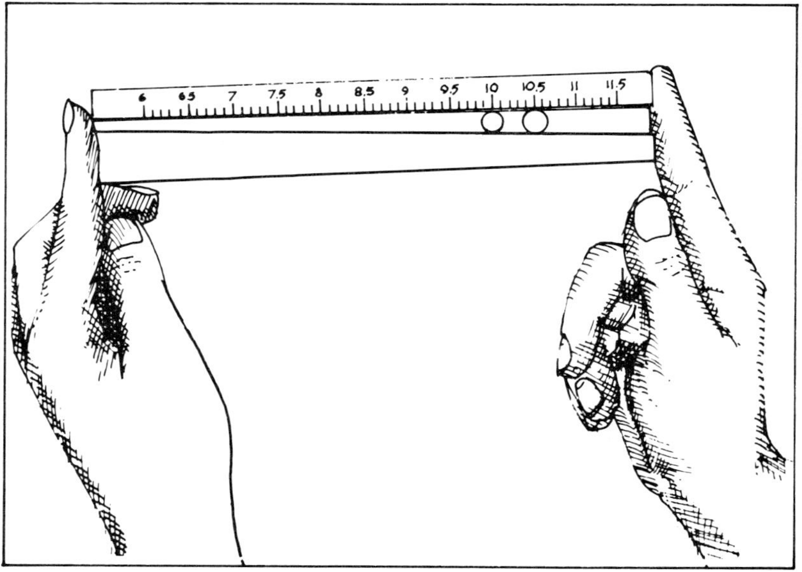

Fig. 11-15. V-groove diameter gauge. The lens is inserted at the widest opening and allowed to slide to its position of rest, where the diameter reading is obtained.

W

warpage: a permanent bending of a hard lens. May also refer to a semipermanent altering of the corneal curvature.

water content: expression of the percentage of water to the total mass of the lens.

wet storage: the use of soaking solution to store hard contact lenses.

wetting solution: solutions that increase the spreading or wettability of liquids on the plastic contact lens by converting the surface of a lens from a hydrophobic to a hydrophilic surface.

X

X chrom lens: a red contact lens designed to aid the individual with partial color blindness.

xerophthalmia: a state of dryness of the eyes; conjunctivitis with atrophy and absent fluid discharge that produces a dry, lusterless condition of the eyeball.

xerosis: drying of the tissues, usually the conjunctiva, seen most clearly when stained with rose bengal stain.

PART THREE

DISORDERS OF THE EYE

CHAPTER 12

DISORDERS OF THE CORNEA AND CONJUNCTIVA

Until the ninth century, visual perception was thought to take place on the surface of the cornea at the pupil. The atomists, early philosopher-scientists of Greece, believed the cornea to be the place of contact between images of the outside world and "the fire within" the soul. One proof of this was the observation that whatever could be seen reflected on the surface of a person's pupil was what that person saw. The Islamic scientists of the ninth and tenth centuries believed that visual perception took place at some location within the optic globe, but without knowing the principles of refraction, they could offer no substantiated theory. Not until Johannes Kepler formulated his laws of optics were the functions of the lens and cornea understood.

Kerato, derived from Greek *keratos* meaning "horn," is the prefix pertaining to the cornea. Because of the firm hard structure of this layer of the eye, which was resistant to surgery and the placing of sutures into its structure for many years, it was felt to resemble a thin slice of animal horn.

Keratitis

Keratitis (*itis* meaning "inflammation") is an inflammation of the cornea (Fig. 12-1). When the conjunctiva is also inflamed, it is called *keratoconjunctivitis.* In *keratoconjunctivitis sicca,* the cornea and conjunctiva react because of dryness (Latin *sicca* meaning "dryness"). In this condition, *filamentary* keratitis may be present in which small filaments of mucus combined with tags of epithelium hang from the corneal surface. The *break-up time of tears,* or *BUT,* measures the time required for the break up of the fluorescein-stained precorneal tear film. The *Schirmer test* described by Otto Schirmer in 1903 is a measure of the amount of tears wetting a filter paper strip in 5 minutes. Both of these tests aid in diagnosing *keratoconjunctivitis sicca (KCS)* or a dry eye syndrome from any cause whatsoever, a condition in which there is insufficient tear production. It occurs with arthritis, in Reiter's syndrome, and in postmenopausal women.

One of the most common problems attacking the cornea is the *herpes simplex*

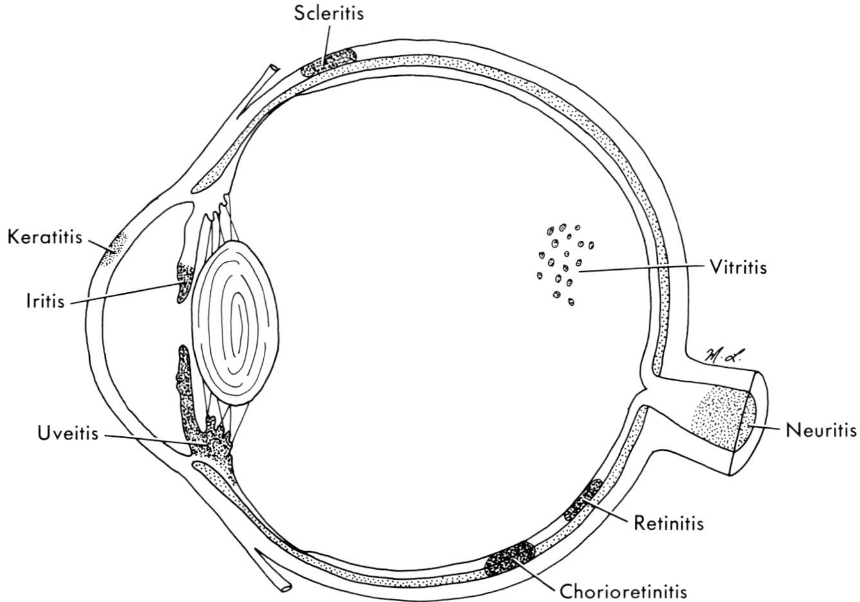

Fig. 12-1. Inflammatory target sites of the eye.

virus type I (Fig. 12-2). Herpes (Greek *herpes,* "creep") is a creeping lesion in the epithelium and is devastating when it infects the corneal epithelium. *Idoxuridine (IDU), trifluridine,* and *vidarabine (ara A)* are used in its treatment. The virus may involve the stroma, giving rise to *disciform keratitis* (disc-shaped edema), *interstitial keratitis* (diffuse widespread inflammation of the stromal layers), or *metaherpetic keratitis (meta,* "after"), in which inflammation and necrosis (death of a part) persist after the herpes virus has been destroyed.

Microbial keratitis is an inflammation of the cornea produced by replicating microorganisms. They are usually exogenous (coming from without) and may be bacterial or fungal, the latter being divided into filamentary *(mold)* or *yeast* types. The inflammation of the cornea from a fungus is called *keratomycosis.*

Marginal ulceration or *ulcerative keratitis* consists of multiple small discrete ulcers located in the periphery of the cornea. *Phlyctenular keratitis* is characterized by single or multiple white nodules of the anterior stroma and epithelium with a leash of parallel vessels and is thought to be caused by a hypersensitivity reaction.

Infiltrates in the cornea are small discrete clusters of cells located deep in the epithelium or the superficial stroma and may occur in a variety of bacterial, viral, or hypersensitivity reactions. *Trantas' dots* are clusters seen in the limbal form of vernal ("springtime") conjunctivitis. *Mooren's ulcer* or *chronic serpiginous*

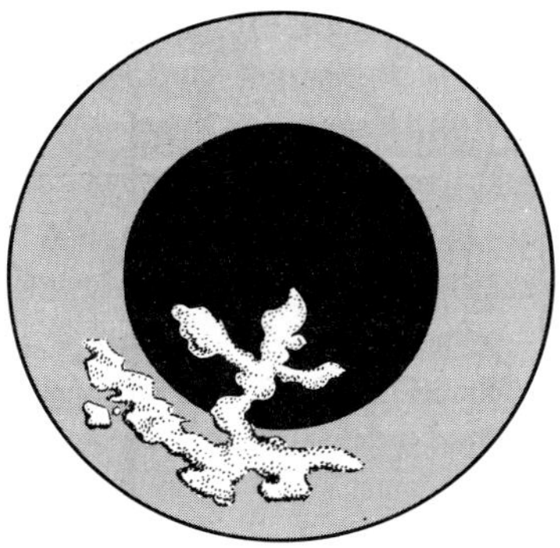

Fig. 12-2. Dendritic figure typical of herpes simplex keratitis.

ulcer (crawling or snakelike) is a progressive degenerative ulceration of the margin of the cornea of unknown cause. A *dellen* is a localized area of dehydration of the cornea with subsequent corneal thinning caused by the tear film in that area not in contact with the cornea. It often occurs adjacent to a raised elevation such as a hard contact lens or follows strabismus surgery.

Corneal dystrophies

Corneal dystrophy (Greek *dys,* "defective" and *trophy,* "nourishment") means defective nourishment of the cornea and belongs to a group of hereditary disorders in which the cornea no longer maintains its normality. Corneal dystrophies may involve any area of the cornea, and an anatomical classification is frequently used.

An *epithelial basement membrane dystrophy,* often called *map-dot-fingerprint dystrophy* because of its similarity in appearance to these identifiable structures, is caused by formation of optic chancres in the basement membrane of the epithelial cells.

Meesman's juvenile epithelial dystrophy is an inherited bilateral progressive disorder in young individuals that results in fine vacuoles or cysts in the epithelium.

In *Bowman's layer,* the second layer of the cornea, *Reis-Buckler ring-shaped dystrophy* occurs in which small, gray, ringlike opacities occur in the subepithelial layer. A number of *stromal corneal dystrophies* exist. Most common are *granular* (sometimes called Groenouw I), *macular* (sometimes called Groenouw II), and *lattice* (sometimes called Biber-Haab-Dimmer). The names in italics represent their clinical description, and the names in parentheses are those of the physicians who first recognized them as clinical entities.

Of the *endothelial dystrophies,* or dystrophies of the endothelium, the most common is Fuchs' dystrophy, often seen in the early stages as corneal guttata (from Latin *gutta,* "drop") because of its droplike appearance.

Corneal degenerations

Degenerations are deteriorations in previously normal tissue as a result of a chemical change or infiltration of abnormal matter. They are frequently associated with aging and do not have any obvious familial tendencies. They may be found in the periphery such as in *marginal furrow degeneration (Terrien's marginal degeneration),* that is a progressive gutter or furrow occurring at the periphery of the cornea which may lead to perforation. A *pterygium* is a fibrovascular wedge-shaped invasive growth from the nasal conjunctiva caused by exposure to sun, wind, and dust and primarily seen in people who live in warm climates (Fig. 12-3). *Band keratopathy* is a band-shaped area of degeneration of the cornea across the exposed palpebral fissure occurring in degenerate eyes, hypercalcemia, and juvenile arthritis (Still's disease).

Keratoconus is a bilateral, degenerative condition of the cornea, which becomes cone shaped with irregular astigmatism. It is treated initially with contact lenses. The *Soper cone lens* is a contact lens with a central steep base curve and a flatter peripheral curve designed and popularized by Joseph Soper of Houston for keratoconus. *Thermal keratoplasty (TKP)* is a method of applying heat to the apex of the cone to flatten it. It is sometimes used in the treatment of keratoconus (Fig. 12-4). *Munson's sign* in keratoconus is noted by the indentation and conical curvature of the lower lid by the cone. It begins to appear in teenagers and

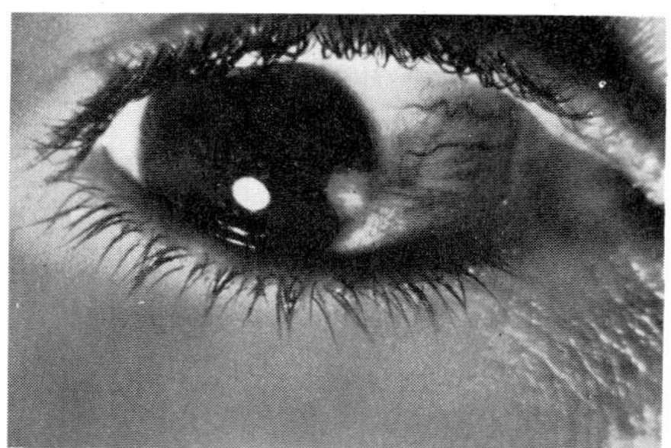

Fig. 12-3. Pterygium.

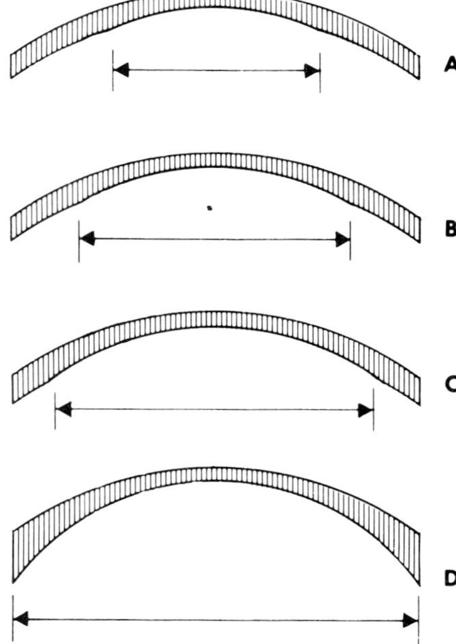

Fig. 12-4. The Soper cone lens. An increase in the sagittal depth can be made by increasing the diameter of the lens. The base curves of **A, B, C,** and **D** are the same.

progresses in severity with time. *Fleischer's rings* are small pigmented rings at the base of the cone seen with slit-lamp biomicroscope. The *keratometer* is an instrument used to measure (*meter,* "to measure") the radius of curvatures of the cornea. The *topogometer* is used to map out the varying radii of the cornea at different points in identifying the highest point of the cone of a patient with keratoconus.

A

abrasion: a limited scraping of the superficial layer of epithelium of the cornea (Fig. 12-5).

acne rosacea: a skin disorder characterized by recurrent skin eruptions, vascularization of the skin, and blepharoconjunctivitis.

acute atopic conjunctivitis: an acute inflammatory reaction coming on a few minutes after a long-term exposure to an allergen to which the patient has become sensitized.

adherent leukoma: adhesion of the iris to a corneal scar.

alkali corneal burn: burn caused by alkali chemicals such as sodium hydroxide (caustic soda), potassium hydroxide (caustic potash), or calcium hydroxide (slaked lime).

aneurysm: an outpouching of a blood vessel.

anterior synechia: an anterior scar usually binding the iris to the angle structures. If the scarring is adherent to the cornea, it is called an *adherent leukoma.*

apical zone: the area of the central cornea that is regular in shape and spherical.

arcus juvenilis: lipid deposition in periphery of cornea in a younger person.

arcus senilis: an annular infiltration of the cornea with lipid material. It is found almost at the corneal periphery separated from the limbus by a clear material and appears as a creamy white ring. The condition does not give rise to symptoms, does not disturb vision, and requires no treatment.

atopy: a term for a hypersensitivity reaction in which specific precipitins are not

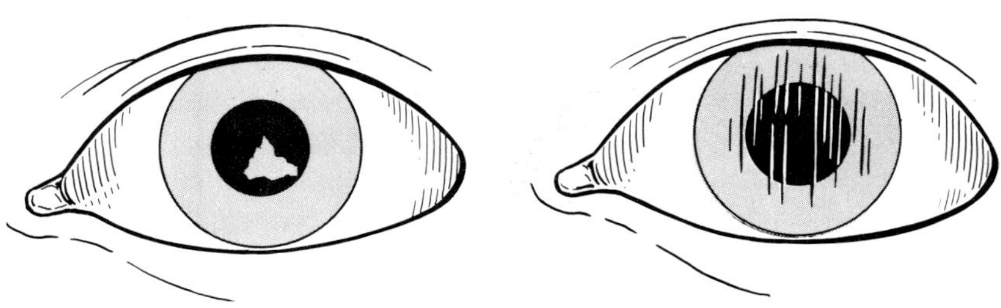

Fig. 12-5. Corneal abrasions.

found in the serum but the formation of specific antibodies can be shown by the sensitization of a normal subject by the injection of serum from a hypersensitive subject.

B

band-shaped keratopathy: a ribbon-shaped opacity that extends from the limbus, usually in the lateral side, across the exposed part of the cornea. It occurs in degenerate and shrunken eyes, in children with infantile polyarthritis, and with trauma. It is a degenerative condition characterized by the development of a lacy band horizontally, largely of subepithelial calcium deposits.

Behçet's disease: recurrent aphthous lesions in the mouth and genitalia associated with uveitis and hypopyon.

Bitot's spots: keratinization of the mucous membrane epithelium of the conjunctiva at the limbus, resulting in a raised spot.

blepharoconjunctivitis: an inflammation of the margins of the lids and conjunctiva. Common causes include staphylococcal infection, seborrhea, and acne rosacea.

blood staining of the cornea: a passage of red blood cells into the cornea following anterior chamber hemorrhage with raised intraocular pressure. The staining of the corneal stroma is associated with an untreated total hyphema and raised ocular tension.

Bowen's disease: intraepithelial epithelioma or squamous cell carcinoma in situ starting at the conjunctiva at the corneoscleral junction and spreading into the cornea.

bullous keratopathy: blisterlike elevations of the corneal epithelium resulting from aqueous humor filtering into the stroma and epithelium. It occurs as a result of a breakdown to the endothelium of the cornea that then allows aqueous to penetrate the cornea. The swelling of the cornea is from endothelium to epithelium with the latter being heaped up into bullae. It is usually the result of long-standing glaucoma coupled with an endothelial dystrophy or endothelial cell loss caused by intraocular surgery. The condition is very painful and results in loss of vision.

C

calcareous degeneration of the cornea: calcium deposition in the anterior layers of the cornea, most commonly seen in band keratopathy.

cellular inclusion bodies: from smears or scrapings, cellular inclusions found by iodine and Giemsa staining may be indicative of trachoma or inclusion conjunctivitis.

chloroquine keratopathy: deposition of chloroquine in the corneal epithelium occurring as irregular light brown streaks or radiating lines in patients taking this drug.

chronic atopic conjunctivitis: a conjunctivitis that occurs in sensitive patients with repeated exposure to a relatively diluted allergen.

Cogan's syndrome: nonsyphilitic interstitial keratitis combined with deafness.

collagen and rheumatoid-related diseases:

episcleral rheumatic nodules: an isolated sterile nodular inflammation.

necrotizing nodular scleritis: an inflammation associated with tissue loss.

scleromalacia perforans: a severe inflammation resulting in herniation of uveal tissue through the sclera.

massive granuloma of the sclera: an inflammation associated with large granulomatous plaques.

congenital endothelial dystrophy: similar to corneal guttata but with larger excrescenses in Descemet's membrane and nonprogressive; dominant inheritance.

conjunctival concretions: minute yellow spots in the palpebrae conjunctiva of elderly people appearing after chronic inflammatory conditions.

conjunctivitis: refers to inflammation of the conjunctiva.

contact dermatoconjunctivitis: an allergic reaction of the skin and conjunctiva caused by repeated contact with a chemical that acts as an allergen (i.e., eye makeup, atropine, topical anesthetics). It is usually bilateral and is characterized by tearing and itching.

corneal dystrophies: bilateral hereditary degenerations of the cornea occurring in the first or second decades of life. Types are:

juvenile epithelial dystrophy of messan: consists of myriads of fine epithelial dots in the epithelium that rarely causes visual problems.

granular dystrophy of the cornea: characterized by the presence of milk-white spots in the superficial stroma in the axial region of the cornea.

lattice dystrophy: consists of minute dots that form lines in the anterior portion of the stroma. Lattice dystrophy can cause epithelial erosions and pain.

Groenouw type II: a hereditary recessive type of stromal dystrophy.

corneal guttata: a degeneration of the endothelial cell layer of the cornea. Corneal guttata is seen as a mosaic of cells with a slit lamp using specular reflection.

corneal fistula: a rupture in the full thickness of the cornea so that aqueous escapes.

cystinosis: deposits of cystine crystals in various parts of the body including the cornea. The appearance of these needlelike crystals in the cornea is pathognomonic for this condition. A fatal autosomal dominant disease of childhood characterized by dwarfism, glycosuria, and the accumulation of cystine crystals in the bone marrow, liver, spleen, and ocular tissues—the cornea, conjunctiva, epithelium, sclera, and the uveal tract.

cystoid cicatrix: a scar with edema fluid making the cornea epithelium bulge as cystic bullae form.

cytology:

polymorphonuclear reaction: characteristic of a bacterial infection.

mononuclear reaction: refers to lymphocytes in preponderance and is characteristic of virus infections (e.g., herpes).

eosinophilic reaction: an eosinophilic cellular response is characteristic of allergic inflammation.

basophilic reaction: runs parallel with eosinophils.

plasma cells: usually found in trachoma.

D

delayed hypersensitivity: caused by prior contact of the tissue with a protein and is the result of the development of antibodies within the cells so that upon exposure to the antigen, an inflammatory reaction causing cellular necrosis occurs.

dellen: a reversible localized area of dehydration with corneal thinning caused by a break in the tear film and often adjacent to a secondary elevation such as a hard contact lens or occurring after muscle surgery. Dellen are shallow ulcers of the cornea occurring near the limbus, usually on the temporal side.

dermoids: cysts composed of stratified squamous epithelium with hair follicles, sebaceous glands, and sweat glands in the cavity wall lining—cavity filled with deratin, hair shafts, and debris (Fig. 12-6).

descemetocele: herniation of Descemet's membrane, the membrane overlying the endothelium, caused by loss of the overlying corneal tissue through ulceration or injury.

disciform keratitis: characterized by the formation of a disc-shaped opacity of the corneal stroma. It frequently occurs as a sequela to herpes simplex keratitis.

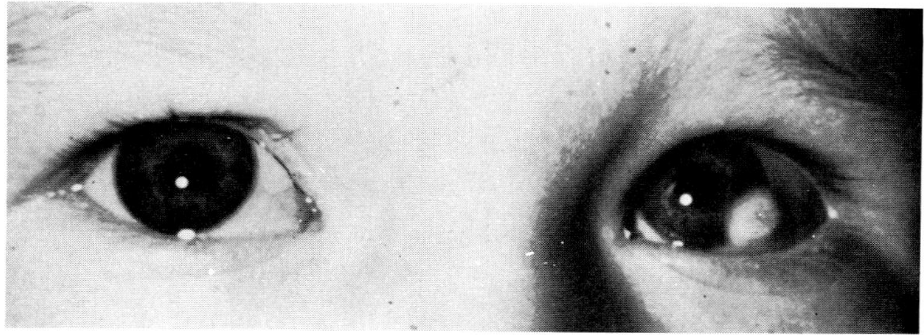

Fig. 12-6. Congenital dermoid of the limbus.

E

E. coli: a gram-negative rodlike bacterium and a normal inhabitant of the bowel. It may contaminate the conjunctiva.

ectasia: a stretching of the tissues. It is found in buphthalmos or high myopia. In the latter, the sclera is stretched to cause a posterior staphyloma.

endogenous: disease derived from internal sources. They may be blood borne such as metastases, derived from an allergy such as vernal conjunctivitis, or part of a general disease, i.e., diabetes.

epidemic keratoconjunctivitis (EKC): an acute inflammatory disease caused by an adenovirus and producing round or oval white infiltrates in the adult cornea.

epithelial bedwing: corneal edema of the epithelium.

epithelial slide: a process in which the cells surrounding a recently injured abraded area of the cornea migrate to cover the defect.

exogenous: disease that is derived from external sources such as thermal, radiation, mechanical, chemical, or parasites.

exposure keratitis: ulceration of the exposed part of the cornea, most commonly caused by seventh nerve palsy. The lid is no longer able to close properly or blink, leaving the cornea exposed during the day and in sleep. It occurs in all conditions where there is inadequate closure of the lids, i.e., lagophthalmos caused by thyroid disease.

F

Fabry's disease: a hereditary disorder caused by alpha-galactosidase deficiency resulting in a deposition of lipid. The lipid is deposited in the cornea in a typical whorl-like pattern.

folds in Decemet's membrane: appears as double-contoured bright lines formed by two parallel linear reflexes and appear in both traumatic and inflammatory conditions of the cornea.

follicular conjunctivitis: refers to a viral infection of the conjunctiva that produces follicles, discharge, redness of the conjunctiva, and regional adenopathy of the preauricular node.

folliculosis: formation of follicles without inflammatory signs occurring in children. It may be a response to an infection elsewhere besides the eye.

fungi: primitive undifferentiated plants that abound in the soil and in the air. They live as parasites whenever there is an organic material, either vegetable or animal.

G

ghost vessels: empty blood vessels remaining after corneal invasion by vessels that were filled with blood.

gonococcal bacillus: a bean-shaped, nonmotile, gram-negative coccus that produces venereal types of conjunctivitis in newborn infants and children.

H

hay fever: the most common type of atopic conjunctivitis affecting approximately 3% to 5% of the population. Other forms of allergic sensitivity are usually present affecting the nose, nasal sinuses, and bronchioles.

herpes virus: a virus that affects the face, cornea, lips, and genitals. In the eye, the typical lesion has an arborizing pattern (the dendrite) that tends to be recurrent and eventually causes corneal scarring.

herpes zoster ophthalmicus: a virus affecting the skin over the distribution of the fifth nerve, which may produce corneal ulcers, iritis, and secondary glaucoma. If the tip of the nose is involved with blisters, the nasociliary branch is affected and thus the eye can be involved. The most common nerve involved in the ocular region is the supraorbital nerve, which affects the upper lid, forehead, and scalp.

heterogeneous donor material: a graft from an individual of a different species.

homogeneous donor material: a graft from an individual of the same species.

Hudson-Stähli lines: pigmented lines of cornea that occur after trauma (alkali burns) or with many degenerative corneal conditions. It is a brown pigmented line in the cornea caused by the deposit of intracytoplasmic iron.

Hurler's disease (gargoylism): condition characterized by abnormal mucopolysaccharides and manifested by dwarfism, depressed nasal bridge, cloudy cornea, retinal degeneration, enlarged spleen and liver, and mental retardation (Fig. 12-7).

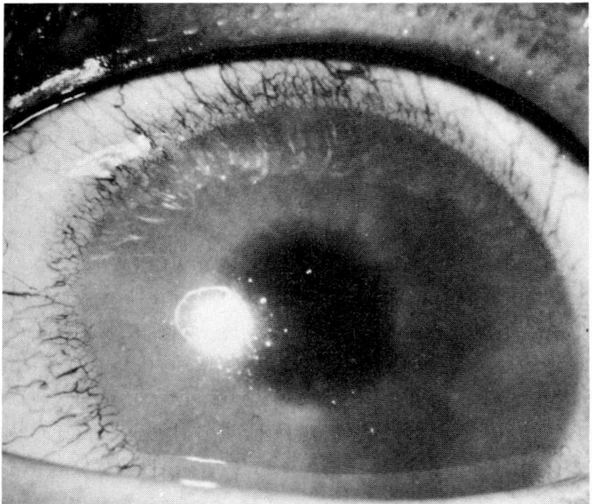

Fig. 12-7. In Hurler's syndrome the corneas show a diffuse cloudiness throughout all layers. (From Donaldson, D.D.: Atlas of external diseases of the eye, Vol. III. Cornea and sclera, ed. 2, St. Louis, 1971, The C.V. Mosby Co.)

hydrops: a swelling of the cornea caused by accumulation of aqueous fluid from the anterior chamber.

hyperemia: refers to the dilatation of blood vessels in the conjunctiva. This can be caused by irritation, allergy, inflammation, or infection.

hypersensitivity: a state in which the tissues react by an abnormal and injurious response to foreign substances (allergies).

immediate type: an inflammatory response that occurs 2 days after exposure to the same protein.

hypopyon ulcer: a corneal ulcer accompanied by a collection of inflammatory cells in the anterior chamber to produce a level. The hypopyon is sterile as long as Descemet's membrane is intact.

I

IDU: 5 iodo-2′-deoxyuridine—the first antiviral drug used against herpes keratitis. It competes with thymidine in the synthesis of DNA.

inclusion conjunctivitis: a benign follicular conjunctivitis of venereal origin caused by the TRIC virus affecting the palpebral conjunctiva. It usually resolves without scarring or visual loss. It has two clinical forms: in newborn infants and in adults derived from venereal contacts or swimming pools.

interstitial keratitis: indicates an inflammation of the corneal stroma. It is common in syphilis.

iron lines: iron deposition in the epithelial layers.

iron-ferry line: iron deposited at the margin of a filtering bleb.

iron-Fleischer ring: iron deposited in keratoconus.

iron–Hudson-Stähli line: iron deposited in a horizontal line.

iron-Stocker line: deposit of iron at advancing edge of a pterygium.

K

Kayser-Fleischer ring: copper deposits at the extreme periphery of the cornea in Descemet's membrane as seen in hepatolenticular degeneration or Wilson's disease. It is pathognomonic of this condition.

keratic precipitates (KP): inflammatory deposits on the back surface of the cornea. Usually seen after a bout of iritis.

keratitis: An inflammation of the cornea. See *specific condition.*

keratectomy: removal of the anterior portion of the cornea.

keratoconjunctivitis sicca: a dry eye that may be caused by local disease of the conjunctiva (xerosis—pemphigoid or vitamin A deficiency) or a decrease in the secretions of the main and accessory lacrimal glands.

keratoconus: a bilateral condition occurring in young people characterized by thinning and ectasia of the cornea. It causes visual loss because of irregular astigmatism that occurs as the disorder progresses.

keratoconus fruste: an aborted form of keratoconus often seen in families with keratoconus and resulting in only minimal central thinning and slight asymmetric astigmatism.

keratoglobus: a forward protrusion of the cornea that may be congenital or developmental.

keratomalacia: softening of the cornea, often occurring in severe vitamin A deficiency.

keratopathy: pathology of the cornea. See *specific condition.*

Koch-Weeks conjunctivitis: previously termed pink eye. It has been a serious cause of blindness of epidemic proportions in North Africa and the Middle East. It is rare in Western Europe and North America.

Krukenberg's spindle: accumulation of pigment on the back of the corneal endothelium in the shape of a vertical spindle that occurs from breakdown of iris pigment. It is seen in pigmentary glaucoma, in trauma, after iritis, and in diabetes.

L

leukoma: a whitish opacity of the cornea.

lipid keratopathy: a nodular yellow corneal infiltrate that follows an old corneal injury.

M

macula: a moderately dense scar of the corneal stroma with a well-defined border.

marginal degeneration of the cornea: a noninflammatory bilateral degeneration of the cornea resulting in the formation of a gutter or furrow in the periphery of the cornea.

McCarey-Kaufman medium (M-K medium): a tissue culture–soaking medium for storage and preservation of corneal tissue.

megalocornea: abnormally large (over 13 mm), stationary cornea usually caused by congenital glaucoma but may be congenital or developmental.

membranous conjunctivitis: an exudate that permeates the epithelium of the conjunctiva so that attempts to remove it leaves a raw and bleeding surface (in diphtheria).

microcornea: a small cornea of 10 mm or less.

mitosis: multiplication of surviving epithelial cells by division to cover an epithelial defect.

Mooren's ulcer: a chronic superficial ulceration occurring in elderly people starting in the corneal periphery. The ulcer has an undermined border and may be progressive to involve the entire cornea.

multinucleated giant epithelial cells: virus particles that are present in herpes simplex, zoster, and vaccinia.

N

nebula: diffuse cloudlike opacity with indistinct borders. It is usually found after corneal trauma or inflammation.

neuroparalytic keratopathy: corneal changes secondary to interference with the sensory nerve supply of the cornea. It can occur with brain tumors or after cutting the fifth nerve (for tic douloureux). It occurs after any neurological lesion that destroys the integrity of the fifth nerve.

nodular episcleritis: a nonspecific inflammation of the sclera characterized by the appearance of nodular inflammatory foci.

nummular keratitis: characterized by disc-shaped infiltrates in the superficial layer of the corneal stroma.

O

ocular pemphigoid: a chronic disease in which there is replacement of the submucous tissue by newly formed connective tissue that contracts. It causes dryness of the conjunctiva and cornea caused by loss of mucous-secreting glands.

ophthalmia neonatorium: conjunctivitis occurring in the newborn infant that can cause damage to the eyes through infection of the cornea. The causes are manifold but the most common are venereal and *Staphylococcus aureus.*

P

pannus: any ingrowth of fibrovascular tissue between epithelium and Bowman's membrane. It can be seen with pterygia, trachoma, or vernal conjunctivitis.

papillary conjunctivitis: a conjunctivitis characterized by raised inflammatory nodules with new formation of capillaries growing into the epithelium. This type of inflammatory response is seen with vernal catarrh or giant papillary conjunctivitis, an allergic sequela of contact lens use.

pemphigus: a lethal disease of relatively rare incidence characterized by the formation of bullae within the skin and mucous membranes. It can affect the conjunctiva.

penetrating keratoplasty: a window of a full thickness of opaque cornea is removed and replaced by a corresponding piece of transparent donor cornea.

pharyngoconjunctival fever: an acute and highly infectious illness characterized by fever, pharyngitis, and nonpurulent follicular conjunctivitis.

phlyctenular keratoconjunctivitis: an infection occurring mainly in children as an allergic response by the corneal and conjunctival epithelium to some endogenous toxin to which it has become sensitized.

phthisis cornea: a shrunken scar.

pinguecula: a yellowish triangular patch formed by a degeneration of connective tissue, situated in the bulbar conjunctiva on either side of the cornea. It is thought to be caused by aging and exposure to ultraviolet, wind, or dust.

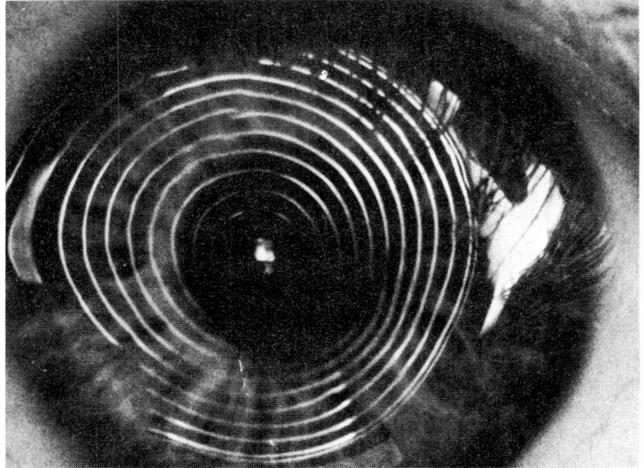

Fig. 12-8. In keratoconus Placido's disc shows rings that are distorted and irregularly spaced in the left eye. (From Donaldson, D.D.: Atlas of external diseases of the eye, Vol. III. Cornea and sclera, ed. 2, St. Louis, 1971, The C.V. Mosby Co.)

Placido's disc: a device composed of a series of rings that examine the corneal surface to detect irregularities and asymmetry (Fig. 12-8).

pneumococcal bacillus: a diplococcus that is enclosed in a capsule and produces a conjunctivitis similar to streptococcal infections.

pneumococcal ulcer: a gray-white ulcer caused by infection by bacillus pneumococcus, showing a tendency to creep in one direction.

posterior polymorphous dystrophy: a corneal dystrophy composed of irregular grayish white opacities in Descemet's membrane.

pseudomembrane: a collection of cells on the conjunctiva forming a membrane that is easily peeled off leaving the epithelium intact *(Streptococcus).*

Pseudomonas pyocyaneas: a gram-negative slender rod producing two pigments—a bluish pyocyanin and a yellow fluorescein. It proliferates in a fluid medium and can easily cause endophthalmitis once it has gained access to the interior of the eye.

pterygium (wing): a triangular invasion of the cornea, usually on the medial side, by a fibrovascular bundle of connective tissue.

punctate keratitis: small discrete superficial opacities and staining areas of the corneal epithelium, probably viral in origin.

pyocyanea (bacillus): a bacteria commonly found in the intestinal tract and frequently in the skin, ear, and nose and capable of producing a devastating infection when it invades broken corneal epithelium. It thrives on a wet medium.

pyocyaneal ulcers: characterized by their rapid course, the primary involvement of the cornea, and the rapid spread of the anterior chamber, a large hypopyon and the pus that is frequently greenish in color.

R

recurrent corneal erosion: a recurrence of an epithelial breakdown weeks or months after the initial injury. Usually occurs with organic agents such as paper or fingernails.

Reiter's disease: characterized by urethritis, conjunctivitis, and polyarthritis.

retroillumination: light is focused on deeper structures, such as the iris, while microscope is adjusted to study the cornea. Best method of showing fine corneal edema.

Riley-Day syndrome (familial autonomic dysautonomia): reduced or absent tears, corneal anesthesia, and corneal ulceration associated with decreased sweating. Occurs primarily in Jewish children.

rosacea (acne): an inflammatory skin disease that can cause recurrent inflammations of the cornea, conjunctiva, and lids (blepharitis, recurrent hordeolum). It also produces a thickening and vascularization of the skin with acnelike pustule formation.

rust ring of the cornea: a ring of siderosis that forms in the corneal epithelium as a result of oxidization of an embedded metallic foreign body.

S

salmon patch: central area of intense vascularization that occurs in interstitial keratitis with the confluence of all blood vessels at the center of the cornea.

Salzman's nodular degeneration: elevated white or yellow corneal area that is usually superimposed on a region of old corneal injury especially at the edge of pannus. It is a slowly progressive degeneration occurring unilaterally in an eye previously affected by keratitis.

sclera: the white inert supportive structure of the eye. It is collagenous and avascular.

sclerosing keratitis: inflammation in which the cornea becomes white and opaque, resembling the sclera.

seborrhea (sebum, grease): a condition characterized by greasy skin, scales on the scalp, forehead, and lids, and the presence of a yeastlike fungus *Pityrosporum ovale.*

Sjögren's syndrome: refers to a keratoconjunctivitis sicca, arthritis, and dryness of mucous surfaces generally in the body.

***Staphylococcus* bacillus:** a spherical gram-positive aerobic organism that causes frequent infection of the lids, corneas, and conjunctiva. It is a common cause of ophthalmia neonatorum.

staphylococcal allergic keratoconjunctivitis: caused by sensitization to the exotoxin of this organism. It produces a severe ulcerative and infiltrative keratitis.

staphyloma (a bunch of grapes): stretching of a corneal scar or tissue with the incarceration of uveal tissue.

stippling: dotlike staining of the cornea.

streptococcal bacillus: a gram-positive aerobic organism that causes a pseudomembranous form of conjunctivitis.

striate keratopathy: the appearance of linear striae (lines) caused by damage of the corneal endothelium with resultant corneal edema and folding of Descemet's membrane.

subconjunctival hemorrhage: a collection of blood under the conjunctiva.

subepithelial keratitis: subepithelial infiltrates that classically occur with adenovirus infections.

superficial punctate keratitis: a small dotlike epithelial keratitis occurring bilaterally with a chronic remittent course in the absence of conjunctivitis.

symblepharon: healing by fusing together of two opposing surfaces such as the tarsal and palpebral conjunctiva. They are adhesions between the conjunctiva.

T

telangiectasia: a network of abnormal arborizing blood vessels appearing on the skin or eye.

tight lens syndrome (TLS): a syndrome popularized by L. Wilson and co-workers in which an extended-wear lens becomes firmly adhered to the corneal epithelium.

total keratoplasty: transplantation of the entire cornea.

trachoma: a follicular conjunctivitis caused by a virus and producing corneal and conjunctival scarring with severe visual loss. The leading cause of blindness in the world, it is endemic in many parts of Africa, the Middle East, and poor third-world countries. The lid scarring on the tarsal side of the lids is characteristic of this disease. This infectious keratoconjunctivitis caused by *Chlamydia trachomatis* is cause by a TRIC virus.

tubercle bacillus: a thin, curved gram-positive bacillus that is rarely seen today as a cause of conjunctivitis.

V

vernal conjunctivitis: a recurrent bilateral inflammation of the conjunctiva (spring catarrh) characterized by cobble-stoned, flat-topped papillae of the tarsal conjunctiva, a discharge (with eosinophils), and a keratitis. It is seasonal, affects the young, with a high percentage of cases in males.

verrucae (warts): a virus with a long incubation period that causes wartlike lesions on the skin and on the lids.

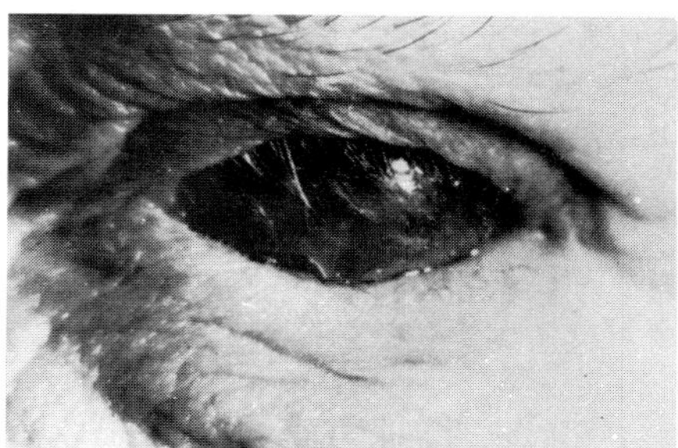

Fig. 12-9. Xerosis, or drying, of the cornea.

vitamin A deficiency: can cause corneal xerosis, keratomalacia, and night blindness. It is caused by a dystrophy of the rods.

W

white limbal girdle of Vogt: a yellowish white opacity forming a half moon–like arc and runs concentrically with the limbus, usually on the nasal side. It is harmless in its significance.

white rings of the cornea: a white ring that is about 0.5 mm in diameter and consists of white dots thought to be calcium or lipid.

X

xerophthalmia: excessive keratinization of mucous membranes including cornea and conjunctiva. It can occur with dry eyes, pemphigus, or Stevens-Johnson syndrome. *See* keratomalacia.

xerosis: a degenerative condition characterized by dryness of the conjunctiva. It is not caused by a decrease in lacrimal secretion. For the most part, it has causes such as atrophy of the conjunctival glands and goblet cells.

xerosis of the cornea: keratinization of the corneal epithelium caused by dryness. In the early phase it causes a burning sensation, which can be treated with artificial tears. In the later stages it can cause corneal scarring. It is detected in its early phase with rose bengal stain, which specifically stains devitalized tissue (Fig. 12-9).

CHAPTER 13

GLAUCOMA

Glaucoma is derived from the Greek word *glaukos,* meaning bluish gray, which is how the eye appears in advanced stages. Hippocrates and the ancients used the term for both cataracts and glaucoma in which a grayish or greenish appearance replaced the normal black pupil. Later a distinction was made between opacity of the lens and other conditions that lay behind the pupil, and the term glaucoma was reserved for the latter situation, the nature of which was unknown. It was not until 1709 that Brisseau clearly differentiated between cataract and glaucoma and noted that the greenish color was a minor feature of the condition and that hardness of the eyeball was the main feature. *Glaucoma* is characterized by a sustained elevation of intraocular pressure. The *intraocular pressure (IOP)* is the force per unit area within the eye that depends on the inflow of aqueous in relationship to the outflow of aqueous through the trabecular meshwork. Glaucoma is usually caused by impaired outflow.

Types of glaucoma

There are several types of glaucoma: primary angle-closure, open angle or chronic, secondary, congenital or infantile, angle recession, phacolytic, and pupillary block. A description of each type is as follows:

1. *Primary angle-closure* glaucoma in which the angle of the anterior chamber is narrow and the anterior chamber is shallow resulting in blockage of the angle at the root of the iris and obstruction of outflow from the eye.
2. *Open-angle or chronic glaucoma* in which the angle between the iris and the cornea is open and in which the outflow blockage occurs in the trabecular meshwork.
3. *Secondary glaucoma* arising from specific disorders within the eye.
4. *Congenital or infantile glaucoma* in which the eyes are often referred to as *buphthalmos* because the infant eye is not rigid and distends as a result of elevated pressure and comes to resemble the eye of an ox *(buph,* "ox") (Fig. 13-1).

Specific secondary types include *angle recession glaucoma,* which occurs after trauma, caused by a tear in the ciliary body resulting in a scar in this body.

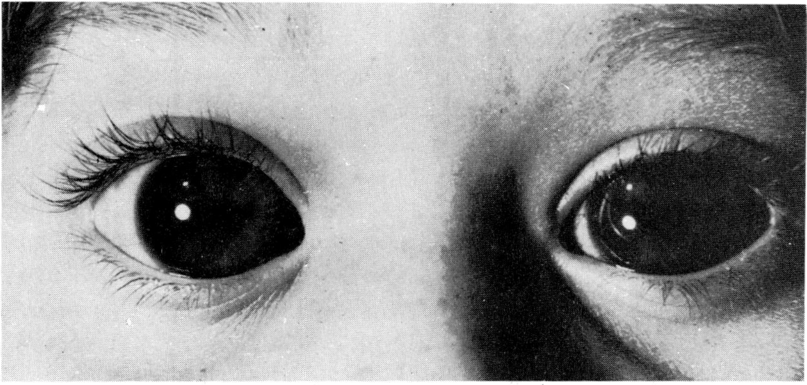

Fig. 13-1. Congenital glaucoma. Note the enlargement of the eyes.

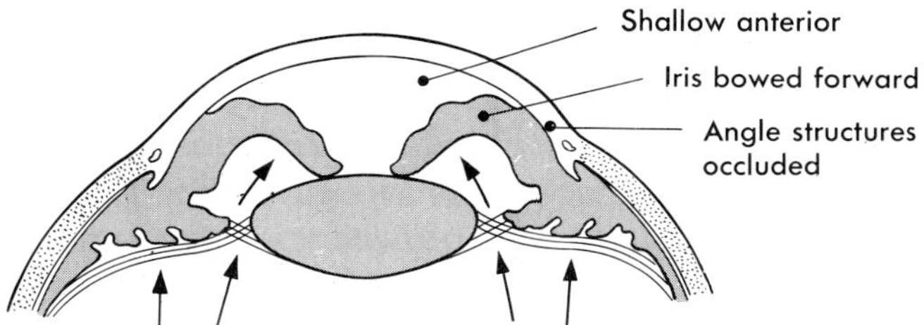

Fig. 13-2. Pupillary block glaucoma. The pressure in the posterior chamber exceeds that of the anterior chamber. The iris is bowed forward (iris bombé) and occludes the angle structures. Without treatment the iris becomes permanently adherent to the angle structures, and intractable secondary glaucoma ensues.

Phacolytic glaucoma is caused by the toxic effect from liquified cortex of the cataractous crystalline lens of the eye (from *phako,* "lens," indicating a lens-induced glaucoma). *Pupillary-block glaucoma* is caused by obstruction of aqueous through the pupil by the lens or vitreous so that fluid cannot pass from the posterior chamber behind the iris to the anterior chamber in front of the iris (Fig. 13-2). *Ocular hypertension* occurs in patients with raised intraocular pressure with no demonstrable visual field loss or optic nerve damage. It is that group of people who have intraocular pressures that are statistically high, but normal, or have early glaucoma with the expectation of further rise in pressure and field loss.

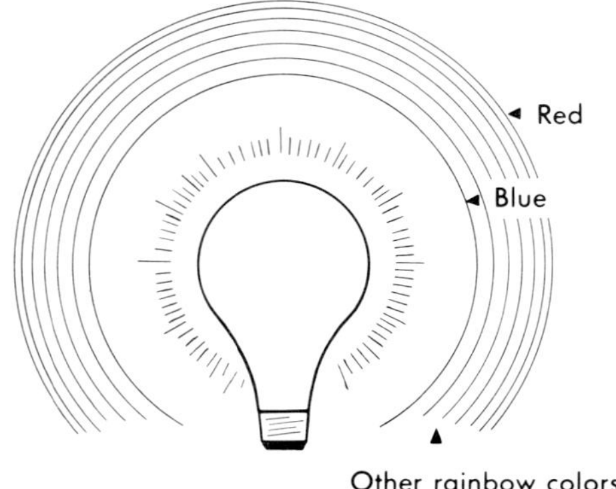

Fig. 13-3. Halos about lights. This is a prominent symptom in angle-closure glaucoma.

Symptoms and signs of glaucoma

Halos are the rainbowlike effect around lights caused by the presence of free fluid in the cornea that breaks up light into its spectral components (Fig. 13-3). *Pain* is a symptom of angle-closure glaucoma resulting from a sudden and drastic high pressure effect within the eye. *Iris bombé* occurs in the pupillary block mechanism when the iris is bound down to the anterior lens capsule or vitreous face by inflammation. Clinically the iris is bowed forward by aqueous trying to pass from the posterior to the anterior chamber.

Sudden visual loss occurs when the cornea becomes edematous; this visual loss is reversible. Gradual visual loss may occur with pressure necrosis, or death, of some of the fine capillaries in the optic nerve; the result is *glaucomatous cupping* in which the relatively flat optic disc takes on the shape of a cup with a small thin rim and deep excavation (Fig. 13-4). *Cupping* is defined as a three-dimensional depression of the optic disc surface relative to the retinal surface; *pallor* is an area lacking the pink color of small blood vessels. The *cup/disc ratio* is the ratio of the horizontal diameter of the cup of the optic disc to the diameter of the disc. Under normal circumstances there is a *physiological* cup, a normal nonglaucomatous cup, caused by the presence of a visible depressed *lamina cribrosa,* a sievelike anatomical structure from which a true glaucomatous cup must be differentiated. *Constriction of the visual field* and *sector-shaped defects* in the visual field occur as a common finding in which the peripheral vision is gradually lost in an orderly and usually characteristic manner with sustained pressure.

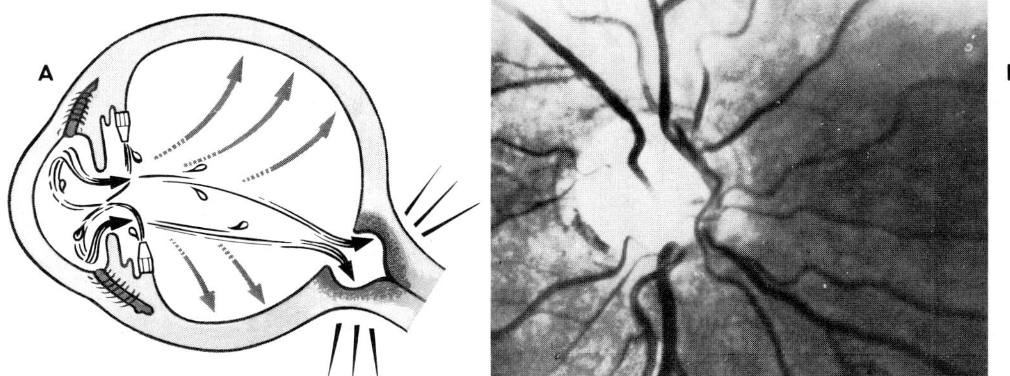

Fig. 13-4. **A,** Increased pressure causes excavation of the optic disc. **B,** Cupping of the optic disc. Note the dip of the vessels as they traverse the temporal margin of the disc.

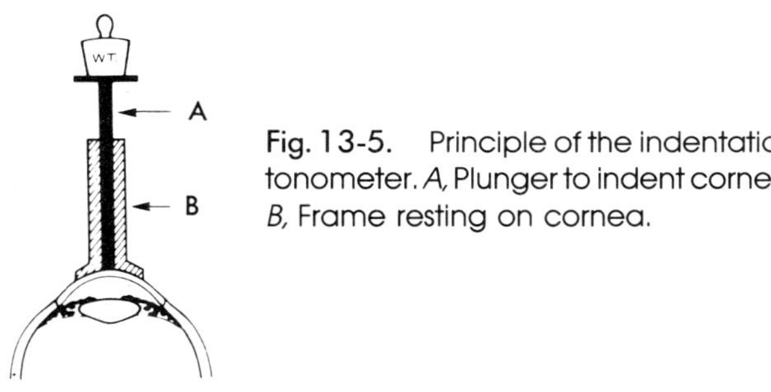

Fig. 13-5. Principle of the indentation tonometer. *A,* Plunger to indent cornea. *B,* Frame resting on cornea.

Tonometry and tonography

To detect glaucoma, a *tonometer* is used to measure *(meter)* the pressure of the eye. In *applanation tonometry,* such as in the use of the Goldman tonometer, the cornea is flattened, and the pressure required to achieve this flattening is a measure of the intraocular pressure. The word applanation originates from the Latin *planare* or *ad planare,* meaning "to flatten." In *indentation tonometry,* such as occurs with the Schiøtz tonometer, the cornea is indented by the footplate of the tonometer (Fig. 13-5). *Tonography* (Greek *tonos,* "that which can be stretched," and Greek *graphos,* "write") is the science of recording the change in intraocular pressure. It measures the change in pressure that occurs when a constant weight is applied to the cornea (Fig. 13-6). The harder the eye, or the greater the pressure, the less will be the indentation of the cornea by the tonometer. This measurement produces a *tonogram,* a recording of the eye tensin, which provides data on the *aqueous outflow,* or the exit of aqueous, through the trabecular meshwork, through Schlemm's canal, and into the episcleral veins. The measurement is known as the *facility of outflow,* and this resistance to outflow can be expressed as a *coefficient (c) of facility of outflow.*

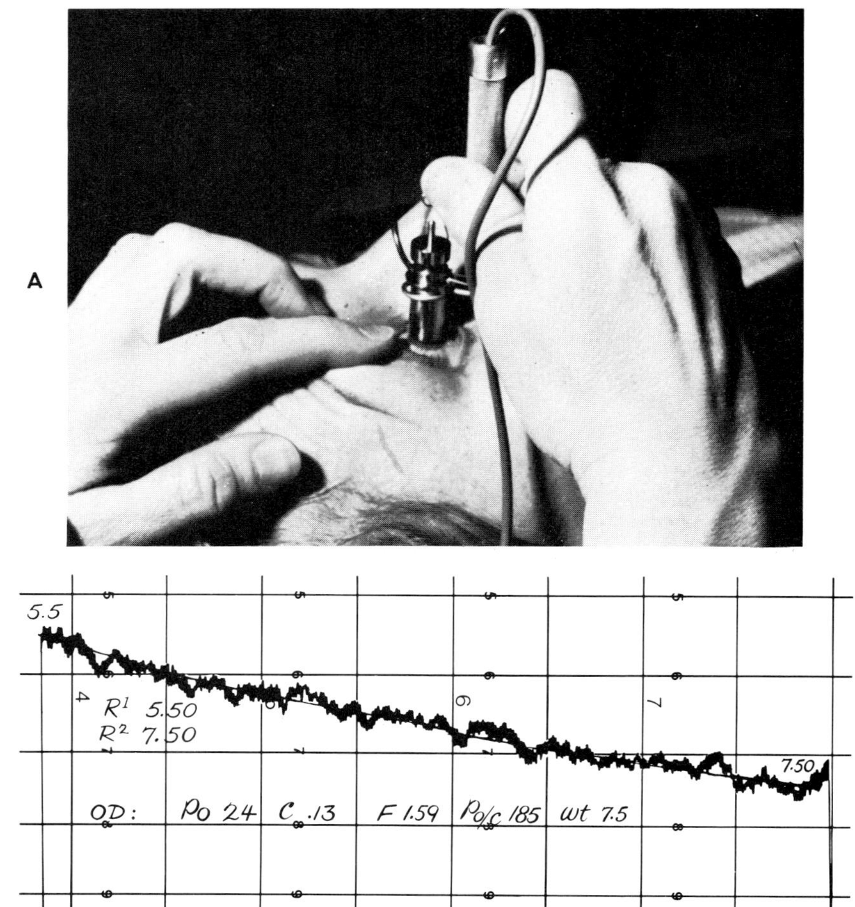

Fig. 13-6. **A,** A constant weight is permitted to rest on the cornea for a measured time, providing a recording of the fall in the intraocular pressure of the eye. **B,** Typical tonogram of a patient with glaucoma. (From Reinecke, R., Stein, H., and Slatt, B.: Introductory manual for the ophthalmic assistant, St. Louis, 1972, The C.V. Mosby Co.)

Ocular examination and surgery

Gonioscopy is derived from the Greek *gonio,* meaning "corner," and from the Greek *scopy,* "examination," and refers to examination of the cornea or angle of the anterior chamber. It is performed with a *goniolens* (Fig. 13-7). *Goniotomy* is a surgical procedure to open the angle and is used in infants for the treatment of congenital glaucoma. *Goniopuncture* is a puncture incision of the angle used in infants.

A *filtering* procedure is one that permits a fistula to form from the anterior chamber to the subtenons or subconjunctival space and filters off the aqueous humor and thus reduces pressure. A *filtering bleb* is an elevated bubble of raised conjunctiva filled with aqueous fluid that flows through the anterior chamber of the eye to the subconjunctival space. The *trabeculum* is the normal filtering structure of the eye that lies in the angle of the anterior chamber and carries fluid to Schlemm's canal. *Trabeculotomy* refers to making a surgical incision in the trabeculum. *Trabeculectomy* is the surgical removal of a portion of the trabeculum to permit filtration of aqueous fluid. *Sclerectomy* is the removal of a portion of the sclera to permit filtration of aqueous out of the eye. *Thermosclerectomy* refers to the making of a scleral fistula by a method of applying heat on either side of a small scleral wound at the site of the posterior limbus. An *iridectomy* is a cutting away *(ectomy)* of a portion of the iris. It may be a *peripheral*

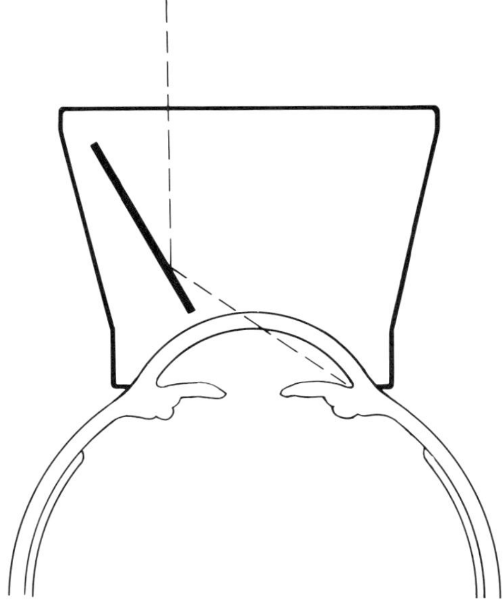

Fig. 13-7. Goniolens. A beam of light is deflected into the opposite angle of the anterior chamber.

iridectomy in which the peripheral portion of the iris is removed or a *sector iridectomy* in which a pie-shaped sector of the iris is removed. It is referred to as *basal* iridectomy if the root or base of the iris is removed.

A

adrenergic agents: these agents act as receptors of the sympathetic nervous system. They are divided into: (1) alpha receptors, which mediate pupillary dilatation, (2) beta receptors: beta-1, results in cardiac stimulation and beta-2 results in relaxation of bronchial and gastrointestinal smooth muscle and vasodilation.

aniridia: absence of the iris, which frequently results in glaucoma. It is usually congenital and is associated with foveal aplasia, cataracts, and rotary and pendular nystagmus.

anterior chamber angle: angle between the iris and the cornea that contains the trabecula and through which the aqueous flows out of the eye.

anterior synechiae: fibrous adhesions of iris to cornea or trabecula in anterior chamber angle. The resultant scar can cause glaucoma.

anticholinesterase agents: inhibit cholinesterase and thereby potentiate the effects of acetylcholine on the parasympathetic end organs. Anticholinesterase agents: physostigmine (eserine), isoflurophate (fluorophyl: DFP), echothiophate iodide (phospholine iodide), and demecarium bromide (humorsol).

aqueous humor: a transparent fluid secreted by ciliary processes into the posterior chamber. It passes through the pupil to the anterior chamber and then to the trabecular meshwork.

aqueous inflow: aqueous produced by active secretion of the epithelium of the ciliary body flows by passive filtration through the blood vessels of the iris and ciliary body.

aqueous outflow: the exit of aqueous through the trabecular meshwork, through Schlemm's canal, and then into the episcleral venous system.

aqueous vein: connects Schlemm's canal to the episcleral blood veins.

automated perimeters: a series of perimeters automated so that they eliminate technician bias and the need for highly trained personnel. They are very standardized, accurate, and with many devices include information storage.

arachnodactyly (Marfan's syndrome): this congenital condition is featured by the presence of congenital glaucoma, dislocated lenses, cardiac abnormalities, musculoskeletal defects, and dissecting aneurysms of the aorta.

arcuate Bjerrum scotoma: a half ring–like visual field defect arising from the disc and extending around fixation.

Axenfeld's anomaly: posterior corneal arcus resulting from bridging filaments from the iris stroma to Schwalbe's line and resulting in glaucoma.

C

carbonic anhydrase inhibitors: agents (acetazolamide) that decrease the secretion of aqueous humor by the ciliary process: acetazolamide (Diamox), methazolamide (Neptazane), and ethoxazolamide (Cardrase).

Chandler's syndrome: includes corneal edema, endothelial dystrophy, stromal iris atrophy, peripheral anterior synechias, and glaucoma.

Cogan-Reese syndrome: consists of iris nodules, peripheral anterior synechias, an abnormal membrane, and glaucoma.

congenital glaucoma: glaucoma that is manifest at birth.

corticosteriod-induced glaucoma: a form of open-angle glaucoma induced by the topical use of steroids.

cup-disc ratio: the ratio of the size of the optic disc to the size of the physiological cup. The larger the size of the cup, the more likely the diagnosis will be glaucoma.

cupping of the discs: the appearance of disc with an excavation usually on the temporal side. It is usually associated with pallor and notching of the disc margin.

cyclocryotherapy: a treatment for glaucoma effected by freezing the ciliary body and thereby diminishing aqueous production.

D

diurnal variations: the variation in intraocular pressure that occurs over a 24-hour period. The pressure is usually highest in the early morning hours between 3:30 AM and 5:30 AM.

drainage angle: the portion of the anterior chamber where the iris and the corneoscleral tissue meet. The term is frequently used in connection with glaucoma because the drainage of aqueous takes place in this region.

E

ectropion uveae: eversion of iris pigment epithelium around the pupil margin.

essential atrophy of iris: rare, progressive, unilateral disease of the iris in which there is a patchy loss of all layers of the iris, leading to a distorted and eccentric pupil and often a secondary glaucoma.

F

facility of outflow: measurement of the volume of aqueous that leaves the eye each minute per each millimeter of tonometer pressure.

flat anterior chamber: potential complication of intraocular surgery characterized by the iris being in direct contact with the cornea and by the virtual absence of aqueous in the anterior chamber.

G

glaucoma field defects: generalized peripheral contraction.

glaucomatocyclitic crisis: a condition that is recurrent, affects one eye in young people between 30 and 50 years of age, and is characterized by inflammation in the anterior segment.

Goldmann lens: lens with mirror to visualize the angle structures of the eye.

Goldmann perimeter: a half-sphere perimeter that is used for both glaucoma and neurological fields.

gonioprism: special type of contact lens with prism that permits examination of the periphery of the anterior chamber or the peripheral retina.

goniotomy: a surgical procedure to treat infantile glaucoma.

H

hyperosmatic agents: systemic agents that cause a drop in ocular pressure. These include oral glycerol, 50% solution; mannitol, 20% given intravenously; and urea given intravenously.

hypertension, ocular: intraocular pressure that is increased above normal but with no demonstrable visual field loss or optic nerve damage.

I

IOP: intraocular pressure (Fig. 13-8).

K

kinetic perimetry: charting the visual fields by moving the target from a non-seeing to a seeing zone.

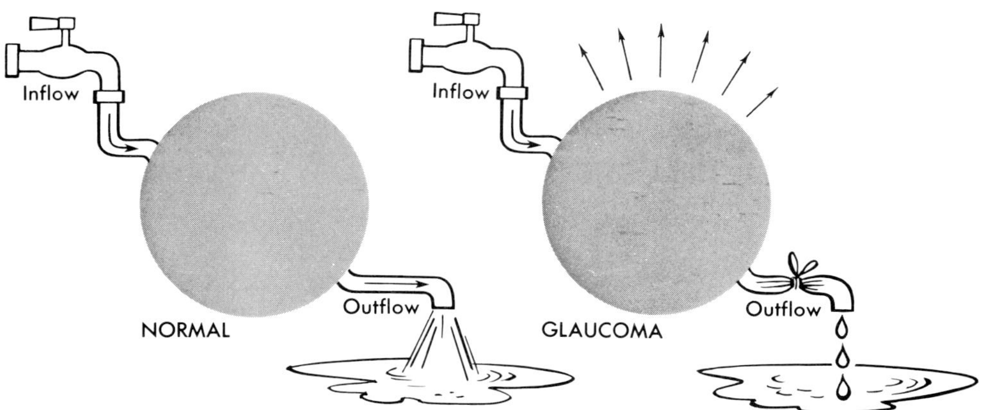

Fig. 13-8. Obstruction of aqueous outflow causes an elevation of intraocular tension.

Koeppe lens: lens which allows the observer to see directly the angle structures of the eye.

L

low-pressure glaucoma: evidence of intraocular glaucomatous damage (cupping of optic disc and visual field defects) with normal or low intraocular pressure.

M

megalocornia: corneal enlargement usually 14 to 16 mm in diameter but without signs of congenital glaucoma.

mesodermal dysgenesis: a basket term representing a group of mesodermal dysplasias of the anterior segment:

posterior embryotoxin: the unusual prominence of Schwalbe's line that stands out like an encircling glass tube inside the limbus.

posterior polymorphous dystrophy: a bilateral dominantly transmitted corneal dystrophy consisting of nodular lesions in the Descemet's membrane.

Rieger's syndrome: refers to features of bilateral hypoplasia of the iris stroma, posterior-embryotoxin, pupillary abnormalities, and frequently glaucoma.

Peter's anomaly: condition characterized by adherent iris attached in a ring-like fashion to the cornea.

microcornea: consists of small corneas (usually less than 10 mm in diameter), shallow chambers, and a tendency to acute glaucoma.

miotics: agents that cause pupillary constriction and increase the facility of outflow of aqueous humor: pilocarpine, 1% to 4%; demecarium bromide (humersol); and echothiophate iodide (phospholine iodide).

mydriatic test for angle-closure glaucoma: test consists of instilling 2 drops of 5% eucotropine or 5% tropicamide (mydriacil) into the conjunctival sac. An 8 mm Hg rise in pressure by the end of 1 hour is considered positive.

N

nasal step: depression of the nasal peripheral portion of the field. A sign of glaucoma.

neurofibromatosis: condition characterized by small skin tumors and café au lait spots on the skin, tiny neurofibromotosis of the iris, and glaucoma. Optic nerve gliomas and skeletal defects are common.

O

ocular rigidity: the resistance of the coats of the eye to deformation or to distention.

P

parasympathomimetic agents: act in the same way as acetylcholine; pilocarpine and methacholine chloride (mecholyl).

Peter's anomaly: adhesions between the central iris and the central posterior cornea resulting in glaucoma.

Pierre Robin syndrome: consists of hypoplasia of the mandible, glossoptosis, cleft palate, congenital glaucoma, high myopia, cataract, and retinal detachment.

pigmentary glaucoma: condition in which pigment granules from the iris and ciliary body flake off and become lodged in the trabecular meshwork and impair the normal outflow of aqueous. The pigment deposits are visible on the endothelium of the cornea or in the trabecula of the angle.

Posner-Schlossman syndrome: recurrent elevated intraocular pressure associated with recurring inflammation of the anterior segment of the eye.

posterior synechia: an adhesion of the iris to the crystalline lens.

profile perimetry: see *static perimetry*.

provocative test: in glaucoma, a test to artificially provoke an elevation of intraocular pressure as a diagnostic test for glaucoma.

pseudoglaucoma: optic atrophy and cupping that resembles glaucoma but is caused by vascular damage rather than increased intraocular pressure.

S

Schwalbe's line: marks the most anterior extension of the trabecular meshwork and the termination of Descemet's membrane of the cornea (Fig. 13-9).

scleral spur: the most anterior internal projection of the sclera.

secluded pupil: a pupil that is bound completely by posterior adhesions (synechiae).

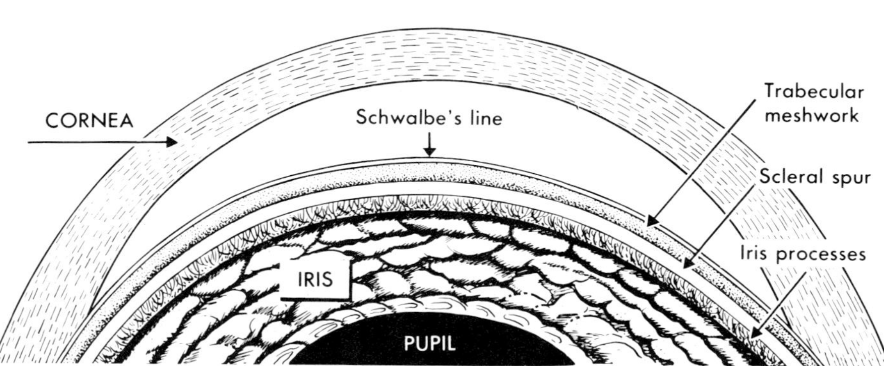

Fig. 13-9. Angle structure as viewed through the goniolens.

Schlemm's canal: lies in the scleral sulcus just anterior to the scleral spur and receives aqueous humor from the trabecular meshwork.

sensitivity threshold: the object is not visible until the illumination is gradually increased and the patient can just see the target.

spherophakia (Marchesani syndrome): this syndrome is characterized by microspherophakia, skeletal deformities, a short build, and mental retardation. High myopia, a tendency to lens dislocation, and angle-closure glaucoma are also present.

Sturge-Weber syndrome: this condition is unilateral and results in a cutaneous hemangioma involving the distribution of the fifth nerve. Also occurring are unilateral glaucoma, mental deficiency, and convulsions.

static perimetry: charting of the visual fields by altering the illumination of a fixed target.

sympathomimetic agents: in general, these agents have an effect similar that to epinephrine or norepinephrine.

T

timolol (Timoptic): this drug is a nonselective beta-$_1$ and beta-$_2$ adrenergic blocking agent. It is the most widely used local agent for the treatment of glaucoma.

trabecular fibers: the fibers that make up the trabeculum or filtering area for the aqueous humor.

trabecular meshwork: the area between Schwalbe's line and the scleral spur over the perforated layers of connective tissue is sheets of the trabecular meshwork. Through these openings flow the aqueous humor to Schlemm's canal.

trabeculum: filtering tissue that lies in the iris-corneal angle through which the aqueous humor passes on its way to Schlemm's canal.

W

water-drinking test: a provocative diagnostic test for glaucoma; the patient drinks 1 quart of water after fasting, and the intraocular pressure is measured every 15 minutes until it stops rising.

CHAPTER 14

STRABISMUS

Strabismus (Greek *strabismos,* "twisted") refers to eyes that are not straight. Strabo, the geographer, was a prominent figure in Alexandria during the Roman times who suffered from a noticeable turn of his eyes. From then on it was popular to call a person with a turn, "Strabo."

Strabismus may be *paralytic* caused by paralysis of a muscle or *nonparalytic.* Strabismus may be *concomitant* (sometimes called comitant), in which the deviation is the same in all directions of gaze, or *noncomitant,* in which there is a greater deviation in one or more directions because of an acquired paralysis of a muscle. In the case of nonconcomitant stabismus, diplopia or double vision may exist.

Pseudostrabismus is a condition in which there is an apparent strabismus to the observer but no true strabismus. It may be produced by the presence of *epicanthal* folds *(epi,* "upon," *canthus,* "angle") that cover the inner angle of the junction of the eyelid. It also may be caused by an abnormal *angle kappa,* the angles formed by the pupillary axis and the visual axis (which usually do not coincide), which may be sufficiently large to produce an optical illusion of a turn (Fig. 14-1).

Ocular motility refers to the movements of the eye in all directions of gaze and to its relationship with its fellow eye. *Orthoptics* (Greek *orthos,* "straight," and *ops,* "eye") is the science that investigates the motor and sensory adaptations of the eyes and deals with training the individual to use both eyes together to obtain comfortable binocular vision. *Orthophoria* is the absence of any tendency of the eye to deviate.

Movements of the eyes together in the same direction are known as yoke movements and include *dextroversion* (right gaze), *levoversion* (left gaze), *supraversion* (upward gaze), and *infraversion* (downward gaze) (Fig. 14-2). *Torsions* are wheel-like movements of an eye along its long axis. If the eye rotates inward, it is called *intorsion. Vergences* are dysjunctive movements of the two eyes in opposite directions. *Convergence* is the act of moving the eye in toward the midline. *Convergence insufficiency* exists when there is insufficient ability to converge the eyes inward for near vision. *Convergence excess* exists when there is excessive motor action in converging the eyes inward so the eyes overshoot at

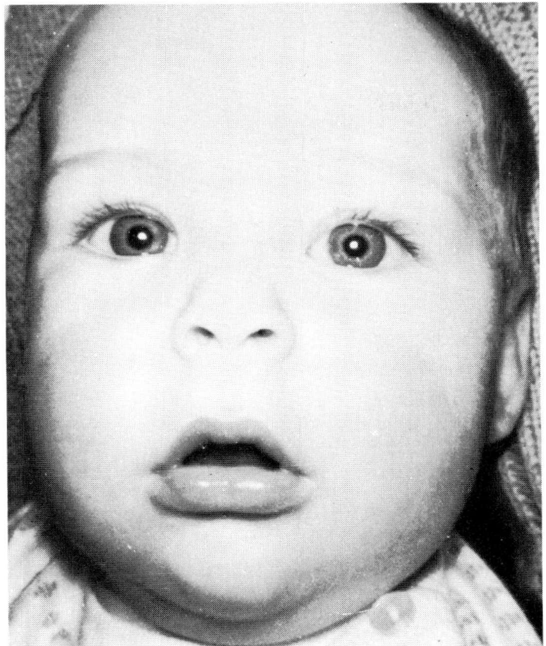

Fig. 14-1. Pseudostrabismus. The right eye appears to turn in because of a wide nasal bridge and epicanthal fold.

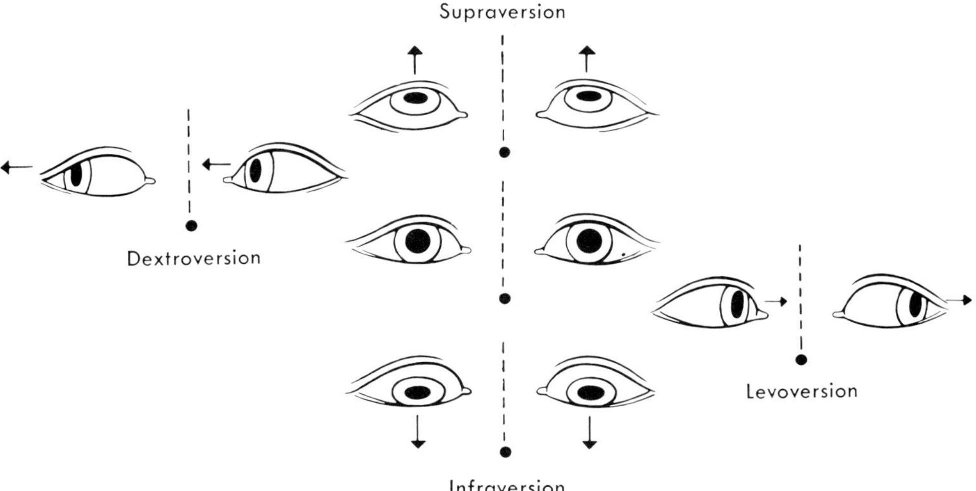

Fig. 14-2. Version movement of the eyes. These are eye movements in which both eyes rotate in the same direction, that is, to the left or right, up or down.

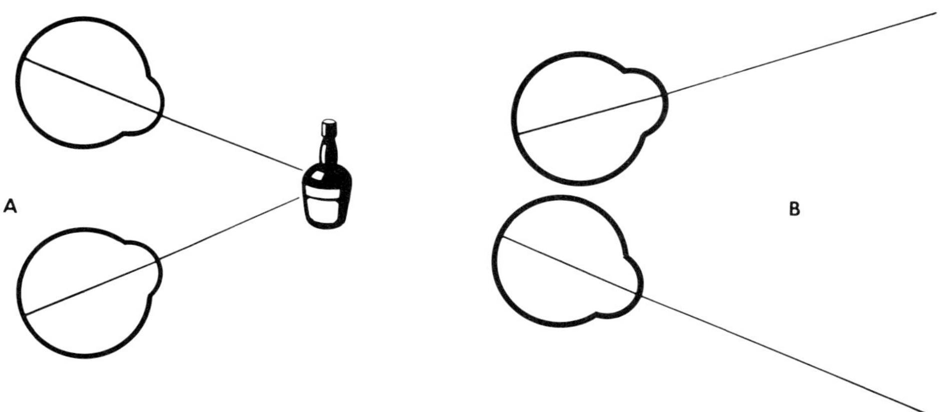

Fig. 14-3. **A,** Convergence. The eyes are turned in toward the midline plane. **B,** Divergence. The eyes are turned out away from the midline plane.

near. *Divergence* is the act in which the eyes move outward from the midline (Fig. 14-3).

Ductions are rotations of one eye when the fellow eye is covered. It may be *adducted* (rotated in), *abducted* (rotated out), *supraducted* (rotated up), or *infraducted* (rotated down).

Heterophoria, sometimes shortened to *phoria,* is a latent deviation of the two eyes held in check by the power of fusion. Fusion is the power exerted by the brain over both eyes to keep the position of the eyes aligned so that both foveae project the same point in space. It is measured by an instrument called the *amblyoscope.* When dissimilar targets are presented to each eye, such as a test target of a rabbit with a tail and one without a tail but with flowers in his hand, the individual will fuse these separate targets and see a tailed rabbit holding flowers. When fusion is interrupted, the deviation can be measured. Phorias must be differentiated from *heterotropia,* sometimes shortened to *tropia.* A phoria is basically a latent deviation of the eyes held in check by fusion. A tropia is a manifest deviation that has occurred because of a lack of fusion. Both *phorias* and *tropias* may be designated by the position of deviation of the two eyes such as *esophoria* or *esotropia* (turning in), *exophoria* or *exotropia* (turning out), *hyperphoria* or *hypertropia* (turning up), or *hypophoria* or *hypotropia* (turning down). *Cyclophoria* is the tendency of the eyes to become misaligned when one eye rotates on its anteroposterior axis because of an abnormality of the oblique muscle.

A syndrome is an ocular abnormality in which the eyes are more esotropic in looking up than down and which takes its name from the shape of an A.

V syndrome is an ocular abnormality in which the eyes are more esotropic looking down than up and which takes its name from the shape of a V. Both A and V syndromes may apply to esotropia or exotropia and are then referred to as *A-esotropia, A-exotropia, V-esotropia,* or *V-exotropia. Monofixation syndrome* is a small-angled strabismus often caused by a small central scotoma in the non-dominant eye and not detected by the cover-uncover test. It is also called a microtropia or monofixational phoria.

Amblyopia (Greek *amblyo,* "dull," and *ops,* "eye") means dimness of vision without any pathological condition in the eye or the brain. The lay person frequently uses the term *lazy eye* to indicate this condition. If it results from the child suppressing the vision of a turned eye to avoid double vision, it is called *suppression amblyopia. Deprivation amblyopia* is loss of vision because of being deprived of the ability to see. Amblyopia also occurs with anisometropia, in which the refractive difference between the two eyes is so great that fusion cannot occur, and the most out-of-focus image is ignored. *Eccentric fixation* occurs when a peripheral area of the macula other than the fovea is used for vision and the vision is relatively poor. The individual is unable to gaze directly ahead at an object of regard. Pointing to a light with the good eye covered, the person with eccentric fixation will miss the light with his finger so the vision is said to be eccentric. *Anomalous retinal correspondence* (ARC) is said to exist when a parafoveal point of one eye corresponds with the fovea of the fellow eye.

Pleoptics is the science dealing with treating eccentric fixation and amblyopia. It was popularized in Europe, but never became widely used in North America. There are two main methods. The Cüppers method (Germany) uses negative afterimages to relocate the principal visual direction of the fovea. The Bangerter approach (Switzerland) is to dazzle the peripheral area of the macula to obliterate the eccentric fixation, and to stimulate the fovea by aiming strong beams of light toward it. *Penalization* is a method of treating amblyopia by forcing the individual to use one eye for distance by medication or optical means. *Occlusion therapy* is a method of treating an amblyopic eye by blocking out all visual impulses to the fellow eye and forcing the use of the amblyopic eye. The success of this method of therapy is drastically reduced after a child is 6 years of age or older. In older children, pleoptics may be used.

Ocular torticollis is an abnormal head tilt adopted to overcome an anomaly caused by a congenital palsy of one or more vertically acting extraocular muscles. *Duane's syndrome* is a congenital ocular disorder of muscles characterized by limited outward movement of one or both eyes, limited inward movements plus retraction of the globe, and narrowing of the palpebral fissure on inward movement of the eye (Fig. 14-4).

A number of well-known laws exist that govern muscle function. *Sherrington's law* is the law of reciprocal innervation and states that when a muscle is stimulated, its opposing muscle is simultaneously inhibited. *Herring's law* states that when

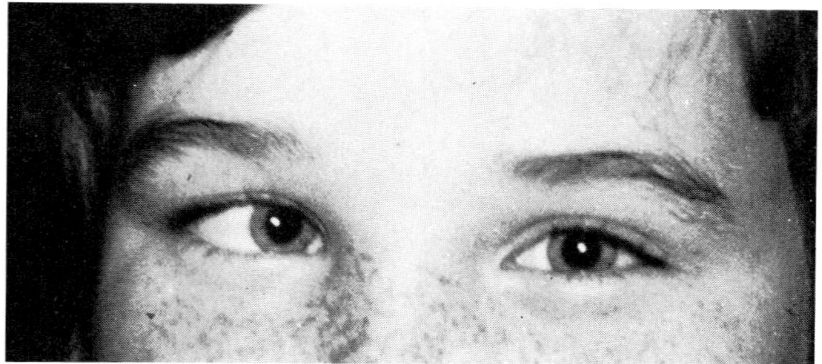

Fig. 14-4. Duane's syndrome. Note inability of left eye to abduct or look to the left when gaze is directed to the left.

one muscle is stimulated, its fellow or yoke muscle of the opposite eye is equally stimulated so that gaze in that direction becomes smooth and even.

The *major amblyoscope* is an instrument for measuring degree of strabismus, assessing grades of binocular vision, and treating suppression amblyopia. The *afterimage* test is a test relying on the ability to see images after a bright-light stimulation is exposed to each eye and is used to detect anomalous retinal correspondence.

Other words related to ocular motility are given in the following glossary.

A

abducens nerve: sixth cranial nerve, which innervates the lateral rectus muscle.

AC/A ratio: the accommodative convergence to accommodation ratio. It may be refractive and a normally limited accommodative convergence or nonrefractive with an abnormal convergence mechanism. The ratio of the accommodative convergence (AC) to the accommodation (A) usually expressed as the quotient of the AC in prism diopters divided by A in diopters.

accommodation-convergence ratio: relationship between accommodation and convergence of two eyes. Some types of esotropia have a high accommodation-convergence ratio, often referred to as the AC/C ratio.

accommodative esotropia: inward deviation of the eyes characteristically more marked for near than far vision and increased by ciliary muscle contraction in accommodation.

A-dellen: a corneal ulcer at the margin of the cornea. It occurs after strabismus surgery usually on the side in which muscle surgery has been done.

advancement: the moving forward of an extraocular muscle for surgical correction of strabismus with the intent of increasing the strength of the muscle.

A-esotropia: a deviation in which the convergence increases on elevation.

A-exotropia: a deviation in which divergence increases on depression.

afterimage test: a test of retinal correspondence using afterimage projections of two flashing lights, one in the vertical direction and one in the horizontal. With normal retinal correspondence, the afterimages superimposed should yield the picture of a perfectly centered cross.

agonist: the contracting muscle that receives primary innervation. For example, the right medial rectus muscle is the agonist when the eye moves inward.

alternating sursumduction: a condition in which either eye deviates upward under cover but returns to its original position when the cover is removed.

amblyopia: loss of vision in an eye without any overt pathological changes in that eye.

angle of anomaly: the difference between the angle of deviation measured objectively with prisms and that measured subjectively with the Lancaster red-green test, Hess screen, and so forth.

angle of convergence: the angle formed between the primary lines of sight of each eye during convergence.

angle of deviation: the angle by which the primary line of sight of the deviating eye fails to intersect the object of fixation subtended at the center of rotation of the deviating eye.

anomalous fixation: the eye uses an area other than the fovea for sighting.

antagonist: a muscle that acts in opposition to another, namely, the agonist muscle. For example, the right lateral rectus muscle is the antagonist of the right medial rectus muscle when the eye is adducted.

A-tuck: a surgical folding of a muscle to strengthen it.

B

Bielschowsky's head-tilt test:

(1) head-tilt test used to differentiate between a superior oblique palsy and a contralateral superior rectus palsy. The patient looks at a target and tilts the head to the suspected superior oblique palsy. If the eye elevates, it is an affirmative diagnosis for a superior oblique palsy.

(2) a head-tilt test designed to help determine the primary paretic muscle when there appears to be a limitation of the superior rectus of one eye and the superior oblique of the other eye. With superior oblique palsy, the deviation increases with the head tilted to the same side as the paresis.

Bielshowsky's phenomenon or sign: a response seen in alternating sursumduction in which the elevated, occluded eye depresses when a filter is placed before the fixing eye.

bifoveal fixation: the alignment of the visual axis of both eyes so that the object of regard falls on the fovea under binocular conditions. The fixated point is simultaneously imaged in the center of each fovea.

binocular vision:
(1) the coordinated use of the two eyes to produce a single mental impression.
(2) ability to use both eyes simultaneously to focus on the same object and to fuse the two images into a single image that gives a correct interpretation of its solidity and its position in space. Grade 1 requires simultaneous macular perception. Grade 2 requires simultaneous macular perception plus fusion. Grade 3 requires simultaneous macular perception plus fusion plus the sensation of depth.

C

concomitant strabismus: nonparalytic strabismus in which the degree of deviation is the same, regardless of the position or movement of the eyes.

confusion: the simultaneous perception of two different objects at the same location in subjective space.

congenital ocular motor apraxia: refers to an eye movement disorder in which conjugate eye movements are impeded through visual or command stimuli. Ocular rotation is done by a compensatory head thrust to bring the eye to the position of regard.

conjugate movements: parallel movements of the two eyes in the same direction, that is, looking to the left or right.

corresponding points: points on the retina of each eye that have the same visual direction so that an object seen by these points is interpreted as arising from the same point in space.

corresponding retinal points: points on the two retina from which images are projected to the same place in space.

cover test: an occluder is placed before an eye to dissociate the eyes.
single cover test: when the occluder is placed over the eye, the opposite eye, if deviated, will take fixation and move to see the target.
alternation: if the covered eye takes up fixation once the occluder is removed, alternation of the deviation has occurred.
cross cover test:
(1) an alternate cover test to exaggerate the deviation by fully dissociating the vision. The cover is moved from eye to eye, and the movement of the uncovered eye represents the total phoria-tropia.
(2) a test for strabismus or heterophoria by covering one eye. The other eye, if deviated, must move to pick up fixation.

cover-uncover test: the eyes fixate on an accommodative target. One eye is occluded. The movement of the eye is noted as the cover is removed. If the eye moves temporally from an inward position, an esophoria would be noted (Fig. 14-5).

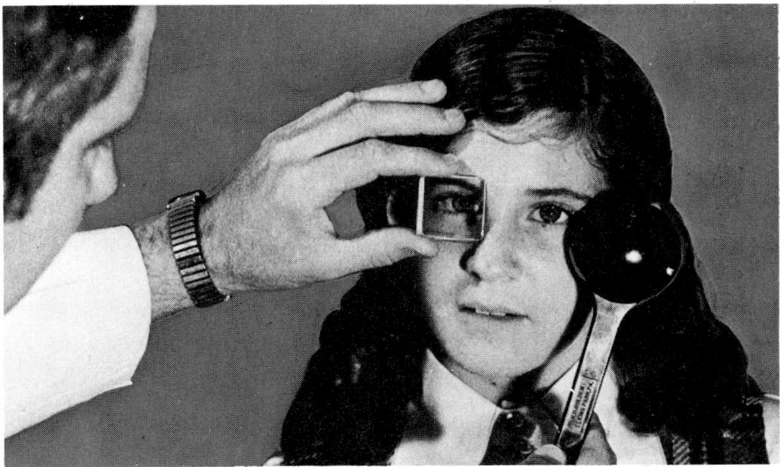

Fig. 14-5. Cover-uncover test. Covered eye is observed as cover is removed. In strabismus the eye may make a correctional move once the cover is removed.

craniofacial desostosis: refers to a developmental anomaly of the face and skull in which there is premature closure of some of the suture lines.

cross-eyes: lay term for strabismus.

D

depressor: a muscle whose action is to turn the eye downward.

depth perception: stereopsis caused by the fusion of slightly disparate images.

deviating eye: the eye that is not straight in strabismus, as distinguished from the "fixing eye."

deviation: bending or turning in another direction, such as the visual axis in strabismus.

primary deviation: ocular deviation seen in paralysis of an ocular muscle when the nonparalyzed eye is used for fixation.

secondary deviation: ocular deviation seen in paralysis of an ocular muscle when the paralyzed eye is used for fixation; the second deviation is usually greater than the primary deviation.

dextroversion: conjugate movements of both eyes to the right.

diplopia:

(1) double vision occurring because the foveas of each eye are not pointing to the same place in space. It is usually caused by a paretic extraocular muscle.

(2) seeing the same object in two locations in space because the object of regard is projected onto the fovea of one eye and a parafoveal area of the other eye.

A condition of seeing double when both maculae are not pointing to the same object of regard.

Duane's classification of squint:

convergence excess: a convergent deviation greater at near than at distance.

convergence insufficiency: a divergent deviation greater at near than at distance.

divergence excess: a divergent deviation greater at distance than at near.

divergence insufficiency: a convergent deviation greater at distance than at near.

Duane's syndrome: an apparent loss of abduction with retraction of the eye with attempted adduction. With adduction, the palpebral fissure narrows. With abduction, the palpebral fissure widens.

ductions: rotation of one eye.

abduction: rotation of the eye temporally.

adduction: rotation of the eye nasally.

deorsumduction: rotation of the eye downward.

sursumduction: rotation of the eye upward.

E

esophoria: a turning in of the eyes when one eye is covered and fusion has been disrupted.

esotropia: a turning in of one eye.

microtropia: a small deviation inward of one eye.

accomodative: an esotropia made worse by the act of accomodation.

euthyscope: a flashing device invented by A. Cüppers used to train eyes with eccentric fixation to learn to project centrally.

excentric fixation: a monocular condition in which a parafoveal point is used for fixation. Usually the vision is very poor, and the projection of that eye to a target is erroneous.

exodeviation: the deviation outward of the line of sight of the nonfixing eye from the point of fixation of the fixating eye.

exotropia: a manifest deviation of the eye in an outward direction.

intermittent: a deviation that is variable and not constant.

extorsion: the corneal meridians tilt away from each other.

F

fixation disparity: a condition in which the fixated object is not imaged on exactly corresponding points, but in which the images still fall within Panum's area so that the object is seen singly.

fixing eye: the nondeviating eye in strabismus.

following movement: a slow eye movement predicated on the speed of the target being followed.

fusion: the amalgamation of similar images from the two eyes to create a fused binocular product.

fusion with amplitude: blending of the similar images from the two foveas into a single perception (grade 2 binocular vision).

fusional reserves: the range of convergence, divergence, and vertical vergence through which binocular single vision can be maintained. This may be measured in degrees or prism diopters.

fusion-free: position of the eyes when binocular vision is suspended by covering one eye or changing the direction of one eye or by changing the image of one eye by using, for example, the Maddox rod. A point of light will become a red linear streak for the eye behind the Maddox rod while the other eye, not covered by the Maddox rod, will see a point of light. Therefore fusion of the two dissimilar images is not possible.

H

haploscope: a mirror-type stereoscope. The object-carrying tubes are turnable on the vertical axis to measure the direction of the z-axis of the eyes, or, depending on fusion, to train positive or negative fusional amplitude or both.

Herring's Law: in a fresh oculomotor paresis, the contralateral synergist of the recently paralyzed extraocular muscle will overact when the paretic eye is fixing. The deviation is greater with the paretic eye fixing.

heteronymous: crossed fields.

heteronymous diplopia: crossed double vision. Occurs with exotropia.

homonymous: uncrossed fields.

homonymous diplopia: uncrossed double vision. Occurs with esotropia.

horopter: the locus of points in space in which the images for a given position of the eyes fall on corresponding retinal points.

I

incomitance: a deviation that differs in degree depending upon which eye is fixating. Usually seen with paretic oculo motor disturbances.

inferior oblique: an extraocular muscle in which contraction primarily causes extortion. Its secondary actions include abduction and elevation.

inferior rectus: an extraocular muscle whose contraction primarily results in depression. Secondary actions include adduction and extorsion.

intorsion: a rotation inward of the cornea.

intrinsic ocular muscles: the muscles situated inside the eyeball, consisting of the ciliary muscle, the sphincter pupillae, and the dilator pupillae.

L

latent nystagmus: a jerk nystagmus arising from occlusion of one eye with the fast component in the direction of the fixing eye (uncovered eye).

lateral rectus: an extraocular muscle the contraction of which causes external rotation.

M

major amblyoscope: a device for the measurement of strabismus, the assessment of binocular vision, and the treatment of suppression and amblyopia. Used primarily with children with strabismus.

medial rectus: an extraocular muscle the contraction of which causes internal rotation.

microstrabismus (microtropia): a small deviation squint of less than 5 degrees with harmonious anomalous correspondence and amblyopia of varying degree in the deviating eye. The fixation may be central or slightly eccentric to the macula, and consequently it may or may not be detected with the cover test.

Möbius syndrome: a bilateral facial and abducens nerve paralysis.

myotomy: an incomplete transverse incision of an ocular muscle to weaken it.

N

normal retinal correspondence (NRC): a condition that exists when the two foveae have a common visual direction and all other retinal areas of the two eyes correspond secondarily.

O

occlusion: the covering of one eye to force the amblyopic eye to perform. This type of therapy is most successful with children under 5 years of age.

occlusion therapy: a treatment to increase the vision of an amblyopic eye by patching the normal eye.

ocular saccade: a rapid eye movement as used in reading.

oxycephaly: refers to premature dysostosis of the craniofacial sutures resulting in a vertical elongation of the head.

P

Panum's fusional area: an area in which slightly desparate points can be fused.

parallax: the displacement of objects relative to each other when the eyes are moved.

phoria: a deviation that is present only by disrupting fusion with a cover test. A latent deviation of the eyes.

pleoptics: a method to train children with eccentric fixation to see directly ahead.

The two major methods are the Bangerter (Switzerland) and the Cüppers (Germany).

pleoptophore: a device that dazzles the periphery of the retina to obliterate eccentric fixation and then stimulates the macula by aiming strong beams of light toward it.

primary position: the position of the eyes looking straight ahead and toward infinity. It is at this position that the normal examination of eye movement begins.

proprioception: the ability to convey to the central nervous system an indication of the posture and movements of the body brought about by impulses (proprioceptive impulses) arising within the body from muscles, tendons, and joints and from the labyrinth of the inner ear. Whether eye muscles have any proprioceptive ability is in dispute. Most authorities do not believe that this function is present in eye muscles.

pursuit movement: foveal fixation on moving targets with speeds of 30 to 50 degrees per second. A slow following movement.

R

recession: a surgical procedure to weaken a muscle by disinserting it and replacing it behind the original insertion.

resection: a surgical procedure to strengthen an ocular muscle by removing a section of it to make it tighter. The muscle is replaced to its original insertion site.

retinal correspondence: corresponding retinal areas in both eyes that perceive the same point in space simultaneously.

retinal rivalry:

(1) occurs when two dissimilar images are presented so they cannot be integrated without confusion. Rivalry develops so that one image is seen and then the other in sequence.

(2) a conflict between the two retinas when two dissimilar images are superimposed; first one image is suppressed and then the other.

S

stereoscope: instrument that permits different pictures to be positioned before each of the two eyes.

superimposition: the ability to perceive two similar images, one formed on each retina, as being superimposed but not mentally fused.

superior oblique: an extraocular muscle the contraction of which primarily causes intorsion. Secondary actions include depression and abduction.

superior rectus: an extraocular muscle; the contraction of which primarily results in elevation. Secondary actions include adduction and intorsion.

suppression:

(1) the act of suppressing one image that is out of focus or doubled.

(2) a condition in which the image of an object formed on the retina is not perceived but is mentally ignored or neglected either partially or completely. An active cortical inhibition used to suppress diplopia—a confusing second image—or to suppress an out-of-focus image. Children with strabismus suppress the image of their deviating eye to avoid seeing double.

sursumduction:

(1) rotation of one eye upward.

(2) turning upward of the eyes; a gaze movement.

synergists (yoke muscles): two muscles, one in each eye, that move the eyes in the same direction; for example, right lateral and left medial recti.

synoptophore: stereoscope-like instrument used in orthoptic diagnosis and treatment.

T

tenotomy: a severing of all or part of a tendon; performed to decrease the function of a muscle in the surgical correction of strabismus.

tropia:

(1) a deviation that is constant with both eyes looking at a target.

(2) a manifest deviation of the eyes.

V

V-esotropia: an esotropia deviation that converges on depression.

V-exotropia: an exotropia in which the divergence increases on depression.

vergence: movement of the two eyes in opposite directions.

convergence: rotation of the eyes toward one another.

divergence: rotation of the eyes from one another.

versions: a corresponding movement of two eyes.

dextroversion: looking to the right.

levoversion: looking to the left.

sursumversion: looking up.

deorsumversion: looking down.

visuscope: a device to diagnose eccentric fixation designed by Dr. Cüppers of Germany.

W

wall-eyes: a lay term indicating one eye that deviates outward (exotropia).

Y

yoke muscles: those muscles that work together to produce a given ocular gaze movement, that is, a left lateral rectus and right medial rectus to look to the left.

Yoke muscles

Right eye:	*Left eye:*
medial rectus	lateral rectus
superior rectus	inferior oblique
superior oblique	inferior rectus

CHAPTER 15

DISORDERS OF THE RETINA AND VITREOUS

Anatomy

Retina is derived from the Latin word for "net" because the retina, composed of *rods* and *cones,* acts as a net to gather the light rays for transmission to the brain. The *rods* and *cones* are named after their characteristic shape as either rodlike or conelike. The cones are concentrated in the *macula* (Latin *macula,* "spot"), which was originally considered a blemish or sun spot. It is sometimes called the *macula lutea* from Latin *lutea* meaning "yellow" because of a visible yellow spot that is seen when the retina is examined grossly in a pathological specimen. The macula is the area of the retina devoid of blood vessels. The center of the macula is the *fovea centralis,* from Latin for "small pit" or "depression," because the fovea clinically is a central depression in the macular area (Fig. 15-1).

Vitreous is derived from the Latin word for "glass" because of its transparent characteristics and its resemblance to the transparency of glass. It is sometimes referred to as vitreous humor after the Latin *humor,* meaning "moist." There was a time when all the liquids or areas of moisture in the body were referred to as humors. Supposedly the nature of these body fluids gave rise to the temperament, disposition, and personality of an individual and thus were said to affect the individual's "humor." The vitreous was widely held to be a refracting agent acting along its interface with the crystalline lens until Father Scheiner, using Johannes Kepler's geometric theories, proved in 1625 that an inverted image of the seen object is formed on the retina.

Abnormalities of position

When the retina becomes *detached* it is not truly a detachment of the complete retina, but rather the pigment layer of the retina remains attached to the choroid while the rest of the retina detaches from it. In fact, a retinal detachment is a splitting of the retina in which the anterior nine layers detach from the posterior

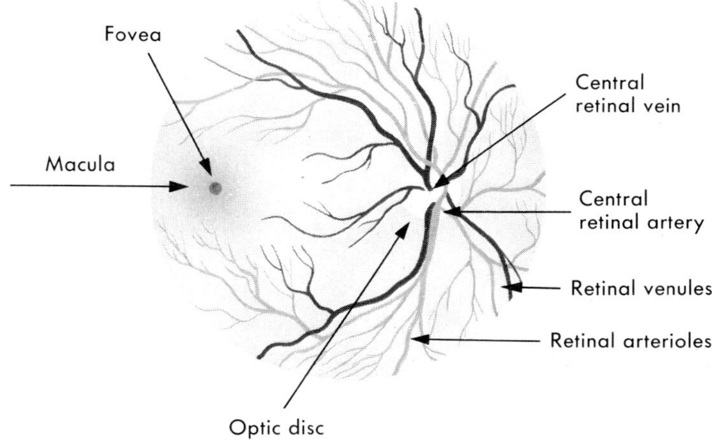

Fig. 15-1. The macula is the area devoid of blood vessels in the retina and contains specialized cone receptors.

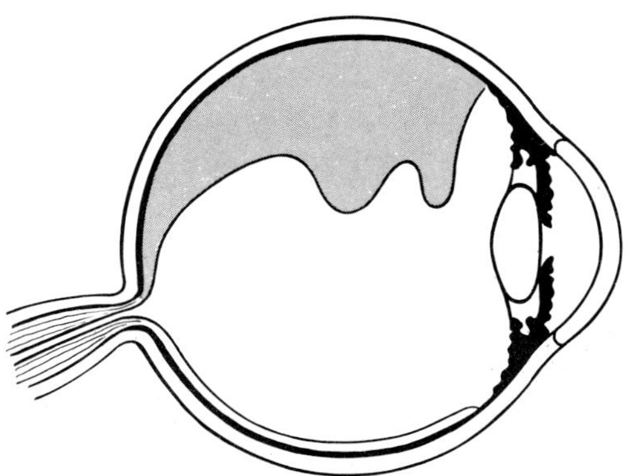

Fig. 15-2. Retinal detachment.

pigment layer. The detachment occurs when the vitreous wedges itself between the two split layers (Fig. 15-2). *Retinoschisis* (Greek *schisis* "to split") is a true splitting of the retina more anteriorly without detachment. If there is a localized blister elevation, the term *macrocyst* or *giant cyst of the retina* is frequently used. *Rhegmatogenous detachment* (Greek *rhegma,* "hole") is a detachment in which there is a retinal hole or tear resulting in watery fluid that enters behind the retina. *Nonrhegmatogenous detachment* is a detachment with no holes or tears;

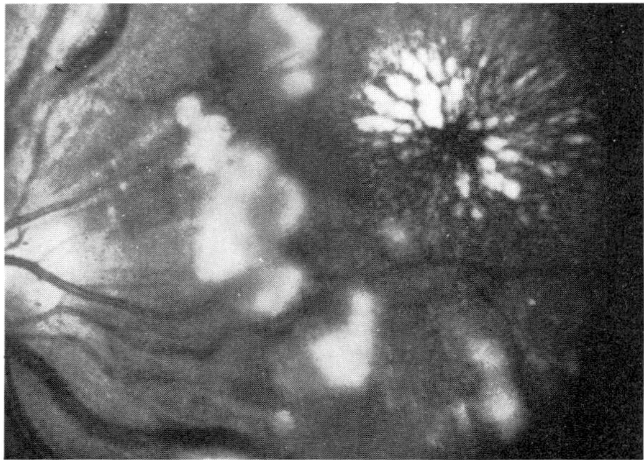

Fig. 15-3. Hypertensive retinopathy advanced with cotton-wool exudates and macular star.

it may be caused by traction pull on the retina, by fluid leaking under the retina from the choroid, or by a malignant melanoma (Fig. 15-3).

The detachment may be classified as *aphakic detachment* if it occurs after cataract surgery or *pseudophakic detachment* if it occurs after an artificial lens implant procedure. *Vitreous detachment* or *separation* may occur in which the vitreous becomes separated from the retina.

Abnormalities of vessels

Arteriovenous crossings occur where an arteriole crosses over a vein. *A-V nicking* occurs when the arteriole wall compresses the vein and an indentation is noted in the vein when examined with the ophthalmoscope. *Narrowing* of an arteriole may be generalized along its complete course, or there may be focal narrowing, called *focal constrictions.* Localized areas of constriction of the arterioles occur primarily in young patients with hypertension. *Tortuosity* of the vessels is a situation in which either the arterioles or veins of the retina have an increased waviness. *Copper wire arterioles* is the clinical condition in which the arterioles lose their normal rosy appearance and take on a metallic copper-wire appearance. It is a sign of arteriosclerosis. In more advanced cases of arteriosclerosis they may become *silver-wire* in appearance. *Sheathing* of vessels may occur in which white lines appear alongside the vessel walls and parallel the vessel course. *Aneurysms* of the retinal arterioles are *microaneurysms* (small aneurysms) and are outpouchings of diseased arterial wall. They have sharp margins as opposed to small hemorrhages, which have blurred edges. *Thrombosis* is an occlusion of the vessel by a clot.

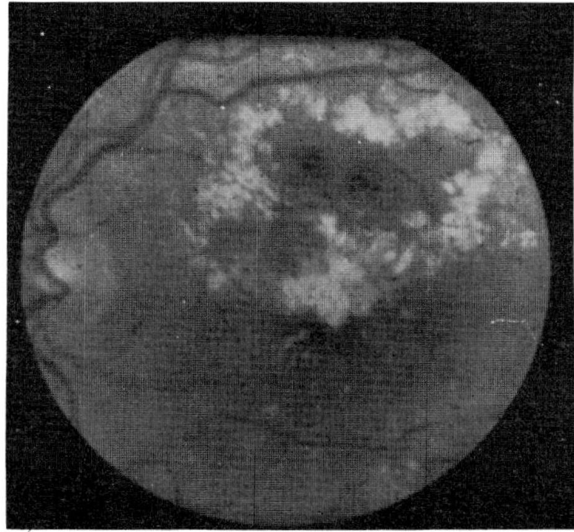

Fig. 15-4. Clusters of small, hard exudates, small blot hemorrhages, turgid retinal veins, and microaneurysms are commonly seen in the posterior portion of the eyes of people with diabetes.

Retinopathies

Retinopathy is a general term denoting any pathological occurrence in the retina. It is usually associated with systemic or general body disorders such as diabetes, hypertension, anemia, or leukemia.

Central serous retinopathy is a clinical condition in which there is a loss of vision caused by the sudden accumulation of circumscribed edema in the macula. It used to be called *central angiospastic retinopathy* because of the possible association with spasm of the macular vessels with resulting hypoxia and escape of fluid through the capillaries. This condition results in the distortion of central vision.

Retrolental fibroplasia or *retinopathy of prematurity* is an obliteration of developing blood vessels in an immature retina initially caused in the premature newborn by a high concentration of oxygen. The high oxygen content causes profuse new blood vessel formation, especially in the periphery of the retina. These fibrovascular tufts may eventually progress to form a retrolental (behind the lens) membrane and cause a detached retina as a result of traction and contraction. If the condition is bilateral it can result in blindness of the child. It is uncommon now that the pathogenesis is better understood.

Arteriosclerosis found in the retinal arterioles is a thickening of the lining wall of an artery as may occur in hypertension (Greek *sclera,* "hard," and Latin *osis,* "full of"). *Exudates* (Latin *ex,* "out," and *sudare,* "to sweat") are substances that filter through the walls of living cells. They may be hard or waxy exudates, sometimes called *edema residues* as seen commonly in diabetes. *Hard exudates* (Fig. 15-4), which are caused by lipid infiltrates in the deeper layers, may be found in the macular area, in which their radiating deposits form the picture of a *macular star*. *Soft exudates* of the cotton-wool type are commonly seen in hypertension. These descriptive notes are related to their ophthalmoscopic appearance in the fundus. *Cotton-wool exudates* are tiny infarcts (oxygen-deficient areas) in the inner retinal layers. They appear as whitish gray fluffy areas with feathery edges.

Hemorrhages that occur in retinopathy may be referred to as *punctate (punctum,* "a point") or may be the *dot* or *blot* variety depending on their ophthalmoscopic appearance. Hemorrhages may be *preretinal* if they are in front of the retina and deep to the vitreous (Fig. 15-5). *Neovascularization (neo,* "new") is the formation of new vessels that may arise on the retina or may proliferate into the vitreous.

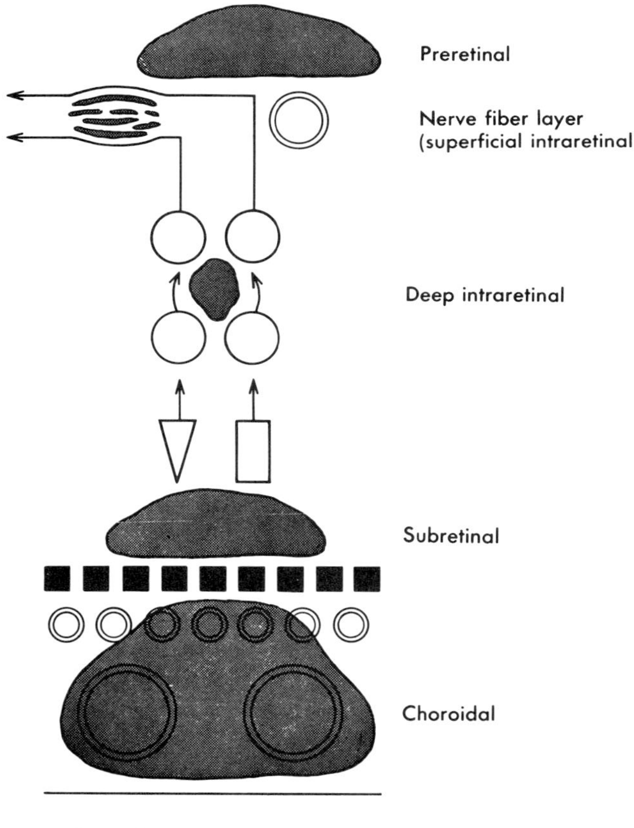

Fig. 15-5. Preretinal hemorrhage lying in front of retina. Note the location of intraretinal, subretinal, and choroidal hemorrhages.

Central retinal artery closure produces a *cherry-red spot* in the macula, resembling a red cherry because of the surrounding area of retinal edema, which appears gray. This makes the macula, which receives its nourishment from the choroid, stand out in relief as a bright, red spot. *Circinate retinopathy* (Latin *circum,* "circle") is a circle-shaped collection of exudates in the macular area. *Drusen* are large hyaline deposits lying on Bruch's membrane of the choroid. They are seen with the ophthalmoscope as yellowish, often pigmented elevations. *Vitelliform* degeneration of the macula is derived from Latin *vitellus* meaning "egg yolk," after the clinical appearance in the macular area, which resembles a fried egg. *Angioid streaks* (from Greek *angi,* "vessel") are pigment striations in the ocular fundus giving the appearance of a vessel, which are caused by breaks in the elastic layer of the choroid. *Retinitis pigmentosa* is a progressive degeneration of the neuroepithelium, primarily rod degeneration, and migration of the retinal pigment from whence it derives its name. This condition belongs to the group called *tapetoretinal degenerations,* its name derived from Greek *tapetum,* "carpet," and referring in zoology to the choroid of eyes in cats and other animals from which Theodore Leber, who coined the name, believed the condition arose. It belongs to a class of *abiotrophies,* a group of disorders believed to result from atrophy caused by defective vitality and premature degeneration, and now considered to be part of *hereditary degenerations.*

Inflammatory changes

Vitritis is an inflammation *(itis)* of the vitreous. *Chorioretinitis* is an inflammation of the retina and choroid. *Asteroid hyalitis* is a condition in which calcium-lipid opacities in the vitreous give a cluster or star effect of white floating balls when viewed with the ophthalmoscope (common in diabetic people). *Synchysis scintillans* is a degenerative vitreous condition in which shiny cholesterol crystals float freely within the liquified vitreous cavity.

Other definitions related to retina but exclusive of tumors, which are covered elsewhere, are listed here alphabetically.

A

acute multifocal posterior pigment epitheliopathy: a disorder of the fundus usually occurring in young females and characterized by irregular, flat, subretinal creamy or yellow lesions. It may be caused by localized occlusion of the choriocapillaris.

aged macular degeneration: A term to indicate macular disease that occurs primarily in the elderly. It is the most common cause of legal blindness in people over the age of 60.

Amsler grid: A field test to show defects in central vision caused by macular disease.

angiomatosis, retinal: retinal blood vessel growths. The combination of retinal vascular tumors (angiomatosis retinae) and vascular tumors of the medulla and spinal cord is known as *von Hippel-Lindau disease.*

angioscotoma: extension of the normal blind spot because of local blocking of vision by a large retinal vessel.

B

Bardet-Biedl syndrome: condition that is characterized by mental retardation, obesity, hypogenitalism, polydactyly, and pigmentary retinopathy.

Batten-Mayou disease: juvenile amaurotic idiocy characterized by retinal pigmentary changes because of abnormal deposition of gangliosides inside the retina.

Behçet's syndrome: recurrent hypopyon, uveitis, and retinal vasculitis associated with aphthous lesions on the buccal and genital mucosa.

Berlin's edema (commotio retinae): grayish or milky swelling of the posterior pole of the retina, usually following a contusion of the eye.

Best disease: an autosomal dominant central retinal degeneration characterized by an ophthalmoscopic appearance of an egg fried sunny side up in the macula and later a scrambled-egg appearance when vision deteriorates.

Bielschowsky-Jansky disease: condition characterized by retinal pigmentary changes secondary to the deposition of lipopigments in the retina.

Bourneville's disease: syndrome of mental deficiency, tuberous sclerosis, and adenoma sebaceum.

branch vein occlusion: obstruction of a branch of the central retinal vein.

butterfly dystrophy: dystrophy of the fovea characterized by pigmentation localized in the deeper layers of the central retina in the form of a butterfly.

C

chloroquine retinopathy: retinal pigmentary changes characterized by a "bull's eye maculopathy" in patients taking large doses of chloroquine.

choked disc: passive swelling of the optic nerve caused by increased intracranial pressure.

choroidal hemangioma: a benign vascular tumor of the choroid.

choroidal neovascular membrane: abnormal vascular channels found in the aging macular degeneration syndrome. Clinical signs include subretinal blood or subretinal lipid exudates.

choroideremia: an hereditary atrophy of the choroidal coat of the eye frequently leading to loss of vision.

circinate retinopathy: a ring of fatty deposits creamy in color surrounding the macula.

Coat's disease: a chronic exudative retinopathy occurring between retina and choroid of unknown cause.

commotio retinae: see *Berlin's edema.*

conus of optic disc: a condition in which the choroid and retinal pigment epithelia do not extend to the optic disc, allowing the sclera to be observed ophthalmoscopically at its margin.

crescent myopia: a crescent-shaped visible area of sclera surrounding the optic disc in myopia.

cysticercosis: an inflammatory cyst in the eye caused by the larvae of the pork tapeworm.

cystoid macular edema: See Irvine/Gass syndrome and macular edema.

cytoid body: retinal microinfarction synonymous with soft exudate.

cytomegalic inclusion disease: a viral illness that may cause a retinitis characterized by retinal pigment epithelial changes, sheathing of vessels, and retinal hemorrhages. The retina may be involved in newborn children or in severely debilitated patients.

D

Dalma's sentinels: pigment clumps in the infratemporal vitreous that herald underlying juvenile retinal dialysis.

detachment, retinal: see *retinal detachment.*

diabetic macular degeneration: the leading cause of decreased vision in the elderly diabetic person.

diabetic retinopathy: a vascular disorder of diabetics characterized by microaneurysms, hemorrhages, and proliferative retinopathy. It is the leading cause of blindness in patients under 60 years of age.

diffuse drusen: extension of soft drusen, important because eyes with these diffuse changes are at risk to develop serous detachments of the retinal pigment epithelium, choroidal neovascularization, and disciform scarring.

disc: the ophthalmoscopic view of the optic nerve head.

disciform degeneration of central retina: secondary type of central retinal degeneration arising from subretinal neurovascularization.

disinsertion of retina: retinal dialysis or separation at the ora serrata in which the sensory retina is separated from the retinal pigment epithelium.

Doyne's honeycomb dystrophy: disorder characterized by drusen of Bruch's membrane that involve predominantly the posterior pole.

drusen: hyaline nodules of the lamina vitrea of the choroid, very commonly present but rarely disturb vision.

E

Eales' disease: vasculitis of the retinal vessels characterized by recurrent retinal hemorrhages.

electroretinography: a method to measure the resting potential between the electropositive cornea and the electronegative retina of the eye. It is a mass response of the retina.

Elschnig's spot: a black isolated spot of pigment with a surrounding yellow or red halo seen in the choroid in patients with hypertension.

embolism: usually a circulating bolus or atheromatous debris that blocks any blood vessel in the body.

entopic phenomena: sensations perceived for mechanical reasons within the eye; for example, the floaters and flashes caused by retinal detachment, or by contusion.

F

Fabry's disease: a whorl-like corneal dystrophy and tortuous retinal vessels caused by an inborn error of metabolism and characterized by skin eruptions.

fat emboli: emboli consisting of fat that lodges in the retinal vessels. This may follow fractures of the long bones or chest bones.

folds, retinal fixed: connective tissue folds in the internal limiting membrane, which may occur in patients with retinal detachments and diabetic retinopathy.

Fuchs' black spot: area of proliferation of the retinal pigment layer in the central retina; occurs in degenerative myopia.

G

gliosis: astrocytic scar proliferation on or within the retina.

Grönblad-Strandberg syndrome: presence of angioid streaks in patients with pseudoxanthoma elasticum.

H

Harada's disease: bilateral uveitis, often with extensive detachments usually occurring in Oriental people.

hard drusen: yellowish white ophthalmoscopically visible lesions that are pinpoint sized and act as window defects on fluorescein angiography.

histoplasmosis: a common endemic fungus inflammatory condition resulting in uveitis and characterized by punched-out depigmented areas in the retinal periphery and lesions in the macula.

hole, retinal: break in the continuity of the sensory retina so that there is a communication between the vitreous cavity and the potential space between the sensory retina and the retinal pigment epithelium.

Hollenhorst plaques: small, glistening yellow spots situated at the bifurcation of retinal arteries, usually caused by emboli from an atheromatous plaque of the carotid artery.

hypertensive retinopathy: vascular disease of the retina associated with general high blood pressure.

I

idiocy, amaurotic (Tay-Sachs disease): a hereditary disorder of metabolism affecting mainly Jewish people and resulting in the accumulation of lipidlike material. In the retina the material accumulates in the ganglion cells, resulting in the classic macular cherry-red spot.

Irvine-Gass syndrome: cystoid macular edema occurring after a cataract extraction.

J

Jensen's choroiditis: chorioretinitis adjacent to the optic disc.

K

Kuhnt-Junius macular degeneration (senile disciform macular degeneration): a specific type of hemorrhagic macular degeneration affecting the elderly that results in loss of vision and functional blindness (vision less than 20/200).

L

lacquer crack: breaks in Bruch's membrane of the choroid usually found in very myopic people.

laser: initials for *l*ight *a*mplification by *s*timulated *e*mission of *r*adiation. This is a device for producing an intense coherent beam of light.

laser-argon: a laser photocoagulating device with light wavelengths between 4880 and 5145 angstroms, which has a smaller spot than the standard xenon laser and a greater spectral absorption by hemoglobin.

laser-ruby: a laser photocoagulating device with light wavelengths of 6943 angstroms.

lattice degeneration: a form of peripheral retinal degeneration characterized by atrophic thinned retina and altered retinal pigmentation.

Laurence-Moon-Biedl syndrome: condition characterized by mental retardation, hypogenitalism, spastic paraplegia, and retinitis pigmentosa.

M

macular degeneration: an age related change in which the specialized cones of the macular area are subject to atrophy usually by an underlying arteriosclerotic process (Fig. 15-6).

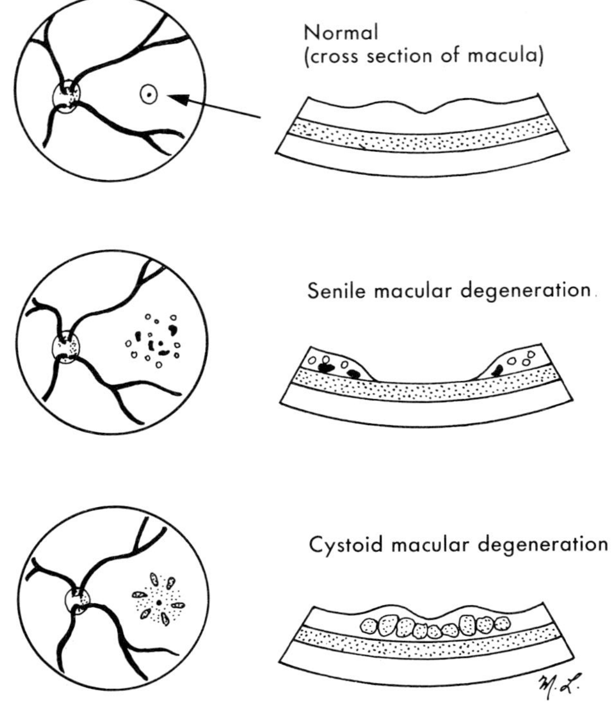

Fig. 15-6. Pathological processes affecting the macular area.

macular edema: the abnormal leakage of macromolecules and ions from retinal capillaries into the retina. The macromolecules are largely lipoproteins and gain access to the extravascular space with edema fluid. It causes distortion and loss of vision.

macular hole: a breakdown of the internal limiting membrane of a macular cyst to yield a hole. It causes marked loss of vision.

macular star: deposits in the macular area. The star pattern is related to the physical properties of the foveal neuroretina in which there are large spaces between the inner segments of the retinal receptors that are radially arranged.

medullated (myelinated) nerve fibers: the retinal nerve fibers are myelinated, and the myelinated fibers are seen ophthalmoscopically as an opaque white patch with feathery edges.

myopic degeneration: a high degree of myopia that affects the retina and that may lead to permanent loss of vision caused by cracks in the macular region.

O

ocular toxocariasis: see *toxocariasis, ocular.*

Oguchi's disease: autosomal recessive night blindness found almost exclusively among the Japanese.

onchocerciasis: a parasitic infection common in tropical areas. A common cause of blindness in Africa.

optic papillae: The visible head of the optic nerve.

optic pit: a small circular or triangular pit about one third of the diameter of the optic disc and seen in the optic disc. It may be associated with macular edema.

P

pallor of disc: paleness of the optic disc suggestive of optic atrophy. Pallor can result after inflammation of the optic nerve, vascular ischemia, or loss of tissue from such diseases as multiple sclerosis or Leber's hereditary optic atrophy.

pan retinal photocoagulation: ablation of the periphery of the retina to stop the progress of the proliferative phase of diabetes.

papilla of Bergmeister: glial (connective tissue) remnant of the hyaloid system in the region of the optic disc.

papilledema: passive swelling of the optic nerve usually caused by raised cerebrospinal fluid pressure.

papillitis (optic neuritis): inflammatory swelling of the optic disc.

pars planitis: a peripheral uveitis characterized by a primary inflammation of the peripheral retina and vitreous base, which results in a preretinal and intravitreal fibroglial proliferation.

persistent hyperplastic vitreous: abnormality arising from failure of the hyaloid system to regress. It is visible in the child's pupil as a white mass. May be confused with retinoblastoma.

phakic cystoid macular edema: condition caused by the involvement of macular capillaries by an obstructive or inflammatory vascular retinal disease (diabetes, venous occlusion, uveitis).

phakoma: a small grayish white tumor in the retina.

phakomatoses: group of hereditary diseases characterized by the presence of spots, tumors, and cysts in various parts of the body; types recognized as associated with ocular findings are tuberous sclerosis, Bourneville's disease, von Hippel-Lindau disease, von Recklinghausen's disease, and Louis-Bar syndrome.

photocoagulation: the treatment of ocular disease that depends on the absorption of light by pigmented tissues and the conversion of light energy into heat energy.

Purtscher's retinopathy: edema and hemorrhage of the retina secondary to severe crushing injury.

R

retinal detachment: a space where the retina has pulled away from the underlying choroid tissue.

retinal exudates: hard exudates, fatty exudates, chronic edema residues used to denote those retinal deposits with fatty components free within the retina together with lipid-filled macrophages.

retinal vein occlusion: obstruction of the central retinal vein by a thrombosis. Branch retinal vein occlusion is an obstruction in a branch vein. These conditions are very prone to occur in diabetes.

retinitis proliferans: neovascularization accompanied by a fibrous component extending into the vitreous. Occurs in diseases such as diabetes and retinal vein occlusion.

retinoblastoma: the most common cancer of children's eyes. It may be bilateral and can lead to death or blindness. This cancer is primary and derived from retinal tissue.

retinopathy, diabetic: changes in the retina caused by diabetes mellitus. Usually universal after 30 years of the disease.

retrobulbar neuritis: inflammation of optic nerve occurring without involvement of optic disc. Most common prelude to multiple sclerosis.

retrolental fibroplasia: disorder of premature infants under 1500 g weight exposed to high concentrations of oxygen. This condition can result in mild peripheral retinopathy to full proliferative retinopathy leading to blindness. Other associated features include total retinal detachment, retrolental membrane formation, and severe myopia.

rhegmatogenous retinal detachments: these are retinal detachments associated with retinal tears.

Roth's spot: retinal hemorrhage with a white center as seen in subacute bacterial endocarditis.

S

Siegrist's streaks: chains of pigmented flecks that lie linearly along the course of a sclerosed choroidal vessel in patients with hypertension.

soft drusen: type of drusen with fuzzy edges and a tendency to become confluent. They are larger than hard drusen.

solar burn: an irreversible burn to the macula from unprotected viewing of the sun usually during an eclipse.

Sorsby's pseudoinflammatory macular dystrophy: a hereditary condition that is associated with an acute loss of central vision and an inflammatory-like macular lesion.

staphyloma: a thinned sclera that bulges backward. Most commonly found in persons with high myopia and axial myopia.

Stargardt's disease: a bilateral symmetrical progressive macular dystrophy occurring in young people that eventually leads to the loss of central vision.

subhyaloid hemorrhage: hemorrhage between the sensory retina and the vitreous body; a fluid level is often present.

subretinal neovascular membrane: vascular membranes deep to the retina that appear as a grayish pigmentation. Can be treated with lasers.

sunbursts: areas of retinal pigment epithelial hyperplasia that are seen in sickle cell retinopathy.

sympathetic uveitis: bilateral diffuse uveitis that occurs from 2 weeks to many years after a penetrating or perforating eye injury. The uninjured eye can develop severe uveitis in "sympathy" to the primary injury. It is an autoimmune disease that involves serious injury to the uveal system.

syneresis of vitreous: liquifaction of a portion of the vitreous humor. Normally it is a gel. Often associated with visible floaters.

T

Taenia solium (pork tapeworm): if the eggs of this tapeworm are ingested, the larvae develop into a cyst, and the infestation is referred to as cysticercosis. It can invade the interior of the eye.

Tay-Sachs disease (amaurotic idiocy): a metabolic disorder of gangliosides that is characterized by a cherry-red spot at the macula. It causes blindness and mental retardation. See *idiocy, amaurotic.*

telangiectasis: term used to denote retinal vascular disease of unknown cause in which there are large dilated vascular channels within the retina associated with edema. Included within this definition are Coats' disease, Lebers miliary aneurysms and hereditary telangiectasis.

toxocariasis, ocular: infestation by visceral larva migrans, which is a parasite originating from *Toxocara canis,* a nematode whose natural host is the dog. It is capable of producing uveitis.

toxoplasmosis: a widespread infectious disease from the protozoal organism *Toxoplasma gondii* that produces retinochoroiditis both as a congenital and as an acquired disorder and has a predisposition to affect the macular area.

transillumination: a method to illuminate the presence of a solid tumor by passing a strong light over an accessible area of the sclera.

V

venous stasis retinopathy: a vascular disorder caused by slow blood flow as a consequence of reduced central retinal artery pressure, i.e., diabetic retinopathy.

vitrectomy: removal of a portion of the vitreous by excision or suction. It is done most often to remove vitreous during a cataract extraction.

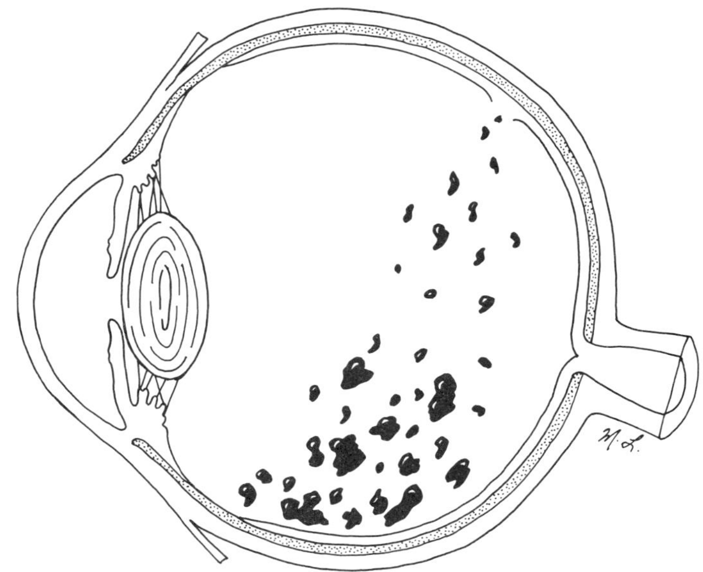

Fig. 15-7. Retinal tear with vitreous hemorrhage.

vitreous detachment: a collapse of the vitreous body occurring in eyes with aphakia, peripheral uveitis, diabetic retinopathy, branch vein occlusion, or retinitis pigmentosa. It also is found in myopic people and after blunt trauma.

vitreous hemorrhage: a hemorrhage lying in the vitreous cavity (Fig. 15-7).

vitreous traction: the pull on the retina by the vitreous.

Vogt-Koyanagi syndrome: bilateral uveitis, associated with absent lashes, baldness, and disturbance in hearing.

von Hippel-Lindau disease: see *angiomatosis, retinal.*

W

window defects: findings present with fluorescein angiography tests, i.e., hard drusen exhibit hyperfluorescence as late fading.

CHAPTER 16

OCULAR TUMORS

Tumor (Latin *tumor,* "a swelling") was a term used by the ancients and continued until modern times to mean any swelling, the nature and origin of which were unknown. The word *tumor* is now restricted to use for swellings arising from new growths.

The term *neoplasm* (Greek *neos,* "new," and *plasma,* "form") are new forms or new cells that proliferate to form a new tissue or tumor. A tumor may be either *malignant* (from Latin *malignus,* "evil") or *benign* (from Latin *benignus,* "kindly"), the former being life threatening and thus capable of causing death, whereas the latter is not, being innocent and nonfatal, and although it may grow, it is not capable of producing death and tends to be localized. *Carcinomas* (Greek *karkinos,* "a crab" or "creeping") are malignant tumors.

Tumors of the eyelid

On the eyelid skin *basal cell carcinoma,* sometimes called *rodent ulcers,* occur frequently and arise from the basal epithelial cells (Fig. 16-1). They spread locally but do not *metastasize* or spread to distant sites. Less commonly, *squamous cell carcinoma,* more malignant tumors arising from the *squamous* cells of the epithelium, have the potential capability of spreading via the bloodstream to distant sites (Fig. 16-2).

Xanthelasma (Greek *xanthas,* "yellow," and *elasmos,* "a metal plate"), or *xanthoma,* are yellowish fatty deposits that arise from blood vessels and may be associated with high cholesterol levels (Fig. 16-3). A *papilloma* is a benign epithelial outgrowth over a fibrovascular cone (Fig. 16-4). It may be *pedunculated* (hanging with a stalk) or may be *sessile* (broad-based). *Hemangiomas* (Greek *haima,* "blood," and *angioma,* "tumor of vessel") are growths of blood vessels and may be benign or malignant (Fig. 16-5). *Keratoacanthoma* is a benign elevated lesion with a central crater filled with keratin, which may be confused with a basal cell carcinoma. A *verruca* is a wart, an elevated lesion of skin caused by a virus; the word verucca is derived from the Latin word for a steep place (Fig. 16-6).

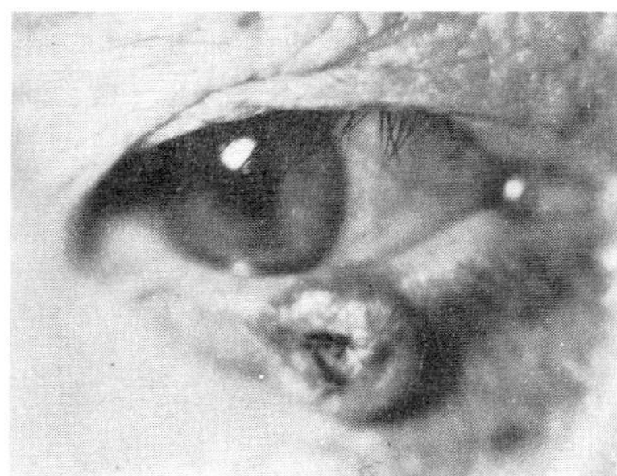

Fig. 16-1. Basal cell carcinoma of eyelid.

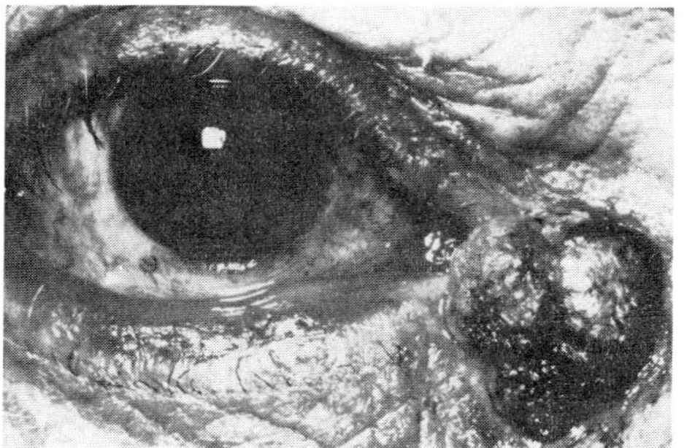

Fig. 16-2. Squamous cell carcinoma of skin over lacrimal sac.

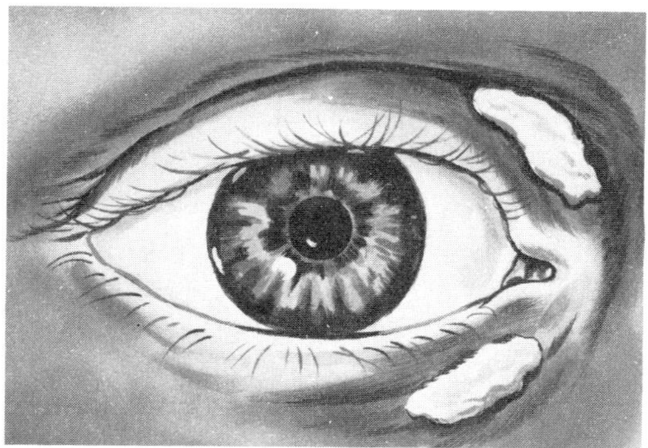

Fig. 16-3. Xanthelasma.

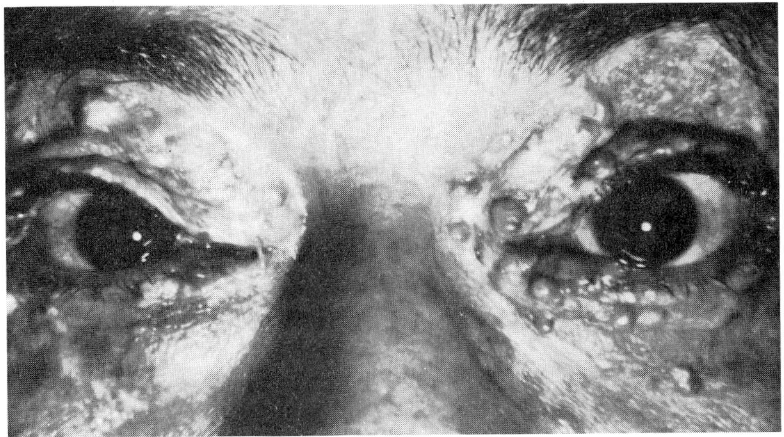

Fig. 16-4. Multiple papillomas of eyelids.

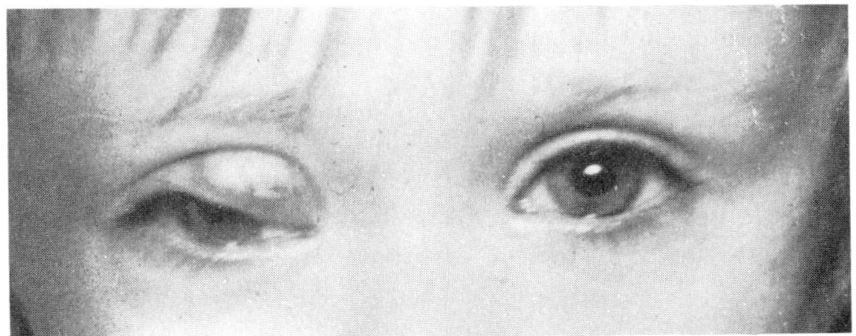

Fig. 16-5. Hemangioma of eyelid.

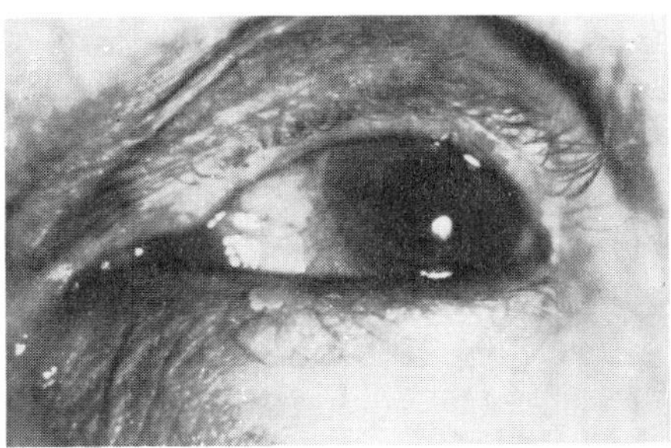

Fig. 16-6. Verruca of lower eyelid.

Tumors of the interior of the eye

Melanomas are tumors that contain melanin or pigment and may be benign or malignant (Fig. 16-7). They may arise in the iris, ciliary body, or choroid. *Retinoblastoma* are malignant tumors arising in infants and young children from undifferentiated retinal cells, sometimes referred to as *gliomas* of the retina. They may give rise to *leukocoria,* or white pupil (Greek *leuko,* "white," and *kore,* "pupil"). The cells of a retinoblastoma may be undifferentiated or arranged in *rosettes,* rings of columnar cells arranged around a central lumen. The retinoblastoma is the most common malignant ocular tumor of children.

Tumors of the optic nerve

Gliomas are malignant tumors of nerve cells occurring in brain, spinal cord, and retina and also arising from the optic nerve cells. The word is derived from the Greek word for glue and refers to the supporting or binding cells of the central nervous system from which they arise. *Meningiomas of the optic nerve* are tumors that arise from the *meninges* (Greek for membrane or outer lining of the optic nerve) and cause compression damage to the optic nerve fibers.

Tumors of the lacrimal gland

The lacrimal gland, which secretes tear fluid, may become involved with tumors such as (1) *lymphomas,* or tumors composed of lymph cells; (2) inflammatory *pseudotumors,* or false tumors, which have the characteristics of a tumor but are inflammatory in origin; or (3) *epithelial* tumors, derived from epithelial cells. The latter may be *mixed tumors* composed of both epithelial cells and connective tissue elements. These may be either benign or malignant. Some of these epithelial tumors are also referred to as *adenoid cystic carcinoma,* named after the characteristic small round cystic foci containing mucin; if the cells take on a cylinder shape, the tumors are then referred to as *cylindroma.*

Tumors and lesions of the orbit

Pseudotumor of the orbit is an inflammatory condition resembling a tumor of the orbit with all the clinical signs of a true tumor. A *mucocele* is a walled, epithelial-lined sac, often arising from the sinuses. A *dermoid of the orbit* is a cyst, that is, a lesion containing embryonic remnants of skin derivatives such as squamous epithelium, hair follicles, and sebaceous and sweat glands along with accumulated sebum. *Neurofibromas* are proliferations of Schwann cells, which frequently progress and lead to disfiguration. *Hemangiomas* are common tumors

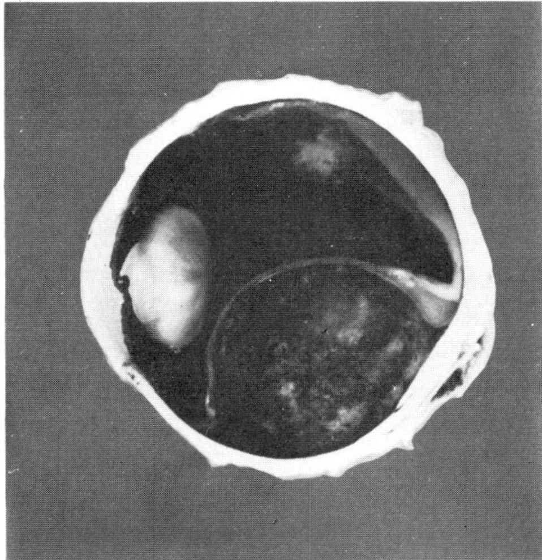

Fig. 16-7. Malignant melanoma of the choroid.

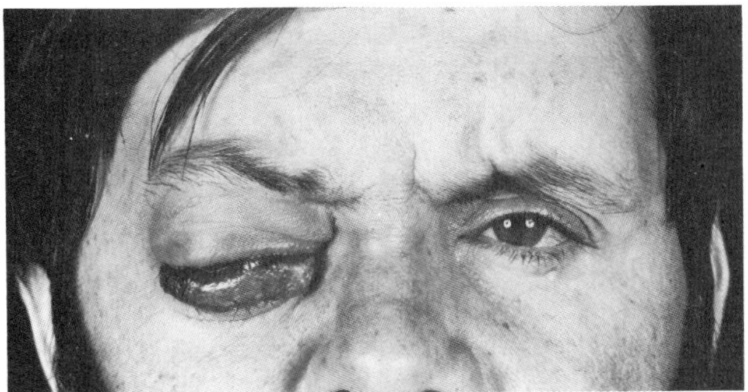

Fig. 16-8. Carotid-cavernous fistula.

of the orbit arising from blood vessel cells. They may be benign or malignant.

Rhabdomyosarcoma is a malignant neoplasm related to the striated muscle and arising from the muscle masses in the orbit. *Liposarcoma* is a malignant tumor related to fat or adipose tissue. *Carotid-cavernous fistula* is a communication between the carotid artery and the cavernous sinus arising from trauma, which may be confronted with an orbital tumor (Fig. 16-8). An orbital *aneurysm* is a vascular enlargement of an artery in the orbit.

Some definitions of other tumors and some words related to tumors arising in the eye and adjacent tissues are listed in the following glossary.

A

acquired melanosis: acquired pigmentation of the basal layers of the conjunctival epithelium.

adenocarcinoma: malignant tumor in which the cells are arranged in a glandlike fashion.

astrocytoma: tumor of the central nervous system formed by astrocytes.

B

Bowen's disease: a disorder consisting of single or multiple intraepidermal squamous cell carcinomas that grow slowly and spread in a superficial, centrifugal manner about the limbus and that are locally invasive.

Broders' grading: a grading of epithelial malignancy from 1 to 4, based on differentiation of cell types.

C

calcifying epithelioma of Malherbe: firm subcutaneous nodule covered by normal skin typically occurring in young adults.

Callender classification: system used to classify ciliary body, iris, and choroidal malignant melanoma (spindle A, spindle B, epitheloid, mixed, and necrotic).

capillary hemangioma: congenital tumor composed of capillaries and usually bright red, solitary, and smooth. Typically begins within the first years of life and characteristically regresses spontaneously.

carcinoma in situ: intraepidermal squamous cell carcinoma.

cavernous hemangioma: tumor of blood vessels in which large vascular spaces are lined by endothelium.

congenital ocular melanocytosis (melanosis oculi): diffuse nevus of conjunctiva.

congenital oculodermal melanocytosis (nevus of Ota): deep nevus of skin associated with a nevus of conjunctiva and diffuse nevus of uvea.

D

dermoid cyst: cyst lined by epithelium with skin appendages (hair follicles, sweat glands, and so on) and filled with keratin. Usually attached to the periosteum of the orbit.

dermolipoma: congenital benign lesion, usually occurring under the bulbar conjunctiva at the external canthus; this lesion is composed of the elements of skin plus fat.

dictyoma: see *medulloepithelioma.*

E

epithelioma: tumors of epithelial origin, namely, squamous cell and basal cell subtypes.

F

follicles, conjunctival: raised nodules of conjunctiva surrounded by blood vessels, which may be seen in patients with viral conjunctivitis.

Fuchs' adenoma: benign nonvascular proliferation of nonpigmented ciliary epithelium generally located at the pars plana of the ciliary body.

G

granuloma: benign nodule, such as a chalazion, that occurs as a result of a localized inflammation of the sebaceous glands. It can cause iritis and inflammatory tumors of the orbit.

H

hemangioma: tumor arising from endothelial cells and most frequently seen in the choroid.

Hodgkin's disease: a disease of the reticuloendothelial system that affects predominantly the lymphatic elements, the lymph nodes, and the spleen.

hyperkeratosis: thickening of the keratin layer. At times, this may be a precancerous transformation of tissue.

I

iris nevus syndrome: an acquired diffuse nevus of the iris that may cause glaucoma by extending into the drainage angle.

J

juvenile xanthogranuloma: a disorder characterized by multiple raised orange skin lesions; the eyeball, meninges, and testes may also be involved.

K

Kaposi's sarcoma: tumor consisting of capillary clusters in a stroma of malignant spindle-shaped cells.

L

leukemia: a malignant tumor of blood cells that produces widespread retinal hemorrhages.

leukocoria: any pathological condition, such as retrolental fibroplasia, that produces a white reflex in the pupillary area.

leukoplakia: clinical term used to describe whitish plaques of slightly elevated tissue. May be precancerous.

lymphangioma: tumor composed of lymph-filled spaces, often involving the orbit. Some people consider the lymphangioma to be varices.

lymphoma: malignant tumor of the reticuloendothelial system.

M

malignant schwannoma: malignant tumor of peripheral nerves arising from Schwann cells.

medulloepithelioma (dictyoma): congenital tumor of nonpigmented ciliary body epithelium. These tumors may be benign or malignant.

meibomian cyst: chronic cyst of the meibomian gland of the eyelid.

melanocyte: cell that produces melanin and is found in dermal tissues.

melanophage: cell that has the ability to phagocytose or ingest melanin.

melanosis: condition characterized by abnormal deposits of melanin or pigment.

molluscum contagiosum: viral infection of the skin around the eyelid that causes a dome-shaped swelling with an umbilicated center.

N

neurilemoma: encapsulated benign tumors of peripheral cranial or sympathetic nerve sheaths composed of Schwann cells. They may have a solid appearance (Antoni A) or there may be a mucoid degeneration (Antoni B).

neuroblastoma: malignant tumor of the nervous system, one type of which is the retinoblastoma, or tumor of the retina.

neuroepithelioma: neuroectodermal tumor of the retina in which the cells arrange themselves in the form of true rosettes.

neurofibroma: tumor composed of proliferating Schwann cells of the peripheral nerves.

nevus: congenital pigmented area of variable size and shape, usually found on face, head, neck, and arms, though no region is exempt.

O

osteoma: tumor arising from bone. Very rare around the orbit.

P

papules: a papillary inflammatory reaction of the conjunctiva consisting of raised nodules (cobblestones) with a central core of blood vessels. The papules most frequently affect the superior tarsal conjunctiva. Vernal (allergic) conjunctivitis is the most classic cause of papillary reaction.

phakoma: a small grayish white tumor in the retina.

phakomatoses: group of hereditary diseases characterized by the presence of spots, tumors, and cysts in various parts of the body; types recognized as associated with ocular findings are tuberous sclerosis, von Hippel–Lindau disease, Recklinghausen's disease, Bourneville's disease, and Louis-Bar syndrome.

pseudoepitheliomatous hyperplasia: benign proliferation of the epidermis that simulates an epithelial neoplasm characterized by marked acanthosis with a moderate inflammatory cell infiltration. It may be seen around areas of chronic inflammation.

R

retinal pigment epithelial hypertrophy: jet-black flat lesion of the retinal pigment epithelium surrounded by a halo.

retrolental fibroplasia: a disease of the retina in the premature infant exposed to increased amounts of oxygen in which the retina becomes partially or completely detached and may be pulled forward against the posterior surface of the lens. It used to be a common form of blindness in children.

S

sarcoma: malignant tumor of connective tissue, vascular tissue, fat, or bone.

sebaceous adenoma: benign tumor of sebaceous glands.

sebaceous cyst: cyst caused by the obstruction of the glands of Zeis, the meibomian glands, or a sebaceous gland associated with a hair follicle.

seborrheic keratosis: tumor that sits like a button on the surface of the skin.

senile or solar keratoses: growths that appear as multiple lesions on the sun-exposed parts of the body. They may be a precursor to basal cell carcinoma.

spindle A: malignant melanoma composed of cells with small spindle-shaped nuclei with a central dark stripe.

spindle B: malignant melanoma composed of cells with spindle-shaped nuclei and distinct nucleoli.

syringoma: benign adenoma of sweat glands that may arise in the caruncle.

T

trichoepithelioma: benign tumor of hair follicles.

V

verruca vulgaris: viral infection of skin that produces a typical wartlike lesion.

X

xanthogranuloma: see *juvenile xanthogranuloma.*

CHAPTER 17

SYSTEMIC DISEASES AND THE EYE

This chapter will highlight some of the more common systemic diseases along with some both common and interesting systemic disorders that have ophthalmic manifestations. The eye participates by involving the anterior segment and the posterior segment of the eye, as well as the orbit in many conditions affecting the body. These involvements are covered in previous chapters, but an understanding of the methodology of these systemic disorders is important, since a whole group of medical terms are used in their diagnosis and treatment.

Understanding the ocular manifestations may be helpful in determining the status of disease processes such as diabetes, hypertension, and infectious disorders. These will be common conditions, as well as some unusual disorders, will be highlighted in this section.

Diabetes mellitus

Diabetes mellitus (Greek *diabetes* "a syphon" + *melitta* "honey sweet urine") is a complex metabolic disorder manifested by the excretion of a large volume of sugared urine. The disease is usually genetically determined and is one of the leading causes of blindness in North America. Although the cause of diabetes is unknown, the basic defect appears to be a relative or absolute lack of insulin. The term *insulin* comes from the German word *insula* meaning "islet" which refers to the islets of Langerhans. The islets are located in the pancreas and are responsible for the secretion of insulin.

There are two clinical forms of diabetes mellitus: *insulin-dependent* diabetes mellitus (IDOM) and *non–insulin-dependent* diabetes mellitus (NIDDM). The major clinical differences between these two types are listed in Table 17-1.

The diabetic may initially present with any of the following symptoms. *Polyuria* (Greek *poly,* "much," + *ouron,* "urine") is the passage of a large volume of urine in a given period. This is the result of spillage of sugar from the blood into the urine that increases the volume of urine. *Polydipsia* (Greek *poly,* "much," + *dipsia,* "thirst") is an increased drinking tendency in an attempt to keep up with the fluid loss. Weight loss, fatigue, and còma may be manifestations of an abnormal sugar level.

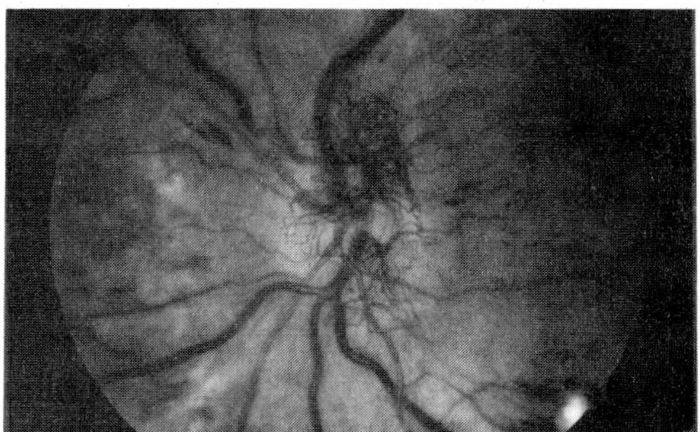

Fig. 17-1. Neovascularization of the disc in a patient with diabetes mellitus. (From the Department of Ophthalmology, Mayo Clinic.)

Table 17-1 Differences between insulin-dependent diabetes mellitus and non–insulin-dependent diabetes mellitus

	IDDM	NIDDM
Defect	Absolute lack of insulin	Relative lack of insulin
Circulating insulin	Very low or absent	Relative lack of insulin
Pancreatic insulin content	<5% normal	Normal to 50% normal
Body habitus	Normal to thin	Usually obese
Stability	Unstable	Stable
Treatment	Diet + insulin	Diet alone or diet + oral hypoglycemic agents

Diabetes can lead to both ocular and systemic complications. The systemic manifestations include most importantly disease of the kidneys, peripheral nervous system, and the blood vessels.

Diabetic eye disease can be classified into *nonproliferative* or *background* stage and a *proliferative* stage. *Nonproliferative diabetic retinopathy* is characterized by: *microaneurysms* (micro + Greek *aneurysma,* "a widening"), which are outpouchings from the walls of the capillaries. *Cotton-wool spots* appear as white retinal patches and are secondary to ischemic damage to the nerve fiber layer of the retina. *Hard exudates* are derived from the serum and appear as yellow deposits in the deep layers of the retina. *Dot, blot,* or *splinter hemorrhages* can be found at various levels in the retina.

Proliferative diabetic retinopathy is probably a vascular response to a hypoxic retinal environment. *Neovascularization,* or new vessel growth, may occur on the disc or on the retina (Fig. 17-1). These fine vessels can easily rupture and result in a *preretinal hemorrhage,* which is located beneath the internal limiting membrane of the retina or a vitreous hemorrhage. The neovascularization is usually accompanied by a fibrous component that can result in shrinkage and lead to a retinal detachment. Occasionally the neovascularization can affect the iris and the trabecular meshwork and lead to obstruction of aqueous humor outflow, which results in a condition called *neovascular glaucoma*.

Laser photocoagulation is the most commonly used treatment for diabetic retinopathy (Fig. 17-2). It is being used to treat macular edema and the proliferative phase of the disease. In macular edema the fluorescein angiogram will demonstrate the microaneurysms and other leakage points which, if the process is not too diffuse, can be directly photocoagulated. In proliferative retinopathy, the technique *panretinal photocoagulation* is used. This procedure utilizes in excess of 1500 *laser burns* that are scattered over the retina and that, if done early in the process of the disease, may result in *regression* of the neovascularization.

The diagnosis of diabetes is made by various laboratory tests. The presence of glucose in the urine should always make one strongly suspicious of diabetes. However, further laboratory support is necessary for establishing the diagnosis of diabetes mellitus, and this can be made by obtaining a fasting blood glucose. A fasting blood glucose is obtained after the patient has fasted for 10 to 12 hours and is positive when it is elevated. If the index of suspicion is high and the fasting blood glucose is normal, the patient should be challenged with a glucose tolerance test. In this test the patient ingests a glucose solution, and then multiple blood samples are drawn over time. The diabetic patient will be unable to lower the blood sugar sufficiently, and the test will be positive.

The treatment of diabetes involves a number of modalities. Diet is of utmost importance with regard to regularity of meals and total caloric intake. Oral hypoglycemic agents are pills that are used to regulate the blood sugar levels in maturity-onset diabetics. The sulfonylureas are the most popular class of drugs and act to stimulate insulin secretion from the pancreas. Since the juvenile-onset

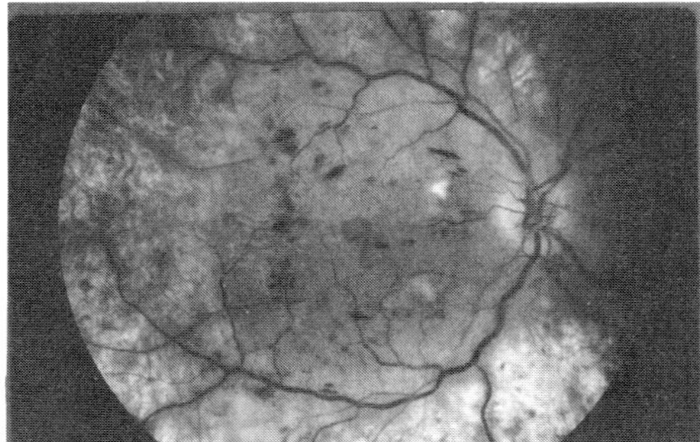

Fig. 17-2. Laser photocoagulation scars can be seen surrounding the posterior pole in a patient with proliferative diabetic retinopathy. (From the Department of Ophthalmology, Mayo Clinic.)

diabetic has little or no insulin stored in the pancreas, this modality would not be effective. Proper control of blood sugar levels may be impossible without the use of insulin. The patient is taught the technique of administering the injection of insulin beneath the skin. The use of a continuous insulin infusion pump provides improved regulation of blood glucose and hopefully will reduce the complications of diabetes.

Thyroid disease and the eye

Graves' disease is characterized by specific ocular features in a patient who is usually hyperthyroid. The disease was named after Robert Graves (1796-1853), a great physician of Dublin who described the classic features in 1835. However the earliest description was by Caler Parry whose work was published posthumously by his son in 1825.

The ocular signs in Graves' disease can be classified by the use of the mnemonic NO SPECS (Table 17-2). Class 1 is characterized by lid changes. Lid retraction (Dalrymple's sign) gives the patient a characteristic "startled" appearance (Fig. 17-

Table 17-2 Classification of eye changes in Graves' disease

Class	Definition
0	*N*o physical signs or symptoms
1	*O*nly signs, no symptoms (signs limited to upper lid retraction, stare, and lid lag)
2	*S*oft-tissue involvement (symptoms and signs)
3	*P*roptosis
4	*E*xtraocular muscle movement
5	*C*orneal involvement
6	*S*ight loss (optic nerve involvement)

From Werner, S.C., J. Clin. Endocrinol. Metab. **44**:203, 1977.

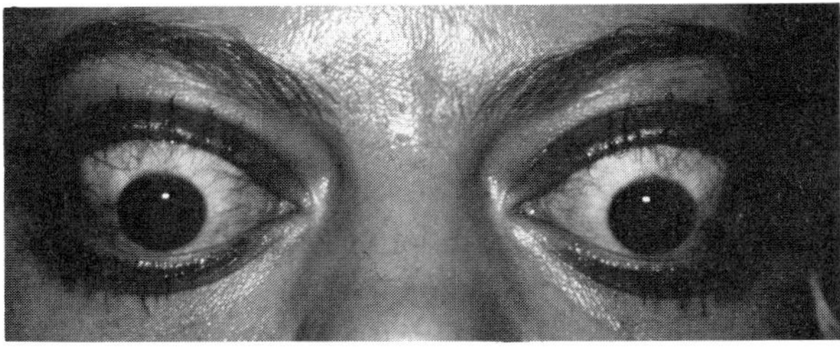

Fig. 17-3. Thyroid exophthalmos. A patient with Graves' disease who demonstrated characteristic signs of lid retraction and proptosis. (From Brian Younge, M.D., Department of Ophthalmology, Mayo Clinic.)

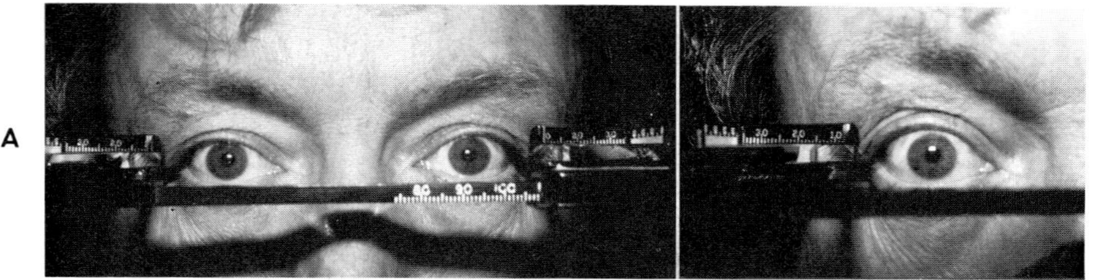

Fig. 17-4. **A,** The Hertel exophthalmometer is used to measure the amount of proptosis. **B,** A higher magnification view demonstrates the ease in which proptosis can be measured with the exophthalmometer. (From Brian Younge, M.D., Department of Ophthalmology, Mayo Clinic.)

Table 17-3 Eponyms for external eye signs

Eponym	Definition
Ballet's sign	Complete immobility of the globe
Boston's sign	Jerky movement of upper lid on downward gaze
Dalrymple's sign	Staring appearance
Enroth's sign	Puffy swelling of lids
Gifford's sign	Difficulty in everting upper lid
Jelliinek's sign	Increased pigmentation of lids
Joffroy's sign	Absence of forehead wrinkling on upward gaze
Kocher's sign	Increased lid retraction with visual fixation
Möbius' sign	Difficulty converging
Rosenbach's sign	Tremor of closed lids
Sainton's sign	Delayed forehead wrinkling after upward gaze
Stellwag's sign	Infrequent blinking
Suker's sign	Weakness of fixation on lateral gaze
von Graefe's sign	Upper lid lag on downward gaze

3). Lid lag (von Graefe's sign) is demonstrated by having the patient look from upgaze to downgaze and noting the relative lag of the lid position to the movement of the globe. Class 2 is characterized by edema of the conjunctiva and lids, conjunctival injection, and swollen extraocular muscles. Class 3 is characterized by exophthalmos (ex "out of" + Greek *ophthalmos,* "eye"), which is protrusion of the eye. In Graves' disease a swelling of the retrobulbar tissues within the confines of a bony orbit that results in the eye being pushed forward. The extent of protrusion of the eye is measured with the exophthalmometer (Fig. 17-4). Class 4 is reached when there is a limitation of eye movement because of the inability of the fibrotic eye muscles to relax. Involvement is most common in decreasing order of frequency of the inferior rectus, medial rectus, superior rectus, and

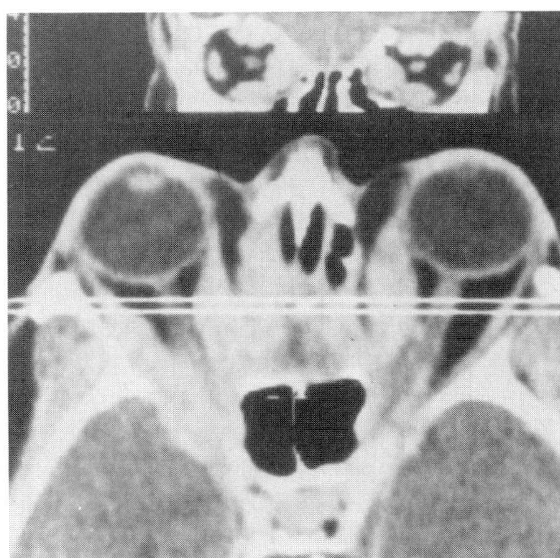

Fig. 17-5. Computed tomographic scan showing thickened extraocular muscles characteristic of Graves' disease. *Above,* a coronal scan: superior-inferior cut; *Below,* a transaxial scan: anterior-posterior cut. (From Brian Younge, M.D., Department of Ophthalmology, Mayo Clinic.)

lateral rectus. This restriction in eye movement can be differentiated from a muscle weakness problem by checking the intraocular pressure when the patient looks straight ahead compared with upgaze. In Graves' disease the tight extraocular muscles press on the globe in upgaze, and the intraocular pressure increases unlike that seen with a nonrestrictive problem. Another means is by the technique of forced ductions, in which a drop of anesthetic is placed onto the eye and then forceps are used to grasp the globe and move it. In Graves' disease the tethered extraocular muscles prevent the free movement of the globe. Corneal involvement occurs in class 5. This is related to drying of the ocular surface, which has been attributed to upper lid retraction, exophthalmos, and a decreased blink rate. Class 6 is characterized by visual loss caused by optic nerve compression from the surrounding swollen orbital tissues. Additional signs are included in Table 17-3, which presents a summary of the eponyms used in describing the ocular signs in Graves' disease.

The diagnosis of Graves' disease is confirmed with the clinical features as described and a computerized tomographic (CT) scan that shows enlargement of the extraocular muscles (Fig. 17-5). The patient is usually hyperthyroid and shows evidence of an enlarged thyroid gland (goiter), fine tremor, increased nervousness, palpitations, loss of weight, increased appetite, warm skin, and a fast heart rate. The hyperthyroidism is confirmed in florid cases by an elevation in the thyroid hormones: thyroxine (T4) and triiodothyronine (T3). In milder cases the diagnosis is more difficult, and the thyroid-releasing hormone (TRH) stimulation test is used.

Treatment of Graves' disease involves attention to the ophthalmopathy and to the hyperthyroidism. Lubrication and ointment can be used for corneal exposure. Muscle surgery can be used to relax the tight fibrotic muscles. Lid surgery making recessing Müller's muscle and the levator palpebras superioris can improve the cosmetic appearance of the patient by reducing the retraction. Systemic steroids, radiation, or both, can be used to decrease the marked congestion. A variety of surgical procedures can be performed to decompress the orbits so as to allow more room for the swollen tissues. A Kronlein procedure is a lateral approach to decompressing the orbit. A transantral decompression is an inferior approach that allows some bulging of the orbital tissues in the maxillary sinus. Decompression procedures are used when the optic nerve is compressed and vision is threatened.

Radioactive iodine can be used to manage the hyperthyroidism by destroying the thyroid tissue. This treatment is simple and involves no surgical complications or hospitalization. The major difficulty is the onset of hypothyroidism after therapy that may be 40% to 80% after 10 years. A subtotal thyroidectomy, a surgical procedure that removes the majority of the thyroid gland, can also be used in the management of hyperthyroidism.

Hypertension

Hypertension is associated with a large increase in morbidity and mortality from various causes. Although there is no sharp dividing line between normal and elevated blood pressure, an adult is considered by many to be hypertensive if arterial pressure is 160/95 mm Hg or higher (15% to 20% of the adult population in North America have values at or above this range). Hypertension results in an increased risk of premature death and vascular disease involving the eyes, brain, heart, and kidneys.

Over 90% of patients with hypertension have no known cause. This is referred to as idiopathic or essential hypertension. The development of hypertension before 35 and after 50 years of age suggests a specific cause. Major known causes of hypertension are discussed below.

Oral contraceptives may be associated with an elevation in blood pressure that is usually reversible after the pills have been discontinued. Diseases of the blood vessels that supply the kidneys (renal vascular disease) can result in activation of the renin-angiotensin system, which results in the release of various substances into the blood that act to raise the blood pressure. Intrinsic diseases of the kidney may also elevate the blood pressure by a variety of mechanisms.

There are specific diseases of the adrenal gland that result in the secretion of a number of substances that can lead to hypertension: 1. Conn syndrome (primary hyperaldosteronism) results in an elevation in serum aldosterone. 2. Cushing's syndrome results in a large output of glucocorticoids. 3. Pheochromocytoma releases epinephrine and norepinephrine into the bloodstream. All of these substances act in different ways to raise the blood pressure.

Hypertension affects all the blood vessels in the body but it is the ones in the eyes that are most readily observable. The eye findings in hypertension can be expressed according to a grading system developed by Keith, Wagener, and Baker of the Mayo Clinic. Four grades of hypertensive retinopathy are considered. Grade 1 consists of mild narrowing and sclerosis of the retinal vessels. Grade 2 changes consist of more marked retinal vessel changes with localized or generalized arteriolar narrowing and retinal arteriolar-venous crossing phenomena (nicking). Grade 3 (Fig. 17-6) comprises grade 2 plus retinal hemorrhages and exudates. The hemorrhages characteristically occur in the superficial or nerve fiber layer of the retina as splinter or flame hemorrhages. Cotton-wool spots, often termed soft exudates, are not true exudates but represent focal microinfarcts to the nerve fiber layer of the retina. Hard or waxy exudates represent lipid-rich collections of plasma deposited in the retina. Grade 4 hypertensive retinopathy consists of grade 3 findings plus papilledema and is seen only in severe cases of hypertension.

Treatment of hypertension depends on the cause. When a cause of hypertension is found, which is the exception rather than the rule, often the patient can be cured of the hypertension by surgery. If, as is usually the case, the cause cannot be determined, treatment is usually lifelong and is designed to prevent the com-

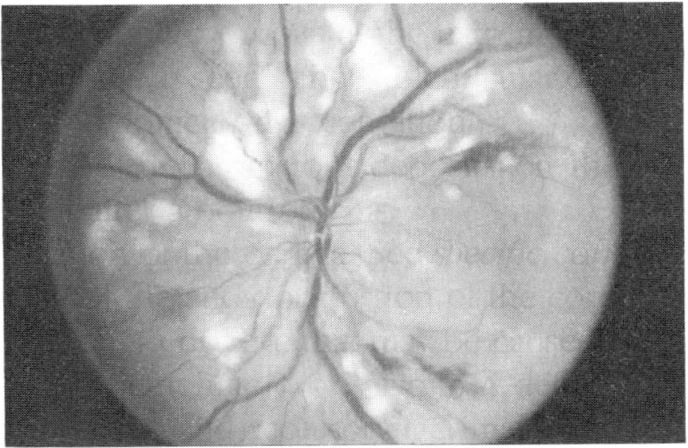

Fig. 17-6. Advanced hypertensive retinopathy (grade 3) with narrowed arterioles, scattered hemorrhages, and cotton-wool spots. (From the Department of Ophthalmology, Mayo Clinic.)

plications of cardiovascular disease, renal failure, and stroke. The aim of the therapy is to control the disease. General treatment measures include a low-salt diet and weight reduction. Therapy with drugs is usually indicated and has two main goals: (1) reduce the blood pressure to normal, and (2) achieve this goal with as little medication as possible.

There are four main classes of drugs that are used: (1) diuretics are used, which act on the kidneys to influence the retention and excretion of electrolytes and fluid. The most commonly prescribed drugs in this class are hydrochlorothiazide and furosemide. (2) Vasodilators are potent drugs that are used only in the treatment of severe hypertension. The most commonly used drugs in this class are hydralazine, prazosin, and minoxidil. (3) Beta-blocking agents are effective in lowering blood pressure by a number of mechanisms. They reduce the output volume of the heart and probably decrease the release of a vasoconstrictor (renin). They may also act on the central nervous system to decrease the blood pressure. The most commonly used drugs in this class are propranolol and metoprolol. (4) Sympathetic inhibitors may act on the central nervous system and/or the peripheral vasculature to decrease the blood pressure. Some of the most commonly used drugs in this class are methyldopa and clonidine.

Infectious disease

Pharyngoconjunctival fever

Infection with a few specific types of adenoviruses (e.g., types 3 or 7) may cause a condition manifested by a sore throat, fever, and a red eye. The disease predominates in children and young adults. The eye findings are typically those of a conjunctivitis with a watery discharge and occasional corneal involvement. The disease usually runs its own course over several weeks. No specific treatment is indicated, and no permanent eye damage results.

Toxoplasmosis (Fig. 17-7)

Toxoplasmosis is a disease caused by the parasite *Toxoplasma gondii.* Infection may be either congenital or acquired (e.g., from raw meat or cat feces). Systemic manifestations are more common in the congenital form and may include intracranial calcification, convulsions, and mental retardation. Ocular disease in the congenital and acquired forms may be manifested by yellow-white retinal lesions and cells in the vitreous and occasionally in the anterior chamber. Diagnosis is confirmed by the indirect fluorescent antibody test, which measures serum antibodies that are directed against the *Toxoplasma* organism. Treatment is indicated if the inflammatory process threatens the macula or optic nerve. Pyrimethamine and sulfadiazine are the most commonly used antibiotics. Clindamycin, which has been evaluated on an experimental basis, has shown favorable preliminary results.

Toxocariasis (Fig. 17-8)

This infection is caused by the parasite *Toxocara canis*. The disease is usually acquired by children who ingest the *Toxocara* eggs that have been excreted by dogs usually in the soil in public playgrounds. Systemic infection usually goes unnoticed. Occasionally the syndrome of visceral larvae migrans results from the spread of the organism throughout the body. The typical features that usually occur at 2 years of age may include: fever, cough, enlargement of the liver (hepatomegaly), and seizures. Ocular involvement is usually unilateral and occurs at

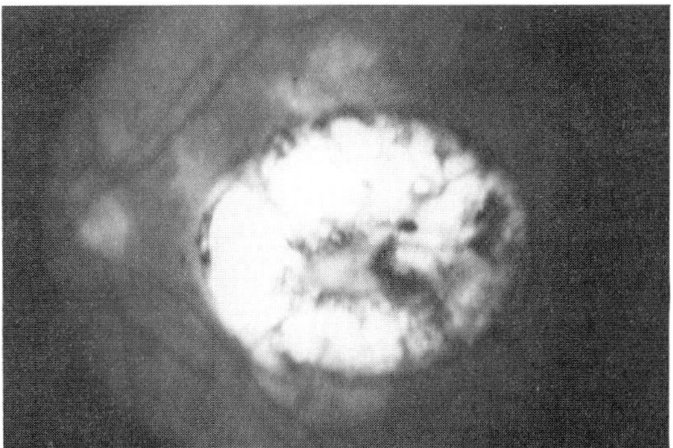

Fig. 17-7. Ocular infection by toxoplasmosis can result in a chorioretinal scar that affects central vision. (From the Department of Ophthalmology, Mayo Clinic.)

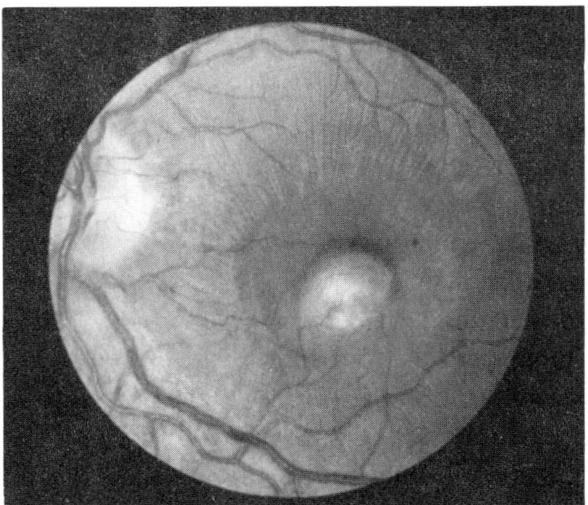

Fig. 17-8. Toxocara can result in a granuloma of the posterior pole. (From the Department of Ophthalmology, Mayo Clinic.)

an average age of 7 to 8 years. The eye findings may include whitish mass lesions (focal granulomas) involving the retina and choroid, inflammation of the vitreous (chronic endophthalmitis), and occasionally the formation of a tubular structure beneath the retina, which provides objective evidence of previous passage of the *Toxocara* worm. Corticosteroids by mouth or by injection around the eye can be administered in the acute inflammatory phase. Laser photocoagulation can be used to kill a live worm outside of the macula if one suspects that it might turn and enter this vital area.

Candidiasis

This infection is caused by a yeastlike fungus referred to as *Candida albicans*. Infection is more common in patients that are critically ill, patients with indwelling catheters, patients that are being treated with steroids or chemotherapeutic agents, or intravenous drug abusers. Systemic infection may involve any organ. Multiple microabscesses may form in the bones, kidneys, intestinal tract, brain, and other areas. Ocular involvement is characterized by fluffy yellow-white lesions that usually start in the retina and spread into the vitreous. Diagnosis is made by the typical fundus picture in the right clinical setting. The blood cultures may or may not be positive. Treatment is with antifungal agents, e.g., amphotericin, which can be administered by the intravenous, periocular, or intraocular routes.

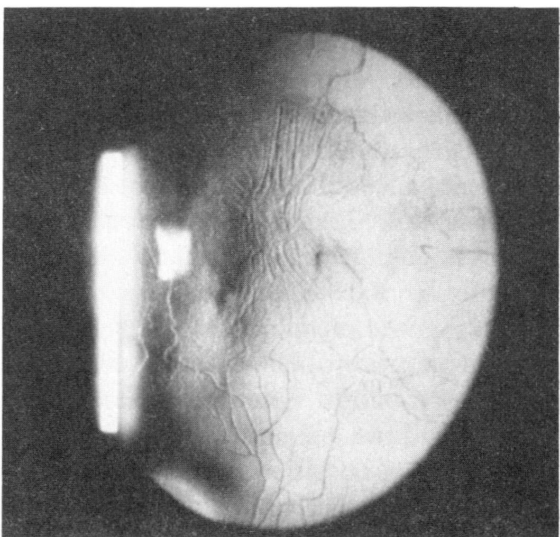

Fig. 17-9. The ingrowth of vessels in the deep layers of the cornea are manifestations of the interstitial keratitis of congenital syphilis. (From the Department of Ophthalmology, Mayo Clinic.)

Syphilis

Syphilis is caused by the spirochete *Treponema pallidum.* The disease was named after Syphilus, the supposed first sufferer from the disease and the hero of the poem *Syphilis Sive Morbus Gallicus* by Girolamo Fracastoro (1530), an Italian physician, astronomer, and poet. The disease may be congenital or acquired. The systemic manifestations of congenital syphilis include saddle-shaped nose, notching of the teeth (Hutchinson's sign), and deafness. The most common eye lesion is an interstitial keratitis (Fig. 17-9), which results from inflammation in the deep layers of the cornea. The inflammatory response usually occurs in the first or second decades of life and is thought to be an immune reaction against the treponemal organism located in the cornea. The other typical eye finding is a chorioretinitis (Fig. 17-10), which gives a "salt and pepper" appearance to the fundus. The treatment of congenital syphilis involves large doses of antibiotics (e.g., penicillin). Topical steroids are used to control the corneal inflammation.

Acquired syphilis does not usually affect the eye. Inflammation involving the lids (blepharitis), iris (iritis), or iris and ciliary body (iridocyclitis) is the most common finding. Less common ocular manifestations include an interstitial keratitis and chorioretinitis.

The laboratory diagnosis of syphilis can be made by the Venereal Disease Research Laboratory (VDAL), which is usually positive in acute infections, or by the fluorescent treponemal antibody absorption test (FTA/ABS), which will continue to be positive throughout the patient's lifetime.

acquired immune deficiency syndrome (AIDS): the occurrence of life-threatening opportunistic infections (e.g., cytomegalovirus, *Pneumocystis carinii, Cryptococcus,* etc.) in persons who were otherwise well and not receiving immunosuppressive therapy. Approximately 75% of patients are homosexually

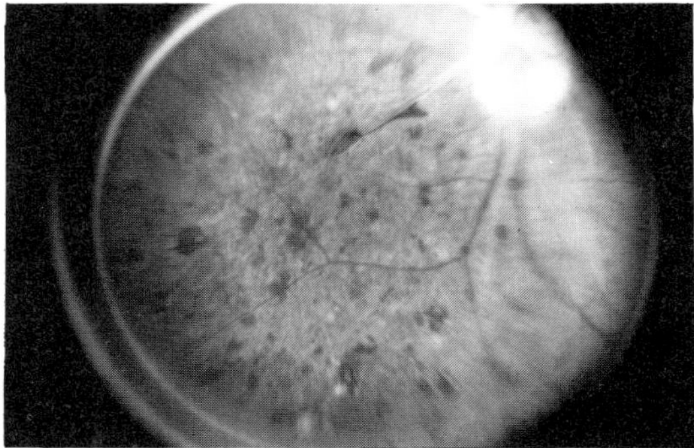

Fig. 17-10. Pigmentary changes of the fundus in a patient with congenital syphilis. (From the Department of Ophthalmology, Mayo Clinic.)

active men; 13% are intravenous drug abusers with no history of homosexuality; 6% are Haitian immigrants who are not homosexual and do not use drugs; 0.7% are patients with hemophilia; and approximately 5% have no apparent risk factor. Ocular involvement may include cotton-wool spots, retinal hemorrhages, retinitis, choroidal granulomas, conjunctivitis, keratitis, and Kaposi's sarcoma, a tumor that may be found on the conjunctiva and eyelids.

C H A P T E R 18

NEUROOPHTHALMOLOGY

The *nervous system* of the human body is that part that receives and reacts to the multitudinous number of stimuli that make humans aware of their environment. This system, made up of the *brain,* the *spinal cord,* and a complex network of *nerves,* coordinates the body's activities and responds to signals from both inside and outside the body. When the area in and about the eye, eyelid, or eye muscle is affected, the subspecialty of neuroophthalmology is involved. *Neuroophthalmology* is that branch of ophthalmology that deals with the nervous system associated with the eye. It is in this area that the neurologist, internist, family doctor, and ophthalmologist interrelate eye findings with systemic manifestations and pinpoint diagnosis both as to site and to pathology and identify an exact area of the brain or tract of the cranial nerves. In this area signs may play a greater role than symptoms because often patients may show ophthalmological signs of increased intracranial pressure or optic atrophy indicative of a brain tumor and yet remain symptomless.

Neuroanatomy

Our knowledge of neuroanatomy began in ancient times during which the brain was always regarded as the seat of intelligence and the master of the body. The anatomy of the eye-to-brain pathways has been studied since these early times. Plato and his followers believed that the optic nerve was a messenger between the eye and the brain, serving as a conduit for a substance called pneuma. Pneuma was thought to travel from the brain to the eyes, where it met and communicated with light outside the body. The anatomists (circum 450 BC) viewed the role of the optic mechanism more passively, believing it received miniature complete reproductions of the seen object. In some ways this resembles some more modern theories of visual mechanics but does not embrace a geometric theory of action. The Romans continued the Platonic tradition of regarding the optic nerve as a transmitter of the energies of the soul, which they believed to reside in the brain. Galen, the Greek physician who lived in Roman times, subscribed to this theory and added considerable anatomical data. Abu Al-Hasab ibn Al-Haytham, also known as Alhasan, proposed in the tenth century that images flowed from the eye to the brain. The electrical nature of nerve transmission, as we now understand it, was discovered by Galvani in 1792 with his famous frog-leg experiment.

The *brain,* weighing about 3 pounds, is the center of the nervous system, coordinating the messages from all areas. From the brain, 12 *cranial nerves* arise. The *ophthalmic area* represents six of the 12 cranial nerves in which the second, third, fourth, fifth, sixth, and seventh all have some role to play. Two of the nerves, the second and fifth, are *sensory,* receiving stimuli, whereas the rest are motor nerves. The second, or *optic,* nerve (Greek *optikos,* "an eye") carries visual impulses to the *occipital area* (Latin *oc,* "back of," and *caput,* "head"), or back of the head, where it is interpreted by the brain. The fifth, or *trigeminal,* nerve (Latin *tres,* "three," and *geminus,* "a twin," thus *trigeminus* means "triplets") has three branches, which carry the sensory fibers of pain and touch to the brain. The other nerves, the third, fourth, sixth, and seventh, are motor nerves along which the brain sends to the eyelid and eye muscles its orders to react. The third, or *oculomotor,* nerve is the chief motor nerve that moves the eye muscles, not only those that move the eye but also those that constrict the pupil. The fourth, or *trochlear,* nerve, derived from the Latin word for "pulley," is so named because the nerve courses through a pulley mechanism in the frontal bone. The name of the sixth, or *abducens,* nerve is derived from its action of leading the eye away from the center, or "abducting" the eye. In addition to this, an *autonomic nervous system* exists, which is outside our conscious or voluntary control and controls functions such as the heart, blood vessels, and glands.

The pupil

The pupil is the center of the iris, the latter structure opening and contracting to permit the pupil to transmit light in the proper amount to form a clear image on the retina. When a pupil is contracted, it is said to be *miotic.* When the pupils of each eye are of unequal size, *anisocoria* is said to occur. The lens acts to provide accommodation for focusing an image at varying distance. Alterations of these two functions occur in a number of neuroophthalmological disorders, and some famous names have been associated with atypical pupils.

Adie's, or *myotonic,* pupil is a type of abnormality in which there is diminished or absent constriction to light stimulation but pupillary constriction to accommodation. *Argyll Robertson* pupil, named after Robertson who first described it in the Edinborough Medical Journal in 1869, is a type of pupil found in syphilis in which direct and consensual light reflexes of the pupil are absent but there is still a brisk response to accommodation for near objects. *Amaurotic pupillary paralysis* occurs in an eye blind from retinal or optic nerve disease in which the pupillary direct reflex is absent, but on stimulation of the fellow eye, the consensual reflex is present. *Horner's syndrome,* described by Johann Horner, a Swiss

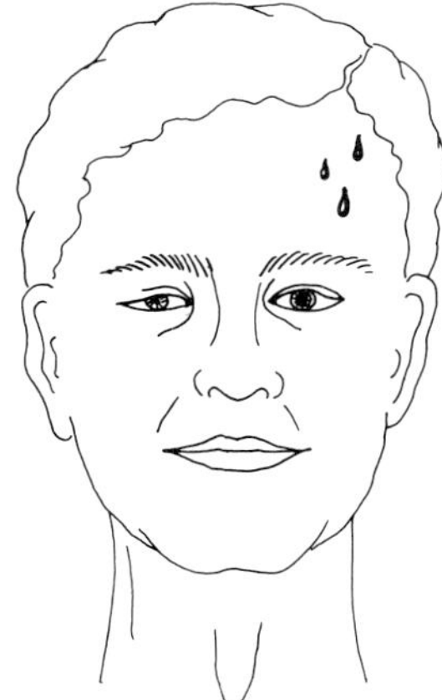

Fig. 18-1. Horner's syndrome: myosis, ptosis, and absence of sweating on the same side of the face.

ophthalmologist, results in a *miosis* (constriction of the pupil) associated with slight *ptosis* (drooping of the eyelid) and apparent enophthalmos and absent sweating on the same side of the face all caused by paralysis of the sympathetic nerve (Fig. 18-1). *Hippus* is spasmodic dilation and constriction of the pupil independent of stimulation with light.

The eyelid muscles and intraocular muscles

Ophthalmoplegia is derived from *plegia,* meaning "paralysis," and so *chronic progressive ophthalmoplegia,* sometimes called *progressive nuclear ophthalmoplegia,* is a progressive paralysis of all the ocular muscles including the elevator muscle of the eyelid.

Ocular muscle palsies, or paralysis, may be *supranuclear* (situated above the ocular nuclei in the upper brain stem), in which condition they are bilateral disturbances such as gaze palsies to one side, yet the eyes are parallel and diplopia is absent; or *ocular* palsies, which may be *nuclear,* involving the nucleus of the nerve in the brain in which there is paralysis of muscles of one or both eyes; *internal,* involving the involuntary muscles that affect the pupil; or *external,* involving the outer muscles that move the eye. The latter results in a loss of parallelism of the eyes and diplopia. *Stem palsies* are caused by lesions affecting the nerve fibers as they pass through the brain and are usually unilateral with dilated pupil and loss of accommodation if the third nerve is involved. Because of involvement of neighboring structures, there are often associated signs and symptoms so that typical syndromes develop.

Benedikt's syndrome is a paralysis of the third nerve on one side with tremor of the face and limbs on the opposite side. *Weber's syndrome* is paralysis of the third nerve on one side with half paralysis of the face and limbs of the opposite side. *Foville's syndrome* is paralysis of the sixth nerve on one side with loss of conjugate deviation of the eyes to the same side, facial paralysis of the same side, and paralysis of the opposite limbs. The *Millard-Gubler* syndrome is similar to Foville's syndrome without the paralysis of the conjugate gaze.

Aberrant regeneration of a nerve following trauma results in misdirection of a regenerating nerve so that it regenerates in the wrong direction. If it involves the facial nerve, it may result in paradoxical facial sweating with eating *(Frey's syndrome)* or tearing with eating *(crocodile tears).* If it involves the third nerve, the pupil may constrict, or the lid may retract when the eye is adducted.

Disorders that may affect the optic nerve

The optic nerve, which extends from the posterior pole of the eye to the chiasm, carries two sets of nerve fibers, the visual fibers and the pupillomotor fibers. The optic nerve reflects disturbances caused by pressure from cerebrospinal fluid, by direct compression of the nerve fibers from new growths, or by toxic or anoxic changes that alter its electrical conductivity. One of the greatest problems in these and other neurological disorders is that similar symptoms and signs are shown by a wide variety of disorders of different causes.

Optic neuritis is an inflammation of the optic nerve. It may be a *papillitis,* an inflammatory process that involves the head of the optic disc that can be seen ophthalmologically, or may be a *retrobulbar neuritis,* an inflammation that lies behind the visible head of the optic nerve and is not seen clinically. *Multiple sclerosis,* a chronic relapsing demyelinating disorder of the central nervous system, is a frequent cause of this condition. Multiple sclerosis follows retrobulbar neuritis in 25% of cases. *Devic's* disease, or *neuromyelitis optica,* is a rare demyelinating disease of the central nervous system that causes bilateral optic neuritis and paraplegia in children.

Papilledema, or *choked disc,* is a noninflammatory congestion of the optic disc associated with increased intracranial pressure (Fig. 18-2). It is most commonly

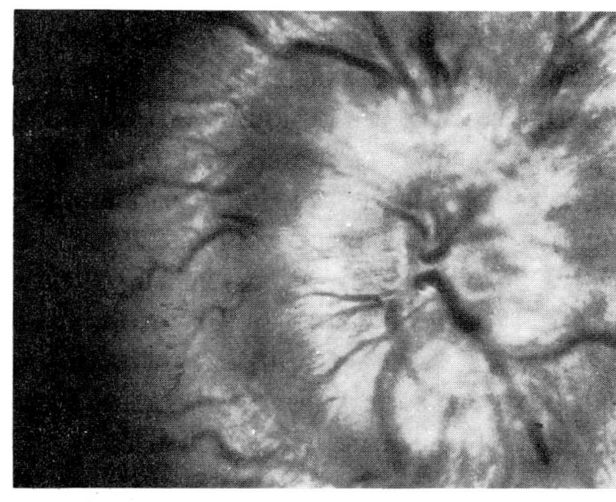

Fig. 18-2. Papilledema.

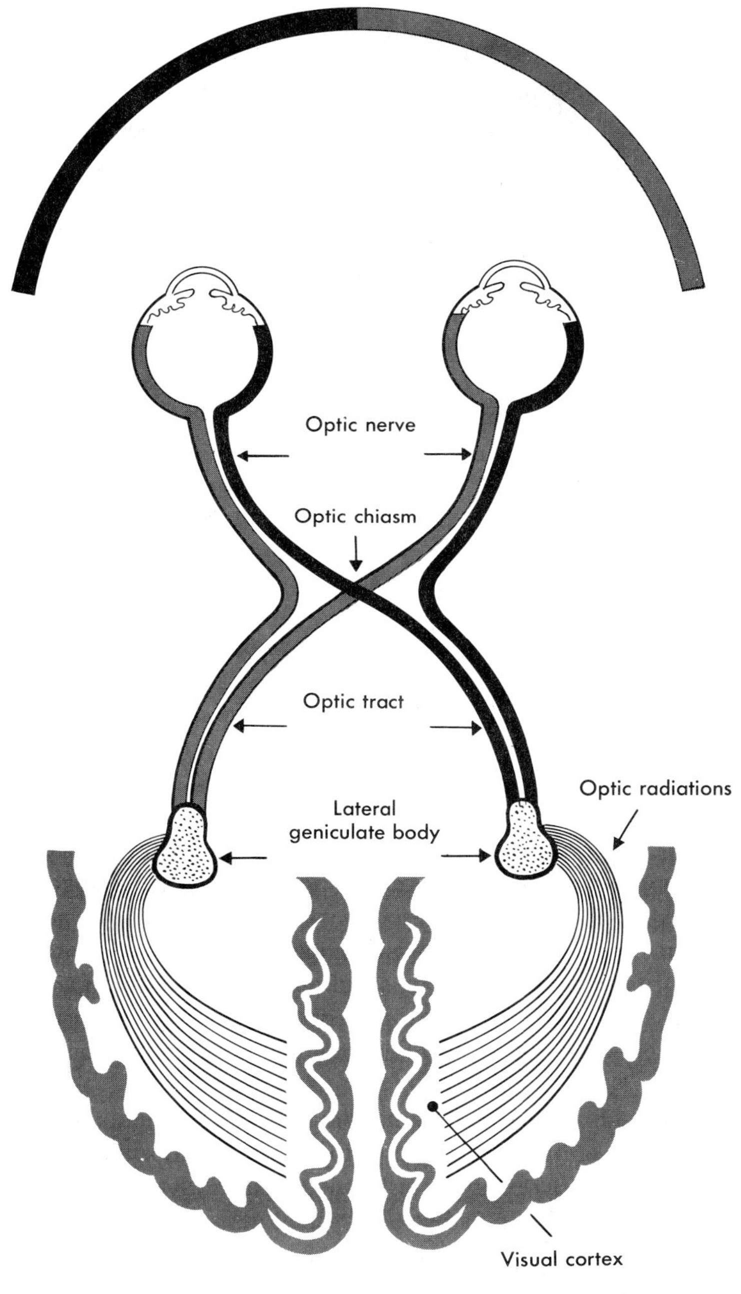

Fig. 18-3. Visual pathway. One half of the visual field from each eye is projected to one side of the brain. Thus visual impulses from the right visual field of each eye will be transmitted to the left occipital lobe.

associated with brain tumors, although other causes include increased production of cerebral spinal fluid and venous sinus obstruction.

Optic atrophy is an implied condition. The optic nerve appears pale, so it is considered to be atrophic, either in that there is tissue loss or ischemia to the nerve or both. Optic atrophy occurs in a variety of conditions from tumors pressing on the optic nerve, to toxic conditions of the eye (quinine or lead poisoning), to glaucoma. Optic atrophy, or withering of the optic nerve, is seen in *Leber's disease,* a rare hereditary progressive form of optic atrophy occurring in young men and appearing as a pale, optic nerve head.

Disorders that may occur along the visual pathways

The *visual pathways* represent the pathways of the nervous system from the origins in the eye to their final end at the occipital area of the brain. Any interruption in this pathway may result in a disturbance in the visual system (Fig. 18-3).

Intrasellar tumors are tumors that lie within the sella turcica. *Pituitary* tumors arising from the pituitary gland are the most common lesions in this area.

The *optic chiasm,* the area of crossing of nasal fibers of the retina and their extension through the optic nerves, is affected not only by intrasellar tumors but also by suprasellar tumors (above the sella), which can cause compression. *Craniopharyngioma* is a common example of the latter arising from remnants of Rathke's pouch along with *meningiomas,* or tumors arising from the meninges, which may create pressure on the chiasm. Such effect on the chiasm gives rise to *chiasmal syndromes,* which classically can identify the location of the tumor when visual field measurements are performed. The timing of a bitemporal hemianopia is the classic field defect that invariably points to a chiasmal syndrome.

The central nervous system

A number of tumors arise in the central nervous system, some common and many rare. An *acoustic neuroma* is a common tumor of the eighth cranial nerve. *Neurofibroma* is a tumor of nerve consisting of proliferation of Schwann cells. *Pseudotumor cerebri* is a condition of benign intracranial hypertension not resulting from tumor but producing many of the symptoms and signs of a brain tumor.

Disorders caused by congenital malformations may result from premature closing of the suture lines of the skull as occurs in *craniostenosis.*

Cerebrovascular accident is a stroke resulting from occlusion, vascular insuf-

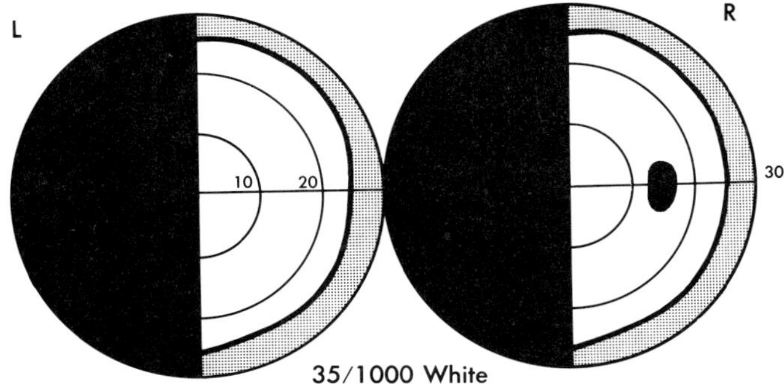

Fig. 18-4. Left homonymous hemianopia.

ficiency, or hemorrhage of an intracranial artery. It may give rise to *hemianopia* (half vision), a term implying seeing out of only one half of the visual field (Fig. 18-4).

Neuroophthalmological investigation

The first recording of the electrical activity of the brain was made by Hans Berger, who invented the *electroencephalograph* in 1928. In 1935 at a meeting of the Physiological Society Adrian and Matthews proved that Berger had in fact discovered the rhythms of the brain through an intact skull.

A number of clinical tests such as the electroencephalogram aid in neurological assessments in arriving at a diagnosis. Some of these tests are described in the following paragraphs.

The *Amsler grid* consists of a series of patterned grids for testing the central 20-degree field at reading distance. It is primarily used to test macular function.

Angiogram refers to x-ray film findings, following the injection of dye into the vascular tree so it can be visualized intracranially and extracranially. *Venography* of the orbit is the radiological investigation of the orbital veins to detect space-occupying lesions in the orbit that may be compressing the orbital veins.

An *electroencephalogram (EEG)* is a recording of the resting activity of the brain. An *electrooculogram (EOG)* is a recording of the resting potential of the eye. An *electronystagmogram (ENG)* is a recording of eye movements. An *electromyogram (EMG)* is the recording of the electrical activity of an extraocular muscle.

CAT scan refers to *computerized axial tomography,* in which serial sections of the brain (or body) are studied by computerized radiographic technique. The abbreviation CAT is formed by the first letters of the technique's name.

Ventriculography is the radiological investigation of the ventricles of the brain to detect a space-occupying lesion in the brain.

Ultrasonography is a test using high-frequency, inaudible ultrasound waves to outline interference patterns in either the brain or eye.

The *edrophonium (Tensilon) test* is an intravenous test using this pharmaceutical agent to diagnose the presence of myasthenia gravis, a disorder characterized by variable ptosis and fluctuating ocular muscle palsies.

Ophthalmodynamometry is a test used to determine the central ophthalmic artery blood flow. Pressure is applied to the eye, then the pulse and blanching of the central retinal artery are recorded. This test is primarily used to detect carotid artery disorders. This test has been replaced by the Doppler test to measure carotid blood flow.

Other neuroophthalmological terms follow in alphabetical order.

A

aberrant degeneration of the third nerve: follows lesions of the third nerve in which nerve fibers originally connected to one muscle grow into the sheaths of another (i.e., nerve fibers to inferior rectus grow into the levator palpebrae superioris so the lid retracts on attempted down gaze).

acoustic neuroma: a tumor of the eighth cranial nerve manifest by vertical nystagmus, papilledema, ataxia, and hearing difficulties.

acromegaly: pituitary tumor producing excess growth hormone and marked by an increase in growth of skeletal tissues of the hands, face, head, and feet. The tumor may result in pressure signs on the optic chiasm.

adenoma: tumor of glandular tissue (e.g., the pituitary gland), which secretes many regulatory hormones such as adrenocorticotropic hormone (ACTH).

Adie's pupil: consists of inability of the pupil to respond to light on near stimuli. The pupil does respond to a fresh 2½% solution of Mecholyl (methacholine chloride). It is usually unilateral, occurring in young women who have absent knee or ankle reflexes.

agraphia (visual): loss of ability to write.

amaurosis: complete blindness.

amaurosis fugax: unilateral, transient loss of vision caused by transient ischemic episodes in the retinal vascular tree. Frequently it is a symptom of carotid artery disease.

amaurotic familial idiocy: Tay-Sachs disease, characterized by a progressive neurological degeneration with the characteristic cherry-red spot at the posterior pole. This disease is a congenital lipid storage disorder occurring with greatest frequency in Jewish children.

amaurotic pupil: characterized by the absence of direct light reaction with preservation of the consensual reaction in a blind eye.

aneurysms: a weakness from an outpouching of an artery or arteriole. Most aneurysms affecting the optic nerve arise from either the internal carotid or anterior cerebral arteries. Microaneurysms of the retinal arteries are common in diabetic patients.

anisocoria: unequal pupil size.

Anton's syndrome: denial of blindness in patients blind from occipital lobe lesions.

aortic arch syndrome: bilateral occlusion of the carotid arteries is seen in Takayasu's disease.

aphasia: inability to speak, while the ability to understand is intact.

aplasia of the optic nerve: failure of the optic nerve to form; it is seen as a rudimentary structure small and pale.

apoplexy of the pituitary: spontaneous hemorrhage in a pituitary adenoma.

apraxia: loss of willed or purposeful movements despite the clinical demonstration of intact motor pathways.

arachnoiditis: inflammation of the basal leptomeninges, which may cause progressive visual loss in the region of the optic chiasm.

arcuate scotoma: characteristically arc-shaped area of blindness in the field of vision; caused by interruption of a nerve-fiber bundle in the retina; most often seen in glaucoma.

area 17: the striate area concerned with the reception of primary visual stimuli in the occipital lobe.

Argyll Robertson pupil: characterized by an absence of the reaction to light by a miotic pupil with preservation of the reaction to near stimulus.

Arnold-Chiari malformation: congenital disorder with herniation of the brain stem through the foramen magnum of the skull.

arteriography: method of outlining the arteries of the brain and other vessels through the injection of an opaque dye.

arteriosclerosis of the retina: characterized by a broadening of the arteriole light reflex, tortuosity of the vessels, spotty occurrence of plaques on the arterial walls, and venous nicking and banking. It is an age-related disease.

arteritis: inflammation of an artery as seen in temporal arteritis.

cranial: chronic granulomatous inflammation of the temporal artery, which may be associated with involvement of the ocular circulation and result in blindness.

ataxia: unsteadiness of gait.

aura: a visual, sensory, or motor sensation that precedes a migraine headache. It usually lasts 15 to 20 minutes.

axon: a nerve.

B

Balint's syndrome: occurs as a result of bilateral disease of the parietotemporal areas and causes loss of voluntary eye movements and loss of visual recognition.

Behcęt's disease: a condition marked by relapsing ulcers of the mouth, eye, and genitalia with chronic uveitis and hypopyon. Optic neuritis is also a frequent feature of this disease.

bitemporal hemianopia: classic bitemporal field defect resulting from compression of the chiasm.

blind spot: the natural blind area of the retina where the optic nerve enters the eye.

bobbing: disordered ocular movements in comatose patients with lower pontine lesions; intermittent rapid downward movement of eyes with slow return to primary position.

Bourneville's disease: synonymous with tuberous sclerosis, a condition affecting the retina. it is often associated with sebaceous adenoma of the face.

brainstem: consists of midbrain, pons, and medulla of the central nervous system.

bruit: audible flow of blood heard with a stethoscope such as occurs in occlusive disease of the carotid artery and in a carotid-cavernous fistula. Bruits are heard whenever there is turbulence in the blood flow.

Buller's shield: a watch glass set in jaconet with the purpose of covering and protecting the eye.

C

café au lait spots: localized area of pigmentation of the skin in Albright's disease, juvenile xanthogranuloma, and neurofibromatosis.

caloric testing: a test performed by placing cold or warm water in the external ear and observing the eye movements to detect neurological lesions.

campimeter: an instrument for determining the integrity of the central field of vision.

carotid-cavernous fistula: rupture of a carotid aneurysm into the cavernous sinus (infrasellar), which causes an increased venous pressure in the sinus; also occurs with dural shunt. Results in severe pulsating enophthalmos.

computerized axial tomography (CAT scan): a radiographic method of outlining any soft tissue mass.

cavernous sinus: a large venous plexus that contains all the oculomotor nerves and the ophthalmic branch of the trigeminal nerve.

cavernous sinus thrombosis: a serious, often fatal, illness resulting from thrombosis of the cavernous sinus adjacent to the pituitary fossa.

cephalic: pertaining to the head or to the head end of the body.

cephalgia: head pain.

cerebral palsy: a term to describe the condition of a mixed group of patients with damage to the nervous system in utero, at birth, or in early life.

cerebrospinal fluid: fluid surrounding the central nervous system.

cervical: related to the neck.

Charcot's triad: nystagmus, intention tremor, and scanning speech, all of which occur as a late sign in demyelinating disease, particularly multiple sclerosis.

chiasm (chiasma): the crossing of the nasal nerve fibers of the retina to form a single bundle of fibers—the chiasm.

choked disc: swelling of the optic nerve, usually visible with the ophthalmoscope.

cholesterol emboli (plaque of Hollenhorst): fragment that breaks off ulcerative atheroma of internal carotid artery and enters retinal circulation. It may be responsible for central or branch retinal artery closure.

cluster headache: severe unilateral head or facial pain that lasts minutes to hours, often associated with lacrimation, nasal congestion, and facial flushing; occurs in clusters over days, weeks, or months.

cogwheel pursuit movements: replacement of smooth following eye movements by jerky following eye movements. It occurs in Parkinson's disease.

coma: a state of profound unconsciousness.

comitance (concomitance): movement of the two eyes in constant relationship for all directions of gaze, usually indicating absence of paralysis of an extraocular muscle.

congruous field defects: visual field defects that are exactly the same in extent and intensity in both eyes; characterizes lesions in the occipital cortex.

convulsions: involuntary abnormal motor movements resulting from a lesion in the central nervous system.

corpus callosum: the major pathway connecting the two halves of the brain. The posterior portion, called the splenium, is concerned with integration of opposite halves of the visual field.

Cowen's sign: jerky pupillary constriction to a consensual light stimulus. A sign of Graves' disease.

cranial arteritis: see *arteritis.*

craniopharyngioma: benign tumor of the stalk from embryonic remnants of Rathke's pouch that connects the pituitary gland to the brain. This tumor can press on the chiasm and thereby destroy it.

craniostenosis: inherited premature closure of the skull suture lines; of ophthalmological interest because of the frequency with which an abnormally shallow orbit develops and because bony construction may cause increased intracranial pressure, papilledema, and cranial nerve damage.

craniotomy: neurosurgical operation involving direct visualization of the brain. Requires performing a "bone flap" to provide an opening to the brain tissue in the skull.

D

degeneration: see *hepatolenticular degeneration.*

demyelinizing: loss of protective myelin sheath of nervous tissue, such as occurs in multiple sclerosis.

demyelinating disease: disorders producing loss of the myelin sheath of a nerve and most commonly caused by disseminated (multiple) sclerosis.

diabetes insipidus: disorder characterized by an abnormally excessive output of urine and by an abnormally excessive thirst. It is caused by disorders in the hypothalamic system.

diabetes mellitus: disorder of carbohydrate metabolism characterized by an elevated blood glucose (sugar) level. Ocular involvement includes cataracts, ocular motor palsies, and retinopathy.

diplopia: double vision, usually caused by a paresis or paralysis of one of the extraocular muscles.

disequilibrium: disturbance of balanced locomotion.

doll's-head reflexes: movement of the eyes from side to side when the head is turned or flexed, occurring in the conscious patient while fixation is maintained and in the unconscious patient without fixation. It is an induced, passive ocular movement created by head movements to differentiate supramuscular disorders from muscular disorders. It is a suprasellar disorder.

drift: involuntary, slow, micro eye movements that occur between flicks or micro saccades.

dwarfism: short stature, such as in pituitary dwarfism; associated with a number of syndromes.

dysautonomia: disorder of the autonomic nervous system that may affect the autonomic supply to the eye (e.g., Riley-Day syndrome).

dyslexia: a comprehensive term denoting inability to read that may be functional or organic.

dysmetria, ocular: a sign of cerebellar disease, consisting of abnormality of ocular movements in which there is an overshoot of the eyes when an attempt is made to fixate an object.

dystrophy: a bilateral inherited disorder.

myotonic: inability to involuntarily relax a contracted muscle, associated with frontal baldness, testicular atrophy, cataracts, and macular degeneration.

oculopharyngeal: involves extraocular muscles and pharynx with associated difficulty in swallowing.

E

Eales' disease: a disease characterized by sheathed and occluded vessels in the retinal periphery, new vessel formation, and retinal hemorrhage.

Edinger-Westphal nucleus: the autonomic part of the third nerve nucleus that gives rise to the pupillomotor fibers.

emboli: debris in the vascular system, which may be lipid, calcium, or fibrin; emboli can occlude the retinal arteriolar system. The prime sources for emboli are the internal carotid arteries and the heart.

encephalitis: inflammation of the brain.

encephalocele: protrusion consisting of herniated brain tissue.

epilepsy: sudden attacks of convulsions or unconsciousness or both.

F

Fisher's syndrome: involvement of extraocular muscles with acute idiopathic polyneuropathy; characterized by oculomotor palsies, areflexia, and ataxia.

fistula: communication between two blood vessels, such as the carotid-cavernous fistula.

flashlight test: test to detect the presence of an afferent pupillary defect, such as Gunn pupil (see Fig. 10-4).

Foster Kennedy's syndrome: optic atrophy in one eye with papilledema in the other eye, frequently caused by an olfactory groove meningioma.

Frey's syndrome: paradoxic gustatory facial sweating as a result of aberrant regeneration of facial nerve following Bell's palsy.

frontal nerve: branch of the ophthalmic division of the trigeminal nerve.

G

Gassian ganglion: ganglion of the fifth, or trigeminal, nerve.

geniculate body: a relay station in the central nervous system for the transmission of visual impulses from the optic tract to the optic radiation of the brain.

geniculocalcarine radiation: a tract of visual fibers that begins at the lateral geniculate body and traverses the posterior end of the internal capsule. One portion of the tract representing fibers of the upper retinal half of the crossed and uncrossed fibers goes directly to the occipital cortex, whereas that group of fibers representing the lower retina passes over the temporal horn of the lateral ventricle before passing to the occipital cortex.

giant cell arteritis: see *temporal arteritis.*

glioma: a tumor arising from nerve tissue of either the optic nerve or brain.

gliosis: astrocytic scar proliferation on or within the retina.

Gradenigo's syndrome: palsy of lateral rectus muscle (sixth nerve) and severe unilateral headache as in suppurative disease of middle ear.

Guillain-Barré syndrome: a neurological syndrome of unknown origin (probably viral) that causes progressive neuromuscular paralysis. The characteristic finding is an increased level of protein in the cerebrospinal fluid without an increase in cellular count. See *polyneuritis.*

Gunn pupil: a pupillary reaction in which, although both the direct and consensual reactions are present, the contraction is not maintained with bright illumination so that the pupil slowly dilates again although the light continues to be directed on the affected eye. This pathological redilation occurs much more rapidly than the normal return in pupil size brought about by retinal adaptation to the light stimulus.

Gunn's jaw-winking phenomenon: congenital ptosis associated with jaw winking. On closing the jaw or chewing, one eyelid winks as a result of aberrant connection of the nerve to the third nerve.

Gunn's pupillary reflex: relative afferent pupillary defect as elicited by the swinging flashlight test. Paradoxial dilatation of the pupil as the light is withdrawn from the sound eye and applied to the affected eye.

H

hallucinations: perception without external stimulus that may occur in every field of sensation. Formed visual hallucinations are composed of scenes, and unformed are composed of sparks, lights, and the like; formed hallucinations characterize temporal lobe disturbances, and unformed visual hallucinations characterize occipital lobe disorders.

hemiatrophy (facial): atrophy or wasting of one half of the face.

hemiplegia: paralysis of one half of the body that may be associated with loss of one half of vision.

hepatolenticular degeneration (Wilson's disease): abnormality of copper metabolism associated with progressive degeneration of the liver, lentate nucleus, and mental retardation along with copper ring in the cornea.

heteronymous diplopia: crossed double vision.

Hollenhorst plaque: see *cholesterol emboli.*

homonomous hemianopia: loss of conjugate fields (i.e., loss of the right or left halves of the visual fields).

homonymous diplopia: uncrossed double vision.

Horner's syndrome: sympathetic nerve paralysis with miosis, enophthalmos, blepharoptosis, and anhydrosis of the face.

Hurler's syndrome (gargoylism): condition with abnormal mucopolysaccharides characterized by dwarfism, depressed nasal bridge, cloudy cornea, retinal degeneration, enlarged spleen and liver, and mental retardation.

hydrocephalus (internal, external): condition characterized by an enlarged ventricular system of the brain resulting from an accumulation of cerebrospinal fluid. The increased amount of fluid intracranially causes atrophy of the brain and possible enlargement of the skull in children.

hypertelorism: excessive width between two organs; in ocular hypertelorism there is increased distance between the eyes that is often associated with mental deficiency and exotropia.

hypophysectomy: surgical removal of pituitary gland.

hypopituitarism: underacting pituitary gland.

I

incongruous field defects: visual field defects that are dissimilar in the two eyes; such defects occur in lesions involving the optic radiation and the visual pathways anterior to the lateral geniculate body.

infectious polyneuritis (Guillain-Barré syndrome): a disorder characterized by an acute ascending paralysis of skeletal muscles, fever, and elevation of protein in the spinal fluid.

internal carotid artery: the artery that gives rise to the ophthalmic artery. The internal carotid artery traverses the cavernous sinus and originates from the aorta.

internal hydrocephalus: any obstruction to the internal flow of cerebral spinal fluid that can cause hydrocephalus (i.e., pinealoma).

internuclear ophthalmoplegia (INO): a combination of eye movement abnormalities attributed to a lesion of the medial longitudinal fasciculus (MLF). In the eye on the side of the lesion, adduction is limited. The other eye shows a jerky nystagmus on gaze to the side opposite the lesion. Convergence may or may not be decreased. If convergence is involved, it is thought that the medial rectus subnucleus of the third nerve is involved. Vertical nystagmus, especially on upgaze, and skew deviation are frequently associated.

iridoplegia: paralysis of the sphincter pupillae muscle of the iris.

ischemia: a comprehensive term covering all forms of inadequate blood supply to the eye.

K

Kearns-Sayre syndrome: chronic progressive external ophthalmoplegia involving the eye muscles and pigmentary tapetoretinal degeneration.

kinetic perimetry: visual field testing with a moving target whose size and luminance remain constant.

L

lamina cribosa: a sievelike portion of the sclera modified to permit passage of nerve fibers out of the eye.

latent nystagmus: a jerk type of nystagmus that is elicited by covering one eye.

lateral geniculate body: termination of the optic tract. As a relay station it transmits visual impulses to the geniculocalcarine radiation destined for the occipital cortex.

Leber's disease: sex-linked form of retrobulbar neuritis occurring at about 20 years of age. It causes optic atrophy and blindness in young men.

M

Marcus Gunn phenomenon: retraction of the upper lid with jaw movement (jaw winking).

medial longitudinal fasciculus: tract that coordinates the nuclei of the extraocular muscles with each other and with other nuclei in the brain stem.

Ménière's syndrome: a disease characterized by vertigo, nausea, vomiting, tinnitus, and progressive deafness.

meningeal hydrops: a condition of young adults most common in obese females that produces headaches, sixth nerve palsy, papilledema, and field defects.

meningioma: a benign tumor attached to and involving the dura mater that slowly expands to cause pressure on the brain and optic nerve pathway. It may result in visual field damage.

methyl alcohol intoxication: general toxic disorder that affects the eye by causing simple optic atrophy.

micro eye movements: small eye movements used in fixation and in position maintenance.

micronystagmus: very fine movements of the eyes normally present at all times.

migraine: a vascular headache, characterized by an aura lasting up to 30 minutes, a positive family history, and one-sided head pain that lasts 1 to 2 hours.

Millard-Gubler syndrome: paralysis of the sixth and seventh cranial nerves and contralateral hemiplegia of the extremities.

Möbius syndrome: facial weakness associated with palsy of the sixth nerve.

multiple sclerosis: a chronic, relapsing, multifocal demyelinating disease of the central nervous system frequently affecting the optic nerve or intrinsic nerves of the eye.

myasthenia gravis: a disorder of the neuromuscular junction characterized by progressive fatigue of the involved muscles with activity, often resulting in ptosis or double vision.

mydriasis: dilation of the pupil.

mydriatic: a dilating agent of the pupil that does not affect accommodation such as phenylephrine hydrochloride (Neo-Synephrine).

myelinated fibers: appear as white fluffy nerve fibers emerging from the disc; their presence is caused by retention of myelination in the retinal axons.

myelinated optic nerve fibers: presence of myelinated fibers in the nerve fiber layer of the retina.

myokymia: involuntary muscle contractions; when it affects superior oblique muscles it causes intermittent, monocular, torsional eye movements.

myotonia congenita: condition characterized by the failure of a contracting muscle to relax. It occurs primarily in children.

myotonic dystrophy: see *dystrophy, myotonic.*

N

neurilemoma: tumor of a nerve.

neuritis: inflammation of a nerve, as in optic or retrobulbar neuritis.

neurofibroma: tumor of a nerve consisting of a proliferation of Schwann cells.

neurofibromatosis (von Recklinghausen's disease): characterized by skin tumors, cutaneous pigmentation, multiple tumors arising from the nerve sheaths, abnormalities of bone, and defective central nervous system; often associated with ocular abnormality.

neuroparalytic keratitis: corneal condition secondary to disruption of the nervous supply of the cornea and characterized by decreased sensation.

nuclear magnetic resonance (NMR): a new technique of medical imaging in which the combined technologies of high magnetic field, radio frequency modalities, and computer manipulation of obtained data are used. The high resolution of the NMR scan makes this technique promising for the future evaluation of orbital and intracranial diseases.

nystagmus: an oscillating movement of the eyeball that may be horizontal, vertical, rotatory, or mixed; it may be congenital or acquired. It may be pendular or jerky.

optokinetic: rapid to-and-fro eye movement when a succession of moving objects traverses the field of vision such as occurs when gazing out of the window of a moving vehicle at a succession of stationary objects (synonym is railroad nystagmus).

pendular: rapid eye oscillations approximately equal in each direction.

rotatory: rapid eye movement partially rotating around the visual axis.

O

occipital lobes: comprise the posterior portions of visual radiation fibers and are concerned with the reception of primary visual stimulus.

oculocephalic reflexes (proprioceptive head-turning reflex, doll's-head eye phenomenon): the passive eye movements obtained as the head is rotated by the patient who is obtunded, unconscious, or unable to fixate. It usually occurs with fresh gaze palsies.

oculogyric crises: spasmodic deviation of the eyes, usually in an upward direction; occurs in Parkinson's disease.

ophthalmodynamometry: a test to determine the systolic and diastolic pressure in the ophthalmic artery by increasing the pressure on the globe until the central retinal artery shows signs of collapse.

opsoclonus: involuntary abnormal eye movement or jerkiness of the eyes that may occur in any direction; found in cerebellar disease.

optic atrophy: pallor of the optic nerve that implies loss of function.

optic foramen: opening in the lesser wing of the sphenoid through which passes the optic nerve.

optic nerve sheaths: a continuation of the meninges of the brain; called the dura, arachnoid, and pia.

optic tract: that portion of the visual conduction system that extends from the chiasm anteriorly to the lateral geniculate bodies posteriorly.

opticomyelitis (Devic's disease): bilateral optic neuritis with transverse myelitis.

optokinetic nystagmus: see *nystagmus, optokinetic.*

oscillopsia: the subjective sensation that the environment is oscillating; related to disorders of the vestibular system; occurs in multiple sclerosis.

osteogenesis imperfecta: a hereditary dominant connective tissue disorder characterized by brittle bones, multiple fractures, blue sclera, and deafness.

P

Paget's disease: bone thickening sometimes associated with angioid streaks and optic atrophy.

papilledema: a swelling of the optic nerve head secondary to raised intracranial pressure (see Fig. 10-1).

papillomacular nerve fiber bundle: nerve fibers passing from the macula to the temporal side of the optic nerve head.

parasellar syndrome: lesion in the vicinity of the pituitary gland causing classic signs and symptoms resulting from the interference of nerves in that region, that is, the third and fourth nerves plus the first branch of the fifth nerve.

parasympathetic: the autonomic nerve system that, in the eye, activates pupillary constriction.

parasympathomimetic: a chemical agent that mimics the action of the parasympathetic nerves, resulting in pupillary constriction.

Parinaud's syndrome: associated with pinealomas and is characterized by an up-gaze palsy, pupillary disturbances, and absence of convergence. The pupils do not react to light but do constrict on near gazing.

parietal lobe field defects: are homonomous and symmetrical; they begin in the lower quadrants of the visual fields on the side opposite the lesion.

past pointing: sign seen classically in cerebellar disorders (see *dysmetria, ocular)* in which the individual points past the indicated spot.

pendular nystagmus: nystagmus in which the oscillations to the right or left are approximately equal in rate and amplitude.

phakomatoses: group of disorders affecting the skin and nervous system including the eye. The most common disorders in this group are Bourneville's disease, neurofibromatosis, Sturge-Weber syndrome, and von Hippel-Lindau disease.

pinealoma: tumor of the pineal gland. It can cause lid retraction and up-gaze palsies.

pituitary adenoma: benign tumor of the pituitary gland; can press on the optic chiasm and thereby cause temporal fluid deficits.

pneumoencephalography: air study of intracranial structures usually used to detect the presence of space-occupying structures.

pontine gaze center (PGC): an area in the pons near the sixth nerve nucleus responsible for conjugate eye movements to the same side.

primary optic atrophy: simple atrophy (e.g., after treatment with methyl alcohol, quinine, ergot, and after retrobulbar neuritis). The visible optic nerve, the disc, appears pale and well defined.

proptosis: protrusion of the eyeball.

pseudopapillitis: nonpathological blurring of optic disc margins as occurs in hyperopia or drusen of the optic nerve without increased intracranial pressure or inflammation of the optic nerve head.

psychogenic: originating in the mind.

psychosis: a severe disease or disorder of the mind, characterized by derangement of the personality and loss of contact with reality.

psychosomatic: pertaining to the mind-body relationship; having bodily symptoms of a psychic, emotional, or mental origin.

R

Raeder's syndrome: Horner's syndrome accompanied by hemifacial pain.

Romberg's sign: unsteadiness of balance when eyes are closed.

S

saccadic eye movements: fast eye movements such as used with reading or elicited with the opticokinetic response.

scotoma: term used to describe an area of visual field loss. For example, an arcuate scotoma may occur in glaucoma, and a central scotoma may occur with macular or optic nerve disease.

scintillating scotoma: a temporary blind area in the field of vision associated with the impression of glittering, shimmering, or silvery lights, often preceding or accompanying migraine.

secondary optic atrophy: the optic nerve is pale, but the perimeter of the nerve is obscured by white glial tissue and the retinal vessels are sheathed (e.g., after papilledema or papillitis).

sella turcica: bony structure upon which the pituitary gland rests. It has a saddlelike appearance.

skew deviation: vertical imbalance of the eyes secondary to brain stem disorders; may give rise to diplopia.

static perimetry: visual field testing with a stationary target whose luminance changes.

Stellwag's sign: infrequent blinking; sign of Graves' disease.

Sturge-Weber syndrome: disorder characterized by a cavernous hemangioma of the face (birthmark). Late glaucoma, mental retardation, contralateral hemiplegia, epilepsy, and intracranial calcification are also manifestations of this syndrome.

subdural hematomas: a collection of blood under the dura that may act as a space-occupying lesion. They usually follow head injuries.

synapse: the anatomical junction between two nerve fibers.

T

Takayasu's disease: a widespread arteritis occurring in Japanese women that causes a deficient blood flow through the carotid arteries.

tangent screen: a fluid tinting device used for measuring the central 30 degrees of the visual field.

Tay-Sachs disease: an abiotrophy affecting Jewish infants who become blind, apathetic, and die within the first few years of life caused by an inborn error of metabolism.

temporal arteritis: a systemic disease of the elderly characterized by highly elevated sedimentation rate and a generalized giant cell arteritis. It is especially likely to occur in the temporal arteries. In the eye, it can cause blindness.

temporal lobe field defects: begin in the upper quadrants and are asymmetrical and homonomous.

toxic optic neuropathies: optic nerve damage caused by toxicity from such drugs as ethambutol, isoniazid, or methyl alcohol.

traction test: test done under anesthesia (local or general) to determine if the restriction of an eye movement is the result of a paralysis or a tethering or entrapment of the muscle. If caused by a paralysis, the eye moves easily; if the involved muscle is trapped or tethered, there is a restriction of eye movement.

transient ischemic episodes: known as transient ischemic attacks (TIA). Temporary loss of vision caused by the interruption of blood flow to the eye.

U

Uhtoff's syndrome: overheating the body or strenuous exercise can worsen the symptoms of multiple sclerosis.

V

venography, orbital: radiological investigation of the orbital veins to detect a space-occupying lesion in the orbit that may be compressing or distorting the orbital veins.

ventriculography: radiological investigation of the ventricles of the brain to detect, for example, a space-occupying lesion intracranially.

von Graefe's sign: lid retraction as in thyroid disease; sign of Graves' disease.
von Recklinghausen's disease: see *neurofibromatosis.*

W

Weber's syndrome: paralysis of the oculomotor nerve producing ptosis, strabismus, and loss of light reflex and accommodation on the same side of the lesion and spastic hemiplegia on the side opposite the lesion.
Wernicke's encephalopathy: syndrome resulting from thiamine deficiency and characterized by dementia, somnolence, ataxia, and oculomotor disturbances.
Wilson's disease: see *hepatolenticular degeneration.*

PART FOUR

SURGERY OF THE EYE

CHAPTER 19

CATARACT SURGERY

Surgical procedures have a language of their own. Most of our vocabulary is derived from either Greek or Latin. Word roots such as *ec,* meaning "out," and *tomy,* meaning "to cut," form the word *ectomy,* meaning "to cut out." This provides the basis for *keratectomy,* to cut out the cornea; *iridectomy,* to cut out the iris; *vitrectomy,* to cut out the vitreous; and *cyclectomy,* to cut out the ciliary body. When *tomy* is used alone in terms such as *keratomy* or *iridotomy,* it means to incise or cut into the cornea or iris, respectively.

The word *cataract* is from the Greek, meaning "something that rushes down" like a waterfall. It was the belief of the ancient Greeks and Romans that something like a grate fell down between the lens and the iris to cause the obstruction. *Couching of a cataract,* an ancient term still referred to, was a practice in Alexandria in the third century BC in which the opaque lens of the eye was depressed back into the vitreous to provide a clear pupil.

The most common form of cataract is *cataract senilis,* senile cataract, which affects older people and is considered a normal consequence of aging. Other types of cataracts are *galactose cataracts, diabetic cataracts, drug-induced cataracts,* and other *metabolic syndrome cataracts.* All of these forms of cataract are thought to be caused by a blocking or altering of enzymes involved in the synthesis of nutrients for the *subcapsular* layer of the lens. This is a layer of cells found on the equatorial surface of the lens capsule, one cell thick, and is the site of reproduction or growth of crystalline lens cells. Other types of cataract that are not enzyme related are *irradiation cataracts* (caused by radioactive irradiation) and various forms of *traumatic cataracts* that follow injury.

Surgery is the only accepted treatment for cataracts. There are two major categories of cataract surgery, *extracapsular extraction* and *intracapsular extraction.* Extracapsular extraction consists of making an opening in the anterior capsule, expressing the lens nucleus through the capsule, and removing it from the eye along with any cortical material, but leaving the capsule. Intracapsular extraction is the removal of the cataractous lens together with its capsule. These procedures may be combined in the treatment of cataracts with the insertion of an *artificial lens,* or *intraocular lens implant,* usually made of polymethylmethacrylate but also available in glass. The artificial lens may have a *haptic* (from

Greek *haptics,* "to lay hold of "), which supports the optical portion of the lens when implanted. After the surgery the state of *pseudophakia* (an eye with an artificial lens) is present. *Phakoemulsification* is a procedure in which the lens of the eye is removed by emulsification by high-frequency ultrasound waves. The term *phacogenic* is used as an adjective when the lens is responsible for causing such conditions as glaucoma.

The lens is covered with a *capsule.* Related surgical procedures include *capsulectomy,* in which part of the lens capsule is excised, and *capsulotomy,* in which an incision in the lens capsule is made. When a lens does not lay in its normal position, it is said to be *luxated* (Latin meaning "dislocated") or *dislocated.* If it is only partially displaced, it is said to be *subluxated.*

Other words related to cataract surgery include:

A

A scan: an ultrasound technique to determine the axial length of the eye to calculate the intraocular lens power required.

aftercataract: opacity of the posterior capsule or opaque lens remnant occurring after extracapsular lens extraction.

akinesia: absence of motor function. An anesthetic injection may be given before eye surgery to produce this effect on the eye and eyelid muscles.

anterior capsule: the anterior or front portion of the capsule that contains the cataract.

anterior capsulectomy: removal of the anterior portion of the capsule containing the lens.

anterior capsulotomy: an opening into the anterior capsule.

aphakic cystoid macular edema: edema of the macular area that occurs in an individual that has had a cataract removed.

aspiration: the removal of material from the aqueous or vitreous humor.

aspiration of lens: a method of cataract removal by breaking up and suctioning off the lens contents.

aspiration portal: an opening in the needle or irrigating aspiration device that usually ranges from 0.2 to 0.3 or 0.5 mm in diameter and is used for cortex aspiration.

automated machines: machines that can mechanically aspirate and irrigate with controlled inflow and outflow.

B

biometric ruler: an A scan used to determine the axial length of the eye.

bridle suture: a suture poised beneath the tendon of the superior rectus muscle to facilitate downward rotation of the globe.

buried sutures: the turning of sutures in the cornea or corneal scleral junctions so the knots are not exposed but buried in the tissue.

C

calibri forceps: a delicate fine-toothed forceps reserved for handling delicate tissues.

cataract: an opacity of the crystalline lens.

cataract nigra: black cataract.

cataractogenic drugs: drugs that can induce cataract formation that is, steroids.

choroidal detachment: a separation of the choroid from the sclera that may follow cataract surgery.

choroidal tap: method used to release the fluid causing a choroidal detachment.

closed chamber: the closure of the anterior chamber during cataract surgery to permit raising of the intraocular pressure to facilitate easier surgery.

closed eye surgery: any surgical technique that reduces the incision while maintaining the normal intraocular pressure.

congenital cataract: a cataract that is present at birth.

coronary cataract: any cataract of the lens cortex. The visible cataract may be spokelike opacities caused by water clefts in the lens cortex or feathery lines.

cortex aspiration: removal of cortical material from the lens of the eye.

cortical cleanup: the removal of all existing cortex.

couching: an ancient surgical procedure of displacing the lens into the vitreous cavity of the eye from the optical axis without opening the eye. It is usually performed by applying manual pressure on the closed eye.

cryoextraction: method of extraction of the lens of the eye using a frozen probe (cryoprobe) that adheres to the lens.

D

dehiscence: a gap in a wound resulting from rupture of sutures or from injury.

diathermy: a form of cautery to coagulate bleeding blood vessels.

dipstick: an instrument to measure the anterior chamber of the eye.

discission: needling of cataract to permit entrance of aqueous humor and absorption of the lens.

dislocated lens: displacement of the lens caused by ruptured zonules.

E

endophthalmitis: an inflammation of the entire eye including the outer coats.

epithelial downgrowth: a downgrowth of epithelium into the anterior chamber that may follow faulty wound healing; may be seen after cataract surgery.

epithelial ingrowth: see *epithelial downgrowth.*

erisiphake: from the Greek *erysis,* "a drawing." A small cup in which suction can be applied to grasp a cataract and its capsule and aid in its removal; an instrument now obsolete.

exfoliation of lens capsule: condition in which the anterior lens capsule degenerates and the sloughed cells appear on the lens surface.

extracapsular cataract extraction: a cataractous lens is extracted by means of first removing the anterior lens capsule, then the contents of the capsule (the lens, cortex, and nucleus) but leaving the posterior capsule intact.

extraction: removal. In cataract surgery, it refers to the surgical removal of the lens.

F

flat anterior chamber: a potential complication of intraocular surgery or penetrating corneal injury; it is characterized by the iris being in direct contact with the cornea, and also by the virtual absence of aqueous in the anterior chamber.

forceps: an instrument for holding tissue or suture.

H

Honan balloon: a balloonlike bag with controlled pressure to apply to the eye to reduce the pressure in a globe before surgery.

hypermature cataract: a cataract in which the lens of the eye becomes white, opaque, soft, and liquid.

hypopyon: the presence of purulent matter in the anterior chamber of the eye. It is usually seen as a yellow or whitish mass inferiorly in the anterior chamber.

I

incipient cataract: a cataract in its early stages of development.

intracapsular cataract extraction: removal of a cataractous lens including the intact capsule.

intraocular: within the eye.

intumescent: describing a swollen part, such as an intumescent cataract.

iridocyclitis: inflammation of the iris and ciliary body.

iridodonesis: a shimmering or tremor of the iris because of lack of support by a lens.

irrigating-aspirating units: an instrument or needle that will aspirate and irrigate at the same time.

iris bombé: the iris is bowed forward and occludes the angle structures.

iris prolapse: the herniation of a portion of the iris through the wound.

iris suture: a suture placed in the iris.

Irvine-Gass syndrome: cystoid macular edema with corneal-vitreous adhesions following cataract extraction.

L

lens dislocation: see *dislocated lens.*

lenticonus: rare abnormality of the lens characterized by a cone-shaped prominence on the anterior or posterior lens surface.

lenticular: pertaining to (or shaped like) a lens.

luxation of lens: complete rupture of the zonular fibers of the lens so that the lens falls into the anterior chamber or vitreous.

M

mature cataract: an opacity of lens of the eye that has become completely opaque.

McIntyre needle: a coaxial aspirating and irrigating needle for cortex removal in extracapsular surgery.

miotic: a drug used to constrict the pupil.

Morgagni's cataract: hypermature cataract in which the cortex is liquefied, permitting the lens nucleus to float within the capsule.

N

nuclear cataract: a cataract largely confined to the central portion of the lens, the nucleus. It is the most common cataract of the elderly.

nuclear expression: the mechanics of expressing the nucleus of the lens out of the eye.

nuclear sclerosis: hardening of the center of the crystalline lens, which causes it gradually to change in color from clear to yellow to brown and eventually leading to loss of vision and cataract formation. It is the most common senile change of the lens.

nylon: a synthetic material used for sutures.

O

O'Brien technique: a local anesthetic block of the facial nerve just anterior to the tragus of the ear to achieve paralysis of the orbicularis muscle.

P

phacoanaphylaxis: a delayed granulomatous uveitis from sensitivity to lens protein liberated by injury to the lens.

phacoemulsification: a technique of emulsifying lens material through the use of high-frequency sound waves.

polishing: a technique for scraping residual cortex and cells from the posterior capsule during extracapsular surgery.

posterior capsulotomy: an opening by surgery or YAL laser into the posterior capsule of the lens.

posterior chamber: space between the back of the iris and the vitreous fovea filled with aqueous.

posterior incision: a scleral incision behind the cornea limbus.

pseudoexfoliation: the production of amorphous, dandrufflike material in the eye. It is called pseudoexfoliation because of its superficial resemblance to true exfoliation of the lens capsule.

R

radiation cataracts: cataracts that are the result of conveying radiation from high-speed neutrons from cyclotron exposure or from atomic blasts.

red reflex: the ability to visualize a red reflex through the microscope or a muscle light as a result of reflection of light from the red choroidal vascular plexus underlying the retina.

retrobulbar: an injection into the muscle cone posterior to the globe to cause anesthesia of the eyes and akinesia of the extraocular muscles.

S

second sight: increase in myopia with improved reading ability, such as occurs in the early stages of cataract.

secondary membrane: a membrane that occurs following extracapsular cataract surgery.

senile cataract: an opacity of the lens occurring in the elderly.

sodium hyaluronate: a viscoelastic substance normally found in many parts of the body but can be made synthetically or extracted from animals (usually from rooster combs).

speculum: an instrument for holding the eyelids apart for exposure of the globe.

spherophakia: small round lens found in patients with certain mesodermal anomalies (Marchesani's syndrome).

sphincterotomy: a surgical incision in sphincter muscle of the iris.

striate keratitis: a form of keratitis in which small or large lines or striae appear on the cornea.

subluxation of the lens: blunt trauma to the eye causing dislocation of the lens by rupture of 25% or more of the zonular fibers of the lens.

sunflower cataract: a cataract resembling a sunflower; seen in Wilson's disease.

super pinky ball: a pink ball used to reduce intraocular pressure before surgery.

surgical keratometry: an instrument or device for measuring the curvature of the cornea at the operating table.

synechia: adhesion between the iris and other parts of the eye.

T

traumatic cataract: a cataract following any injury to the eye.

tumbling: in ophthalmology refers to a technique of intracapsular cataract removal in which the lens is removed by grasping the lower pole of the lens and tumbling it so the inferior portion of the lens is delivered first.

V

vacuuming: removal of the residual cortex cells of the posterior chamber by aspiration.

van Lint technique: an infiltrative diffusion of local anesthetic to achieve akinesia and anesthesia of the eyelids.

visco surgery: the use of solutions, putties, and gels with high viscosity to act as tissue support, for protection, for dissection, and for separation of an intraocular lens from other tissues of the eye.

vitreous loss: the loss of vitreous from the posterior chamber during cataract surgery.

X

X-ray cataracts: cataracts induced from X-rays that have a minimal dosage of 500 to 800 rads.

Z

zonulysis: dissolving of the zonules suspending the lens by a solution of alpha-chymotrypsin instilled into the eye to facilitate cataract extraction.

CHAPTER 20

INTRAOCULAR LENSES

Intraocular lenses are inserted into the eye to replace the human crystalline lens. Intraocular lenses are of an inert substance, usually *Perspex* or *polymethylmethacrylate*. Newer, softer lenses made of *hydrogels* and *silicone* are being investigated. The material required must be *inert*, meaning that it creates no biological irritation and must not be biodegradable. *Biodegradable* means it will degrade in time as a result of contact with the biological fluids or tissues that surround it.

Intraocular lenses are composed of an optical portion called the *optics* of the lens and the *haptics*. The optic portion has a *dioptric power* that permits the focusing of light onto the retina. The *size* of the optics will vary from 5.0 mm to 7.0 mm in diameter.

Haptics is from Greek, meaning "to lay hold of." The haptic refers to the method of holding the optical portion in place in the human eye. The haptic consists of loops made of either *polymethylmethacrylate* or *prolene*. The latter material is a suture material that has been found to be inert and not biodegradable within the human eye. Tantalum and metal loops have disappeared in the manufacture of intraocular lenses because of the adverse reaction they have produced on the human retina. Modern loop designs are usually *flexible* and permit some adjustment within the structure of the interior of the eye.

The shape of the optical portion may be *convex plano*, in which case the anterior portion of the lens is *convex* and the back surface is flat. They may have *reverse optics* in which the back surface of the lens is convex and the front surface is flat. They also may be *biconvex* in which both sides of the optical portion are convex. Some lenses are made *aspheric* in which there is an alteration in power from the center of the lens to the periphery.

Recent designs incorporate an *ultraviolet filter* into the optical portion of the lens. This eliminates wavelengths in the ultraviolet spectrum below 400 nm. Recent designs also incorporate a *laser ridge*. This is a ridge placed on the back surface of the lens in order to minimize damage to the lens that may occur when the YAG laser is used to open a posterior capsular membrane.

Optical portions may have *fenestrations* in which one or more small openings are made within the lens periphery to facilitate the technical movement of the lens within the eye.

Intraocular lenses may be classified according to their position and their method of fixation. They may be classified as to *anterior chamber lenses*, which include lenses that lie in the anterior chamber of the eye. These may be *angle supported*, in which case they are supported in the angle of the anterior chamber, or they may be *iris supported*, in which case they may be attached with or without sutures to the iris. Iridocapsular lenses are lenses that have been fixated to the iris and the capsule. Lenses may lie in the *posterior chamber*, and they may be supported either by *capsular support*, in which case they may be called *in-the-bag lenses* because they are fitted directly into the bag that contained the former crystalline lens. They may be *sulcus supported*, in which case they lie in front of the remainder of the anterior capsule and are supported in the sulcus of the eye. They may be *iris supported*, in which case they lie in the posterior chamber but are entirely supported by the iris. Iris-supported lenses are fast fading from popularity. Other words associated with intraocular lenses include the following:

A

angle-fixated lenses: lenses that are fixated in the angle of the anterior chamber.

angulation: lens loops are angulated so that the optical portion will be angulated backward for posterior chamber lenses and forward for anterior chamber lenses to lessen the incidence of iris irritation and entrapment by the pupil.

aphakia: refers to the absence of any lens within the eye.

B

Binkhorst four loop: historically important lens with four loops for fixation to iris and capsule.

C

capsular fixation: an intraocular lens that is placed within the capsular bag and depends on the capsule for its entire fixation.

cat's eye effect: the development of an irregular pupil that simulates the slit of a cat's eye.

closed loops: loops in which both ends of the loops are maintained within the system of the optic.

creep: the ability of the material to change its shape permanently to conform to its environmental pressure.

D

dialing: a method of inserting and moving an intraocular lens within the eye like the dial of a clock.

dislocation: the movement of a lens, either human or artificial, out of its correct anatomical position.

Drew's syndrome: intermittent touch syndrome; the result of an intraocular lens intermittently touching the cornea and resulting in endothelial cell death, ciliary flush, and cystoid macular edema.

dual lenses: intraocular lenses designed so they can be used in either the anterior or posterior chamber.

E

endophthalmodonesis: the shimmering or tremor of the iris as a result of lack of support.

F

flexible loops: loops that are compressible as opposed to loops that are rigid and firm.

footplate: the peripheral portion of an anterior chamber that lies like feet into the anterior chamber angle.

four-point fixation: refers to the touch of primarily anterior chamber lenses in four places of the anterior chamber angle. There are also some lens designs in the posterior chamber sulcus that provide four-point touch.

I

implant: an artificial insert placed in the eye, socket, or orbit.

implantation: the insertion of any material or substance within another substance.

L

lathe lenses: intraocular lenses that are manufactured by shaping on a machine lathe.

lens exchange: the changing of one intraocular lens for another within a human eye.

lens glide: a thin material placed in the eye to permit the intraocular lens to glide over it and aid in proper positioning.

lens-holding forceps: a forceps designed to hold an intraocular lens for insertion into the eye.

lens removal: the removal of an intraocular lens.

loops:

- ***J loop:*** a loop design similar to the letter "J."
- ***C loop:*** a loop designed like the letter "C." This allegedly places less outward pressure on the more curved loops than does the J loop design.
- ***modified J loop:*** modifications that have been made to the original J loop.

M

McCannel suture: a suture developed by Dr. Malcolm McCannel to correct a dislocation of an intraocular lens.

medallion lens: a lens shaped like a medallion that has been supported to the iris usually by a suture.

memory: the ability of a material to return to its original shape.

mold-injected lenses: intraocular lenses that are manufactured by a molding process.

O

one-piece lens: an intraocular lens that is made of a single material such as polymethylmethacrylate.

one-plane lens: an intraocular lens that lies in one plane.

open loops: loops in which one end is attached to the optical portion and the other end lies freely.

P

phakia: refers to the presence of the normal crystalline lens within the eye.

polymethylmethacrylate: a material used for intraocular lenses because it does not cause tissue reaction.

polypropylene: a material used either as loops on an intraocular lens or as suture material.

posterior dislocation: a lens that is dislocated posteriorly.

power: the strength of an intraocular lens measured in diopters.

primary lens implants: implants that are inserted at the time of cataract surgery.

propellering: the turning within the eye of an anterior chamber lens as a result of the smallness of its size in relation to the diameter of the anterior chamber.

pseudophakia: refers to the existence of an artificial lens within the confines of the eye.

pseudophakos: a false or artificial lens, such as an intraocular lens implant.

pupil block glaucoma: a condition in which the iris bows forward and a secondary rise in pressure occurs as a result of blockage of the aqueous flow from the posterior to the anterior chamber because of obstruction by the intraocular lens at the pupil.

pupillary capture: the condition in which all or part of the iris positions itself behind or in front of an intraocular lens in a position in which it was not intended.

pupillary entrapment: see *pupillary capture.*

pupillary lens: a lens that is held and centered in position by the pupil.

R

repositioning: the positioning of a displaced intraocular lens into its correct position.

resolving power: the quality of the optics of an intraocular lens in resolving lines on a test target.

ridge lens: a lens that has a small raised ridge to permit a gap area between the lens and the posterior capsule. This gap provides safety in preventing lens injury when performing a YAG capsulotomy.

S

secondary lens implants: implants that are inserted as a secondary procedure following cataract surgery.

soft intraocular lenses: intraocular lenses that can be folded and inserted through a small incision. These may be made of silicone or hydrogen material.

sphincter erosion: the development of breakdown of the iris sphincter as a result of iris and pupillary supported lenses.

sunset syndrome: the sinking or dislocation of an intraocular lens (like sunset) as a result of inadequate fixation in the posterior chamber.

T

two-plane lens: an intraocular lens that is designed to lie in a position at two levels within the eye.

U

UGH syndrome: a syndrome of uveitis, glaucoma, and hyphema occurring in an individual with an anterior chamber lens. Rarely it may occur following the implantation of a posterior chamber lens.

W

windshield wiper syndrome: the to and fro movement, similar to a windshield wiper, of a loose intraocular lens in the posterior chamber of the eye.

CHAPTER 21

GLAUCOMA SURGERY

Iridotomy arises from *tome*, to incise or cut, and refers to an incision of the iris. *Iridectomy* arises from *ec* and *tome*, in which *ec* means "out" and *tome* "to cut," so an iridectomy is a procedure in which a portion of the iris is cut out. This may be a *peripheral* iridectomy in which the outer portion of the iris is removed or a *sector* iridectomy in which a pie-shaped sector of the iris is removed. It is referred to as a *basal* iridectomy if the base of the iris is removed.

Other words used in glaucoma include the following:

C

cyclocryotherapy: destruction of a part of the ciliary body by freezing to reduce the quantity of aqueous produced.

cyclodialysis: an operation to reduce the intraocular pressure by forming a pathway for fluid from the anterior chamber to the space between the choroid and sclera.

F

filtering procedure: an operation for the release of aqueous into the subtenon or subconjunctival space by fistulization through the sclera.

flat anterior chamber: potential complication of intraocular surgery characterized by the iris being in direct contact with the cornea and by the virtual absence of aqueous in the anterior chamber.

G

goniotomy: a surgical procedure to treat infantile glaucoma. It includes opening the trabecular meshwork.

I

iridencleisis: a surgical procedure to correct glaucoma in which an incision is made at the corneoscleral limbus and the iris is incarcerated in the wound, creating a filtering wick between the anterior chamber and subconjunctival space.

irido-, irid-: pertaining to the iris.

iridocyclectomy: surgical removal of a portion of the iris and ciliary body; surgery indicated for tumors.

iridodonesis: trembling of the iris on eye movement, such as occurs with loss of lens support as in aphakia, dislocated lens, or pseudophakia.

L

laser iridectomy: a method of using the laser beam for making an opening in the iris to permit fluids to pass from the posterior chamber of the area in front of the iris, the atrium chamber.

laser trabeculoplasty: a method of using the laser beam for shrinking the trabecular meshwork to permit increased outflow of fluid from the anterior chamber to decrease intraocular pressure in glaucoma patients.

lens-induced: caused by the lens; a reaction such as glaucoma, usually by lysis, anaphylaxis, or dislocation of the lens.

P

peripheral iridectomy: procedure in which a section of iris is excised so that aqueous can drain from the posterior chamber to the anterior chamber. Performed routinely in cataract operations and to relieve postoperative attacks of angle-closure glaucoma; also performed as a primary procedure to cure most instances of angle-closure glaucoma.

S

sclerectomy: antiglaucoma operation that permits aqueous to escape through a notch cut from the sclera.

sector iridectomy: the incision of a sector of the iris from its base.

T

thermal sclerectomy: a drainage procedure for glaucoma that uses cautery.

thermosclerectomy: the opening of a cleft in the sclera by applying heat to the edge of the wound; used for glaucoma.

trabeculectomy: surgical removal of a portion of the trabeculum to increase the outflow from the eye.

trabeculoplasty: see *laser trabeculoplasty*.

trabeculotomy: surgical incision of the trabeculum.

trephination: drainage procedure for glaucoma that uses a trephine to excise a corneoscleral button.

CHAPTER 22

CORNEAL SURGERY

Word origins in corneas take their root from the Greek *kerato*, meaning "hornlike," because ancient Greeks believed the cornea resembled a thinly sliced horn of an animal.

When a cornea becomes cone shaped, the condition of *keratoconus*, or *conical cornea*, exists. If an inflammation (itis) affects the cornea, it is called *keratitis*. A corneal transplant is referred to as a *keratoplasty*. A transplant may be *penetrating*, in which full-thickness layers of cornea are replaced with a full-thickness layer from a donor. A transplant may be *lamellar*, in which the outer two thirds of the cornea is replaced. *Refractive keratoplasty*, introduced by José Barraquer in 1949, refers to surgical procedures to modify corneal curvature and alter refractive errors. *Keratomileusis*, derived from Greek words meaning *cornea* and *carving*, incorporates a lamellar section of the patient's own cornea lathed in either a positive or negative fashion and used to correct either myopic or hyperopic refractive errors. *Keratophakia* is a surgical alteration of the anterior radius of curvature of the cornea in which a positive lenticule is cut from a fresh donor cornea and is incorporated within the patient's corneal stroma. This is presently being used to eliminate aphakic refractive areas. *Radial keratotomy* is a surgical procedure in which multiple clocklike incisions are made into the cornea to flatten the cornea and eliminate or reduce the myopic refractive error. *Epikeratophakia* is a procedure designed and popularized by Kaufman and his co-workers in which a lenticule of donor cornea is sutured at the margins to a patient's cornea that is denuded of epithelium. *Keratoprosthesis* is an artificial synthetic cornea that is implanted into the corneal substance for visual rehabilitation in severely scarred corneas in almost blind eyes. It is usually of a plastic material. *Corneal implants* are materials implanted into the corneal stroma to alter the refractive power of the eye.

A surgical instrument used to open the anterior chamber by cutting the cornea is called a *keratome*, from the Greek *tome*, meaning "to incise."

A

alloplastic donor material: an inert graft, either glass or plastic.
astigmatism keratotomy: incisions in the cornea to reduce astigmatism.

autogenous donor material: a graft from the same individual.
autograft: removing and transplanting corneal tissue or any tissue of an individual back to the same individual.

B

blade gauge: a gauge to determine the extension of the blade beyond the guard.

C

coin gauge: a circular gauge designed to measure the depth of a diamond knife beyond its guard.
cryolathe: a lathing machine that freezes and grinds into a cornea.

D

depth gauge: an instrument to determine the depth of a corneal incision.
diamond knife: a blade using a gem-quality diamond as its cutting edge.

F

fixation instrument: an instrument used to fixate the globe.

G

glare: an annoying and undesirable sensation induced by light scattering.
graft:
corneal graft: a donor cornea is transplanted into a recipient eye.
full-thickness graft: a full-thickness corneal button is used.
lamellar graft: a partial-thickness corneal graft.

H

heterogenous donor material: a graft that is taken from an individual of a different species.
heterograft: transplantation from one species such as monkey to another species such as humans.
hockey stick: an instrument shaped like a hockey stick used to estimate the depth of a corneal incision, as for radial keratotomy.
homogenous donor material: a graft from an individual of the same species.
homograft: transplantation from one member of the same species such as humans to another member of the same species. This is the common type of corneal transplant.

K

keratectomy: removal of the anterior portion of the cornea.
keratotomy: any incision into the cornea.

L

laser keratotomy: the use of the laser beam to incise the cornea.

M

macroperforation: a large full-thickness corneal perforation that requires suturing to maintain the anterior chamber.

maladie du greffon: a clouding of the graft as a result of an antigen-antibody reaction.

McCarey-Kaufman medium (M-K medium): a tissue culture–soaking medium for storage and preservation of corneal tissue.

microperforation: self-sealing perforations of the cornea that may occur in radial keratotomy and relaxing incisions.

O

optical centering instrument: an instrument used to mark the visual axis center.

optical zone markers: corneal markers of varying sizes used to outline the optical zone of a cornea.

overcorrection: in radial keratotomy, the creation of more refractive correction than required.

R

radial keratotomy (RK): a surgical procedure in which radial incisions are made in the cornea to flatten the cornea and correct myopic refractive errors.

redeepening: a procedure in radial keratotomy in which radial incisions in the cornea already present are further incised to increase this depth to create more flattening.

relaxing incision: an incision through partial thickness into the cornea to reduce astigmatism.

ruby knife: a blade using a ruby as its cutting edge.

Ruiz procedure: a series of tangential cuts combined with radial cuts in the cornea designed to reduce astigmatism.

S

sapphire knife: a blade using a sapphire as its cutting edge.

superficial lamellar keratoplasty: a transplantation of the cornea, usually no deeper than the stroma, of diseased tissue; it is replaced by a transplanted donor cornea similarly excised.

T

thermokeratoplasty: alternation of the radius of curvature of the cornea by applying heat. Used for keratoconus to flatten by creating a thermal shrinkage to decrease the radius of curvature of the cornea.

T incisions: a relaxing type of incision used to relax in the meridian of steeper curvature of the cornea and reduce astigmatism.

U

undercorrection: in radial keratotomy, the creation of less refractive correction than required.

W

wedge resection: removal of a wedge of corneal tissue, either partial or full thickness. This technique may be used for the correction of astigmatism.

CHAPTER 23

EYELID, LACRIMAL, AND ORBITAL SURGERY

Blepharo is a Greek word meaning "eyelid." Such words as *blepharoplasty* refer to an alteration of the eyelid. *Blepharoptosis* refers to a ptosis or drooping of the eyelids. Repairs to the angle of an eyelid through the angle or canthi is referred to as *canthoplasty*. To open the angle, the procedure called *canthotomy* is performed.

Canthos is from Greek *kanthos*, meaning "angle of the eye." Repairs to the angle of the eye are called *canthoplasty*. Opening the angle of the eye is called *canthectomy*, meaning to incise the angle.

Dacryo is derived frrom the Greek *dakryon*, meaning "tear." *Cyst* means "sac" and *itis* means "inflammation," so *dacryocystitis* refers to any inflammation of the tear sac. *Rhino* refers to nose and *ostomy* is the suffix for opening, so *dacryocystorhinostomy (DCR)* is a surgical procedure in which a communication is made between a tear sac and the nasal cavity to relieve an obstruction in the nasolacrimal duct. *Dacryocysterectomy* is an excision of the lacrimal sac. When the conjunctiva or lining membrane of the eye is joined to the nasal cavity, the surgical procedure called *conjunctivorhinostomy* is performed.

When the eyelid rolls in, *entropion* is said to exist (from *en*, "in," and *tropia*, "to turn"). If the eyelid turns out, *ectropion* exists. Surgical procedures are referred to as *correction of entropion* or *ectropion* and frequently carry the name of physicians who originated the procedures, such as Kuhnt-Szymanowski or Wheeler.

A

acid burn: a chemical burn to ocular tissue caused by acid fluids with a low pH, such as sulfuric acid.

alkali burn: a chemical burn to ocular tissue caused by alkalis fluids with a high pH, such as lime or lye.

avulsion of lids: a shearing of the lid structures through trauma so that the lid dangles like a pedicle flap with little loss of lid tissue.

B

Berke-Krönlein orbitotomy: a lateral approach to the orbit to explore or remove a lesion behind the eye.

Bick procedure: an excision of redundant eyelid tissue at the lateral canthus

Blascovics' operation: an approach through the conjunctiva for the correction of ptosis by shortening the levator palpebrae muscle.

blepharochalasis repair: the surgical excision and repair of redundant eyelid skin.

blepharoptosis repair: the surgical correction of drooping of the upper eyelid.

blow-out fracture of orbit: fracture of the floor of the orbit into the maxillary sinus with prolapse of the intraorbital contents into the antrum. Often associated with enophthalmos, ptosis, inability to turn the eye upward, and infraorbital nerve hypoesthesia.

C

Caldwell-Luc: an approach to the floor of the orbit through the maxillary antrum. An approach sometimes used for repair of blow-out fractures of the orbit.

canthotomy: usually implies a lateral canthotomy, which is the cutting of the outer angle of the eyelid. Performed when widening of the palpebral fissure is required.

chalcosis: retained intraocular copper and its common alloys bronze and brass may cause a sunflower cataract and a Kayser-Fleischer ring in Descemet's membrane. This chemical complex is especially common in Wilson's disease.

chemosis: swelling of conjunctival tissues.

conjunctivoplasty: reconstruction of the conjunctival lining of the eye, with or without grafting.

conjunctivorhinostomy: anastomosis of the conjunctiva with the nasal cavity for improved tear outflow.

crepitus: subconjunctival or subcutaneous emphysema (air) usually derived from fractures of sinuses.

D

dacryocystectomy: excision of the tear sac.

dacryocystorhinostomy (DCR): a communication is made between the nasolacrimal sac and the nasal cavity to relieve an obstruction in the tear nasal duct.

DCR: see *dacryocystorhinostomy*.

decompression, orbital: surgical relief of pressure behind the eyeball, as in endocrine exophthalmos, by the removal of bone from the orbit.

districhiasis correction: surgery to correct the aberrant growth of eyelashes.

E

ecchymosis of the lids: hemorrhage under the skin of the lids caused by contusion—common terminology "black eye."

electrocoagulation: an electric current used to cauterize small eyelid lesions by heat.

electroepilation (electrolysis): a coagulation needle is inserted into a hair follicle to permanently remove misdirected lashes.

enucleation: surgical removal of the entire globe.

epicanthal correction: correction of a fold in the inner angle of the eye.

epilation: the mechanical removal of eyelashes or cilia by the roots, as performed in the removal of misdirected eyelashes.

epiphora: excessive tearing, often caused by blockage of the tear ducts, but may arise from excessive tear formation.

evisceration: the surgical removal of the entire contents of the globe leaving a scleral shell.

exenteration: removal of entire orbit including the globe, eyelid muscles, eyelid, and orbital contents—usually performed for malignant tumors.

F

Fasanella-Servat procedure: an operation for minor degrees of ptosis to raise the upper lid by excising a portion from under the eyelid.

fascia lata frontalis sling for ptosis: fascia lata obtained from the thigh is used to elevate a drooping eyelid.

figure-of-8 suture: a suture repair to close lid defects from surgery or trauma to attain good wound opposition with a simple single suture thread in a figure-8 style.

flap: flaps are used when a recipient bed is not suitable for a free graft or when a defect is too large for a free graft; flaps may be local, open, or single.

Fox's operation: excision of a triangle of tarsus and conjunctiva for the correction of entropion.

free skin autograft: surgery in which skin is taken from one area and transferred and united to another area.

Frost suture: a suture used to keep the eyelids closed to protect the cornea.

G

graft:

full-thickness autograft: a graft of skin or mucus and subdermal tissue that is removed and transplanted.

split-thickness autograft: a graft of dermis only that is removed and transplanted.

gray line incisions: an incision in the lid margin at the gray line to separate the tarsal conjunctiva from the skin and orbicularis.

H

hematoma: hemorrhage into the tissues such as the eyelids.

hyaluronidase: speeding factor used in local retrobulbar injections to aid in the diffusion of the anesthetic.

hyphema: an injury from a blunt object causing blood to appear within the anterior chamber.

J

Jones tubes: pyrex tubes used to restore function of the tear outflow channels.

K

Kuhnt-Szymanowski procedure: a procedure on the lower lids designed to correct a relaxed ectropion by excision of the eyelid in two planes.

L

laceration: a cut or wound of the tissues.

levator resection for ptosis: an excision of the levator muscle to elevate the upper lid. The operation may be done through a skin approach, Berke's skin approach, or through a conjunctival approach, Iliff's conjunctival approach.

O

one-snip operation: a single-cut surgical procedure to enlarge the punctum.

orbital decompression: a procedure usually performed for thyroid exophthalmos when visual loss occurs because of increased orbital pressure. The orbit is decompressed by removing part of the bony wall.

orbital implants: materials that are designed to be left at the time of surgery to replace an eye that is removed so as to provide movement of an artificial shell that is later fashioned six weeks after eye surgery.

orbitotomy: a surgical approach made into the orbit to remove a tumor or to obtain a specimen of lesion for biopsy.

P

pedicle flap: surgery in which a piece of skin, attached at its original base, is rotated to restore position and size of the eyebrow.

S

sac: see *conjunctival sac, lacrimal sac.*

socket reconstruction: repair of a shrunken socket that does not suitably retain an artificial eye.

Stryker saw: a bone saw used in dacryocystorhinostomy to remove bone.
suture sling: the use of a suture to perform as a sling in the correction of ptosis or a drooping canthal angle.

T

tarsorrhaphy: a temporary or permanent surgical union of the upper and lower lid margins. It may be temporal (lateral), nasal (medial), or complete.
three-snip operation: a surgical procedure designed to enlarge the punctum and canaliculus by three cuts.
traumatic ptosis: drooping of the upper lid caused by the cumulative weight of blood or edema fluid in the lid as a result of direct injury to the nerve or to the muscle (levator palpebra superioris) that elevates the lids.
trichiasis repair: correction of misdirected upper or lower eyelashes that scratch the cornea.

U

ultraviolet burns: ultraviolet radiation is the most common form of radiant energy to induce ocular injury. The chief sources are welding arcs, suntan lamps, and carbon arcs. It causes an acute punctate keratitis.

W

Wheeler halving repair: a method of closure of lid defects from trauma or by excision of lid mass by splitting the lids and overlapping the edges.
Wheeler procedure: operation performed for senile entropion.
Wies procedure: operation performed for severe cicatricial entropion.

Z

Z-plasty: an operative procedure used to release and transpose lines of tension by making a Z-shaped incision and transposing the flaps.
Ziegler cautery: scarring by heat; created along the lid margin by electrocoagulation to invert or evert the lid.

CHAPTER 24

LASER SURGERY

LASER is an acronym for light amplification through the stimulated emission of radiation.

Argon and krypton lasers produce powerful light energy when electric current excites argon or krypton gas in the laser cavity. Argon laser is especially suited to treating glaucoma; both types are useful in treating diseases of the retina.

The NdYAG (neodynium yttrium aluminum garnet) laser is a solid-state laser producing a more explosive energy capable of cutting membranes.

Laser energy is delivered through a fiberoptic cable to a slit lamp for treatment to the eye. The operator adjusts for power (watts, joules), spot size (microns), and duration (seconds). The number of shots or discharges is counted for each procedure.

In ophthalmic laser treatment the patient is fully ambulatory; the procedure requires only local or topical anesthetic and no special sterile technique.

Lasers in ophthalmology have revolutionized the treatment of diabetic eye disease. As a result of lasers many cases of glaucoma have been treated without surgery.

A

Abraham iridotomy lens: a modified contact lens with a magnifying button for performing laser iridotomy.

aiming beam: a coincident light beam (may also be a laser) for aiming the laser on target before firing.

argon: the gas in the argon laser cavity from which laser energy is produced when raised to an "excited" state with electrical energy.

B

burst: a "shot" or discharge of the laser.

C

capsulotomy: a hole made in the posterior lens capsule when it becomes opacified and visually obstructive following cataract surgery; performed with the YAG laser.

continuous: this type of laser emits its energy continuously with the operator controlling the duration as opposed to the pulsed laser.

D

delivery system: the optical set-up that delivers laser energy to the eye. This consists of a slit lamp connected to the laser by a fiberoptic cable.

F

foveal avascular zone: the central 500 μ of the fovea and macula, free from blood vessels, which is essential to fine central vision; a common reference point in performing macular photocoagulation.

G

goniophotocoagulation: laser applied directly to abnormal blood vessels in the angle covering the trabecular meshwork (drainage system) in neovascular glaucoma.

H

HeNe beam (helium neon): a low-power red laser beam used in many systems as an aiming beam.

I

infrared: an invisible part of the electromagnetic spectrum ("below red") with a long wavelength.

iridoplasty: alteration of the shape of the iris and/or pupil by direct laser burns to the iris.

iridotomy (laser iridotomy): a hole made in the iris with the laser for narrow-angle or angle-closure glaucoma.

K

krypton: gas in the krypton laser cavity operates on the same principle as the argon laser but produces a yellow or red beam for treating macular disease.

L

laser cavity (or tube): lined with reflective mirrors and containing the gas or solid medium, this cavity is where laser energy is produced through repeated reflection and activation through the medium.

M

macular photocoagulation: treatment of the macular area of the retina for edema or abnormal blood vessels beneath the retina (argon or krypton laser).

membranectomy: cutting of a visually obstructive membrane (usually pupillary membrane) with the YAG laser. The term is sometimes used interchangeably with capsulotomy.

millijoule: one one-thousandth of the unit of energy, the joule.

mode locking: a method of producing a series of very short–duration laser pulses in "trains" as opposed to one longer pulse in the usual q-switched laser.

N

nanosecond: one billionth of a second.

NdYAG: neodynium is incorporated in a crystal of yttrium aluminum garnet as the medium for the NdYAG laser.

O

optical breakdown: when hit with a high-power density discharge from the YAG laser, tissue breaks down into a "plasma" or gas of atoms and electrons.

P

panretinal photocoagulation: treatment of the entire retina except the central portion with the argon laser to prevent growth or cause regression of abnormal blood vessels (neovascularization), as occurs in diabetes or central retinal vein obstruction.

photon: a packet or quantum of light energy.

picosecond: one trillionth of a second.

pitting: marking of an intraocular lens when applying YAG laser to a membrane close behind the lens.

plasma: the short-lined atom and electron gas produced from tissue breakdown with the YAG laser.

power: a measure of energy/time in watts.

pulse train: a series of equally spaced, very short pulses from a mode-locked laser.

Q

quality factor: based on the ratio of energy stored to energy generated.

Q switching: the sudden change of Q of the laser cavity to produce a pulse.

S

spot size: laser beam diameter and therefore size of burn ranging from 500 to 1000 μ.

T

trabeculoplasty: laser treatment (usually argon) to the trabecular meshwork through a gonioscope lens to treat open-angle glaucoma.

W

wavelength: a physical property of light apparent in its color. Violet has a short wavelength, red a long wavelength. Different tissues absorb different wavelengths preferentially, making the various lasers useful for specific purposes.

Y

YAG: yttrium aluminum garnet. The crystal in the "solid-state" YAG laser.

CHAPTER 25

RETINAL AND VITREOUS SURGERY

A *retinal detachment* is a complete or partial separation of the retina from the underlying choroid. When the retina becomes *detached* it is not truly a detachment of the complete retina; rather, the pigment layer of the retina remains attached to the choroid while the rest of the retina detaches from it. In fact, a retinal detachment is a splitting of the retina in which the anterior nine layers detach from the posterior pigment layer. The detachment occurs when the vitreous wedges itself between the two split layers. *Retinoschisis (schisis*, "to split") is a true splitting of the retina more anteriorly without detachment. If there is a localized blister elevation, the term *macrocyst* or *giant cyst of the retina* is frequently used. *Rhegmatogenous detachment* (Greek *rhegma*, "hole") is a detachment in which there is a retinal hole or tear resulting in watery fluid that enters behind the retina. *Nonrhegmatogenous detachment* is a detachment with no holes or tears; it may be caused by traction pull on the retina, by fluid leaking under the retina from the choroid, or by a malignant melanoma.

The detachment may be classified as *aphakic detachment* if it occurs after cataract surgery or *pseudophakic detachment* if it occurs after an artificial lens implant procedure. *Vitreous detachment* or *separation* may occur in which the vitreous becomes separated from the retina.

A

anterior vitrectomy: removal of vitreous and membranes from the area of the pupil (anterior eye).

B

buckling: operating for retinal detachment by resection of a portion of the sclera and implantation of foreign material to indent the outer coats of the eye.

C

cryopexy: freezing treatment using a cryoprobe. The resulting scarring forms a firm adhesion of retina to underlying tissues. It is used, for example, to seal retinal holes.

cryotherapy: treatment by cold usually involving the freezing of the tissue concerned.

D

diathermy: coagulation of tissue by heat to destroy tissue or to create a natural scar such as used in retinal detachment and ciliary body surgery.

E

encircling band: a band of material such as silicone or fascia lata that completely encircles the globe and indents the sclera.
encircling explant or implant: sponge or silicone material encircling the eye for 360 degrees to provide indentation of the full circumference.
explant: a synthetic material made of silicone or sponge that is used in scleral buckling to indent the sclera.

I

intraocular gas or air: gas or air may be injected into the eye after vitrectomy and scleral buckle to maintain the retina in position. The bubble may last several days.

K

Kaufman vitrector: a disposable instrument used to cut and remove vitreous fluid.

M

magnet: used to retrieve metallic foreign bodies from within the eye.
membrane peeling: removal of abnormal tissue from the surface of the retina to relieve traction and wrinkling.

P

panretinal photocoagulation (PRP): complete photocoagulation of the retina except for the central (macular) area.
pars plana vitrectomy: a vitreous removal procedure performed through the pars plana.
peritomy: opening of the conjunctiva near the limbus to gain access to the extraocular muscles and posterior sclera.
photocoagulation: a high-intensity light beam produces a burn to provide an adherence between the choroid and the retina.
posterior vitrectomy: removal of vitreous from the posterior region of the eye behind the lens plane.
PRP: see *panretinal photocoagulation*.

S

scleral buckle: the inversion of the sclera designed to appose the sclera and choroid against the retina.

scleral flap: a partial thickness "trap door" fashioned in the sclera that may be used to cover a surgical opening or bury an implant.

segmental implant or explant: a small section of sponge or silicone creating a local indentation.

silicone sponge explant: a synthetic material made of silicone that is used in scleral buckling to indent the sclera.

subretinal fluid drainage: draining of fluid from under the detached retina by making a small hole through the sclera and choroid. An important part of scleral buckling surgery.

V

VISC: vitreous infusion suction and cutter; an instrument used to cut and remove vitreous.

vitrectomy: surgical removal of vitreous.

vitreous traction: usually refers to a band of vitreous pulling on the retina and causing a hole and/or detachment. Removal of traction bands is one objective of vitrectomy.

CHAPTER 26

STRABISMUS SURGERY

Strabismus (Greek *strabismos*, "twisted") refers to eyes that are not straight. Strabo, the geographer, was a prominent figure in Alexandria during the Roman times who suffered from a noticeable turn of his eyes. From then on it was popular to call a person with a turn "Strabo."

A *tenotomy* is a surgical procedure in which the tendon of the muscle is cut. This was first performed in 1839. In *myectomy*, a portion of the muscle is excised or removed, whereas in a *myotomy* the muscle is cut. A *recession* of the muscle is the setting back of the muscle, derived from the Latin *recedere*, from *re*, "back" or "off," and *sedere*, "to go," so that it is a going back of the muscle. *Resection* is derived from *re*, "back," and *secare*, "to cut," meaning a cutting off of a portion of the muscle. Chapter 14 deals with a strabismus and ocular motility in greater detail.

Other words often used include the following:

A

adjustable sutures: the principle of placing sutures so that they may be adjusted for perfect alignment when the patient is awake and alert.

advancement: the moving forward toward the cornea of the insertional site of a muscle or tendon.

C

cinch: surgery in which a rectus muscle or tendon is split and suture material inserted to shorten a muscle.

E

external route: a route through skin usually reserved for inferior oblique surgery.

H

Hummelsheim operation: transplantation of muscle slips to restore function after lateral rectus palsy.

L

lengthening: a procedure to increase the overall length of a muscle.

M

myotomy: surgical division of muscle fibers without severing the entire muscle. May be called marginal in which marginal cuts are made from one or both sides of the muscle.

O

overcorrection: correcting a deviation beyond the expected amount so the eye turns in the opposite direction.

S

shortening: a procedure to reduce the overall length of a muscle.

T

transconjunctival route: incisional approach through the conjunctiva.

transplantation: the moving of the temporal or nasal half of active muscles to replace paralyzed muscle.

tucking: folding of an extraocular muscle tendon to shorten it and increase its action.

PART FIVE

OPHTHALMIC TESTS AND DEVICES AND MISCELLANEOUS TERMS

CHAPTER 27

OPHTHALMIC TESTS AND DEVICES

Ophthalmology is a highly measurable branch of medicine, because the eye is exposed and visible so that every crevice of the interior can be reached directly or indirectly with lenses, prisms, or ultrasound devices. Also the eye functions as an optical instrument, so the ordinary laws of geometric optics can be applied to this biological camera that has a zoom lens, an automatic shutter, a single vision reflex control, and a focusing device that yields a clear picture with every look.

The basic vision test is virtually an antique; known as *Snellen's chart*, it is still the most widely used test for measuring vision. The letters have been designed to subtend a 5-minute angle to the eye at either 20 feet or 6 meters. The visual record is expressed as the fraction 20/20 or 6/6 in which the numerator reflects the test distance and the denominator indicates the distance at which a person with normal eyesight can see the letters. Therefore the numerator is always the same, either 20 feet or 6 meters, and is referred to as 20 or 6. The bottom lines vary with the degree of acuity. For example, if a person is able to read the 20/20 line at 20 feet, the vision is recorded as 20/20. If the best vision recorded is at 20/50, this means that the person can distinguish only at 20 feet a letter that a normally sighted individual can see correctly at 50 feet. The term 20/20 or 6/6 is an artificial record of a certain type of static acuity. It is measured with the person seated, the eye still, the head motionless, and the object of regard stationary. In real life this is hardly the situation when we look at signs and objects while we walk, jog, or drive a car; the things that we observe with our eyes often are not still, for example, when workers look at conveyor belts and athletes follow fast-moving squash balls, tennis balls, or baseballs. The illumination should be standardized, because the test performed in a lighted room without any controls on the amount of light present will yield a different result than when performed in a well-lit room.

The term 20/40 is a little misleading, because it does not mean that a person with this type of vision has only half the vision of a person with 20/20 vision. The denominator reflects a gradual loss of resolution of the eye, which indicates poorer functioning of the eye. At 20/50 or 20/60 an eye may be designated as partially sighted and at 20/200 as legally blind. These terms relate to function, not to absolute values; a person with 20/200 vision is definitely not blind, since he may have totally intact peripheral vision and may be able to read with magnifying devices and low-vision aids.

Thus the fundamental test and its record result in a limited test of vision that ignores illumination, peripheral vision, near vision, moving vision, or dynamic visual acuity. It has survived because it is simple to do, reproducible within narrow limits, and generally easy to understand. The term 20/20 is vaguely comprehended by nearly everyone, meaning keen vision even to the public.

Other versions of this acuity test are the E *game* in which testing can be done with children or illiterate persons by having them merely indicate the direction of the charted E with their fingers (Fig. 27-1). *Picture charts* are used with children to capture their interest and to avoid mistakes in symbol recognition. *Landolt's*

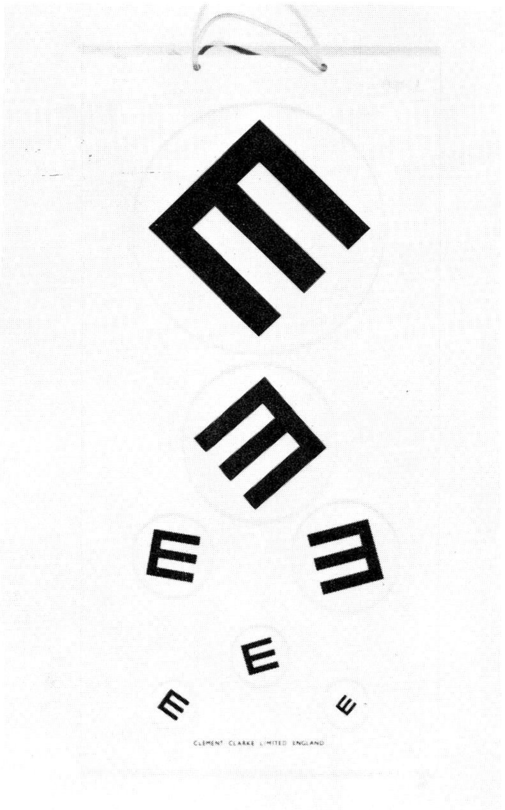

Fig. 27-1. E chart with rotating Es.

broken-ring test is another test for children or illiterate individuals in which they note the position of the break in the ring (Fig. 27-2). *Flash picture cards* are also used for young children because the test distance of 5 or 10 feet is more apt to engage a child's interest than something at a distance of 20 feet.

Near vision testing is done at 14 to 16 inches. A record is made of the smallest type that can be easily read. Most near tests use letters or words, but pictures, numbers, and E's are also used. The most common method used in reading vision is the *Jaeger system*. This system was established by Jaeger in the latter part of the nineteenth century. He fashioned a reading card and arbitrarily assigned numbers to indicate the size of the print. J1 was used to show that the person

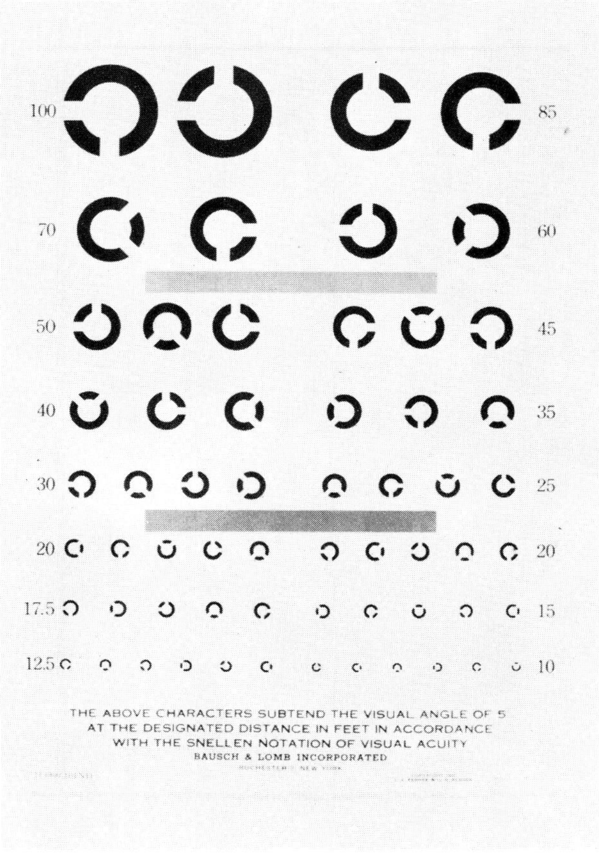

Fig. 27-2. Landolt's broken-ring test.

could read the smallest print, and larger numbers indicated larger print. Other near tests include the *Snellen reading card* (Fig. 27-3) and the *Lebensohn reading chart*. These reading test cards are so versatile that they include recording in the *Jaeger system* and the *printers' point system*. They also display numbers, symbols, musical notes, and letter sizes that equate Jaeger terms with the size of print in the Bible, in newspaper want ads, or in other conventional areas of reading.

The terminology of vision testing must be understood for its application and its limitations. Regardless of the flow of systems, devices, and technology, the first test performed in any eye examination is a vision test for both far and near distance. Without it, the assessment of the function of the eyes is quite meaningless.

The following are ophthalmic tests and equipment used to evaluate the eye or ophthalmic appliances.

A

aesthesiometer: a measuring device using small nylon threads to test the sensitivity of the cornea.

amplitude of accommodation: a test used to measure the focusing ability of the eye from infinity to the closest point that can be seen. The results vary by age with a 10-year-old boy easily having an accommodation of 14 D, where a 50-year-old man would have an accommodation of 2.50 D. The measurement, which is in diopters, is converted from the near point of visibility in centimeters.

Amsler grid: a chart with horizontal and vertical lines for testing the central field of vision for scotomas and detecting macular distortion.

angiography: a diagnostic test in which a substance is injected so that the vascular tree can be examined, for example, the radiographic examination of the retinal circulation can be seen after an injection of fluorescein into the blood vessels of the arm.

applanation tonometer: an instrument that measures the intraocular pressure by the force used to flatten a small area of the cornea. It is the best instrument to measure intraocular pressure because it produces the least distortion of the coats of the eye.

arteriography: visualization of arteries by injection of radiopaque material that can be seen by x-ray enhancement.

astigmatic dial: see *dial, astigmatic*.

automatic refractors: an instrument whose purpose is to provide an accurate assessment of the refractive error of the eye. Automatic refractors may be *subjective* (dependent on patient response) or *objective* (independent of patient response).

Fig. 27-3. Snellen reading cards.

READING CARD--SNELLEN RATING

0.37 M	I walked up the street, gazing about, until near the market house I met a boy with bread. I had made many a meal on bread, and asked him where he got it. I then went to the baker's and asked for biscuit such as we had in Boston. I asked for a three-penny loaf and was told that they had none such. Not knowing	J 2
0.50 M	the difference of money and the greater cheapness I bade him give me three penny worth of any sort. He gave me three puffy rolls. I was surprised at the quantity but took it, and walked off with a roll under each arm. Thus I walked up Market Street as far as Fourth Street, passing by the house	J 3
0.62 M	of Mr. Read, my future wife's father. She, standing at the door, saw me and thought I made a most awkward appearance, as I certainly did. Then I turned and went down Chestnut Street and a part of Walnut Street. Being filled with one of my rolls, I gave the other two to a woman	J 4
0.75 M	and her child. By this time the street had many clean and well dressed people in it, all walking the same way. I joined them and was led into the great meeting house of the Quakers'. I sat down among them and after looking around a while and hearing nothing said,	J 5
1.00 M	I fell fast asleep. This was the first house I was in, or slept in, in Philadelphia. Looking in the faces of people, I met a young man whose countenance I liked, and asked	J 7
1.25 M	if he would tell me where a stranger could get lodging. "Here," said he, "is one place that entertains strangers."	J 8

The above letters are Snellen sizes at the designated distance in meters with Jaeger notations at right

BAUSCH & LOMB INCORPORATED, ROCHESTER 2, N. Y., U. S. A.

71-35-90 PRINTED IN U. S. A.

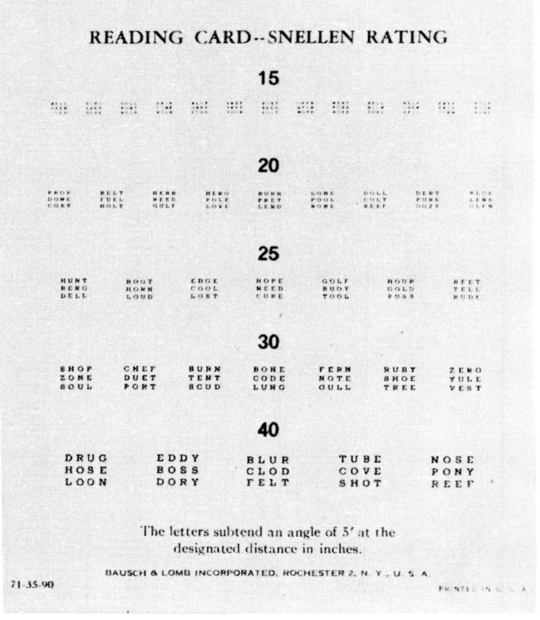

READING CARD--SNELLEN RATING

15

20

25

HUNT	ROOT	EDGE	HOPE	GOLF	HOUR	BEET
BERG	HORN	COOL	NEED	BUOY	GOLD	TELL
DELL	LOUD	LOST	CURE	TOOL	FUSS	RUDE

30

SHOP	CHEF	BURN	BONE	FERN	RUBY	ZENO
ZONE	DUET	TENT	CODE	NOTE	SHOE	YULE
SOUL	PORT	SCUD	LUNG	GULL	TREE	VEST

40

DRUG	EDDY	BLUR	TUBE	NOSE
HOSE	BOSS	CLOD	COVE	PONY
LOON	DORY	FELT	SHOT	REEF

The letters subtend an angle of 5′ at the designated distance in inches.

BAUSCH & LOMB INCORPORATED, ROCHESTER 2, N. Y., U. S. A.

71-35-90 PRINTED IN U. S. A.

B

bar reader: an appliance that provides for the placement of an opaque bar between the printed page and the reader's eye so as to occlude different areas of the page for each of the eyes. A one-eyed person will find the bar an obstruction; a person with binocular vision will not be hampered by the bar. Used for diagnosis and training of binocular vision.

biopter test: a home stereoscopic viewer to measure depth perception.

Bjerrum's screen: a tangent screen to measure the central 30 degrees of the field of vision.

C

caloric testing: a test performed by placing cold or warm water in the external ear and observing the eye movements. Cold water will induce a gaze movement to the opposite side in a normal person.

cheiroscope: a device used for the treatment of suppression.

colorimeter: a color-matching device used to designate an unknown color stimulus by matching it with a known color stimulus. A test for color blindness.

consensual light reflex: constriction of the opposite pupil when a beam of light is directed into the pupil of an eye.

convergence: the act of bringing the eyes together to their closest point. The end point is reached when the person either sees double or one eye drifts outward. The near point of convergence is measured in centimeters (Fig. 27-4).

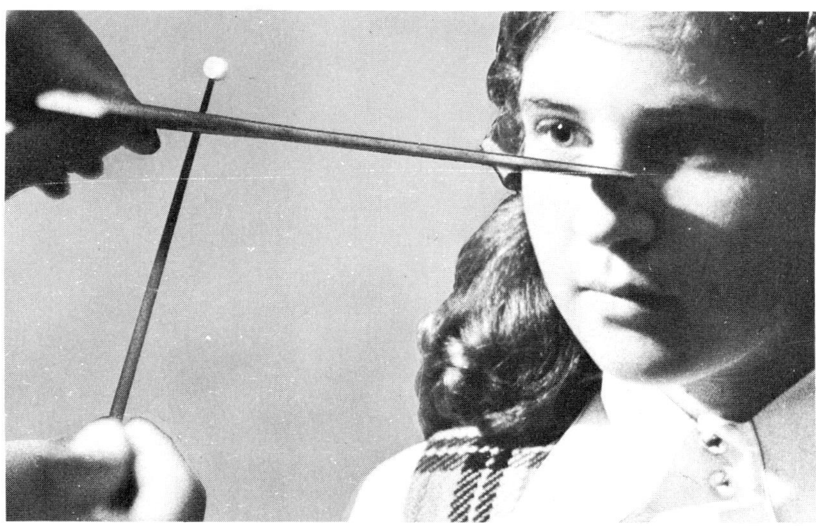

Fig. 27-4. Measuring the near point of convergence.

cover test: a test used to detect strabismus; when the fixating eye is occluded, the eye that is not in proper alignment must make a motion to pick up the target.

cross cylinder: a lens used to measure the power and axis of an astigmatic refractive error. The cross cylinder consists of a plus and a minus cylinder set at right angles to each other with the handle set midway between the two cylinders (Fig. 27-5).

cryophake: a cold probe used to remove a lens or cataract.

D

dacryocystogram: an x-ray photograph of the lacrimal apparatus of the eye, made visible by radiopaque dyes.

dial, astigmatic: a chart or pattern used for determining the presence and the amount of astigmatism.

direct light reflex: contraction of the pupil in the presence of a beam of light with the eye gazing at a distant object. The room illumination should be dim.

distometer: a caliper used to measure vertex distance, which is the distance from the cornea of the patient's eye to the back surface of the lens inserted in the trial frame, phoropter, or glass.

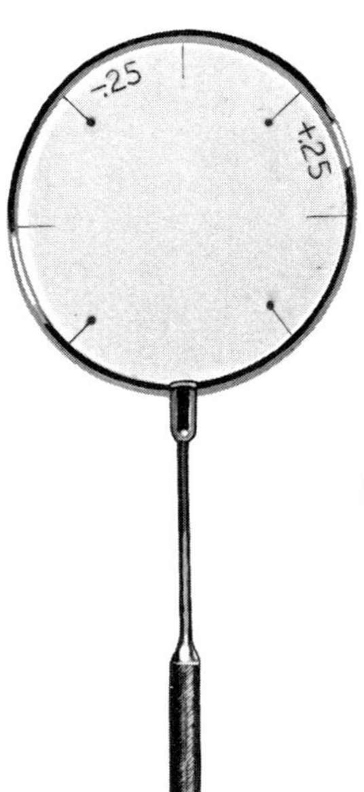

Fig. 27-5. Cross cylinder.

duction test, forced: a test used to establish the presence of restrictive ocular muscle movements in Brown's tendon sheath syndrome, dysthyroid myopathy, orbital blow-out fractures, and double elevator palsy. If passive movement of the eye is restricted, this indicates a mechanical limitation to eye movement, as opposed to the presence of a myopathy or neuropathy.

dynopter: an instrument used to measure ophthalmic artery pressure. An ophthalmoscope is not needed, and the pressure is applied to the cornea, not the sclera.

E

electromyography: procedure in which needles are inserted into extraocular muscles and the electrical activity of the muscles is recorded.

electronic tonometer: an indentation tonometer with the footplate transmitted to an electronic amplifier. The amplified signal activates the meter signal, which yields a pressure measurement similar to the standard Schiøtz instrument. This instrument may be used for tonography measurements.

electro-oculography: a technique in which an electrostatic field is created by means of skin electrodes placed around the eye. The electrical potential difference between the front and the back of the eye is used to detect disorders of the eye.

electroretinography: a test of rod-and-cone function based on the electrical potential that exists between the cornea and retina of the human eye.

euthyscope: a device used to treat eccentric fixation (Cüppers' method) by creating negative afterimages to make the person aware of the proper foveal projection.

exophthalmometer: an instrument designed to measure the forward protrusion of the eye. Types include: (1) the Luedde, a notched ruler that fits into the bony lateral orbital margin with the protrusion measured from the side, and (2) the Hertel, a transverse bar with mirrored carriers on each side inclined at 45 degrees to reflect the scale reading and the apex of the cornea in profile (Fig. 27-6). Comparative measurements are made from the front.

F

Farnsworth-Munsell 100-hue test: a color-hue matching test to diagnose types and degrees of color blindness.

fluorescein angiography: a procedure in which fluorescein dye is injected so that retinal choroidal circulation and iris circulation can be examined and photographed.

fly test: a depth perception test in which the person is given Polaroid lenses and is asked to touch the wings of the fly. A person with normal depth perception will see the wings standing out (Fig. 27-7).

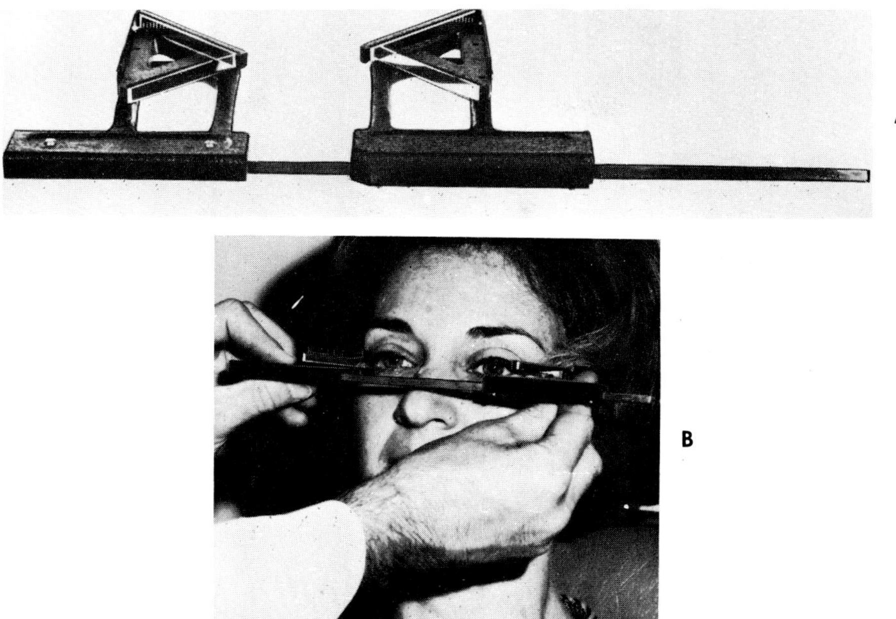

Fig. 27-6. **A,** Hertel exophthalmometer. **B,** Measurement of eye protrusion.

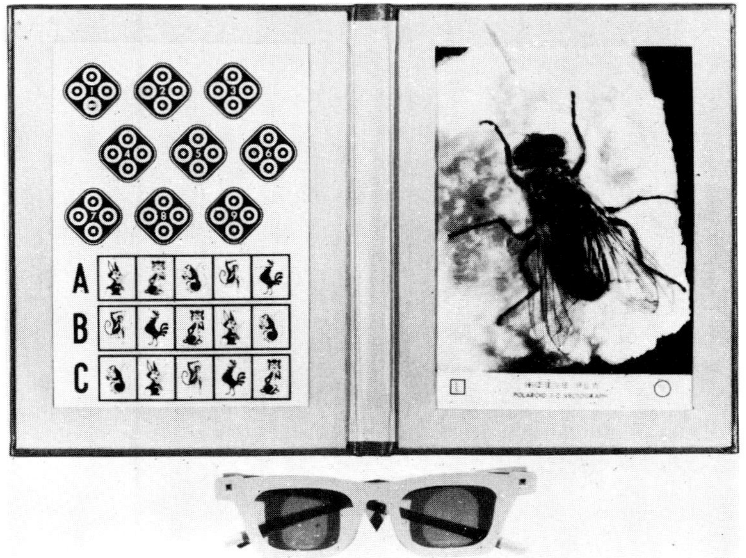

Fig. 27-7. Wirt and fly tests for depth perception.

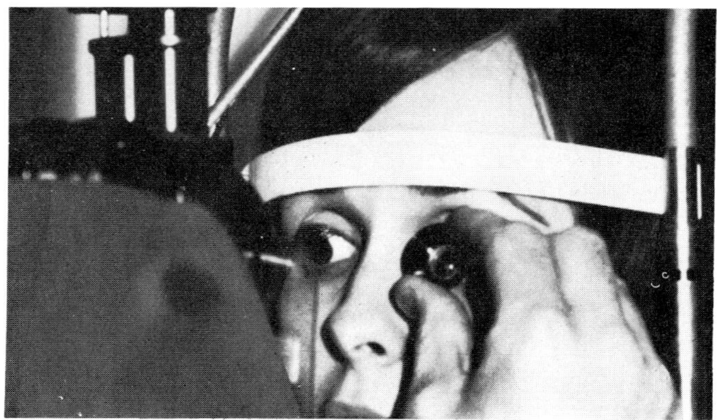

Fig. 27-8. Fundus contact lens.

forced duction test: see *duction test, forced.*

fundus contact lens: a hand-held contact lens placed on the anesthetized cornea to permit the examination of the fundus (Fig. 27-8).

G

Goldmann perimeter: a half-shell perimeter that can examine both central and peripheral fields. Also used for static and kinetic perimetry.

goniolens: a lens used to examine the angle structures of the eye. There are two basic types: (1) a lens that uses mirrors or prisms to see the opposite angle, and (2) a Koeppe lens, which allows the light from the angle structures to leave the cornea. The operative goniolens is similar to the other two except that one side is partially removed to permit access of a goniotomy knife for surgery.

gonioscope: a device consisting of a hand-held microscope and an illuminating system used with a goniolens for viewing the angle structures of the eyes.

H

Halberg trial clip: a device that fits on the patient's glasses and allows an overrefraction to take place. Eliminates vertex distance computations. It is also used to refract young children.

Hertel exophthalmometer: see *exophthalmometer*.

Hess screen test: a test to determine the presence and the degree of strabismus (Fig. 27-9).

Hirshberg test: a screening device to detect strabismus. A light shone in a child's eye should be visible in the nasal spot off the center of the pupil of each eye.

Hruby lens: a −55 D lens designed to be used with the slit lamp to examine the vitreous and retina (Fig. 27-10).

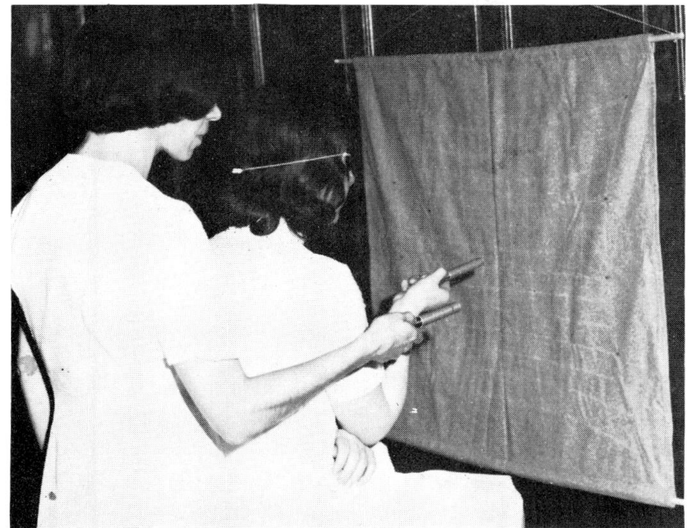

Fig. 27-9. Lancaster screen test used to measure the magnitude of a muscle imbalance.

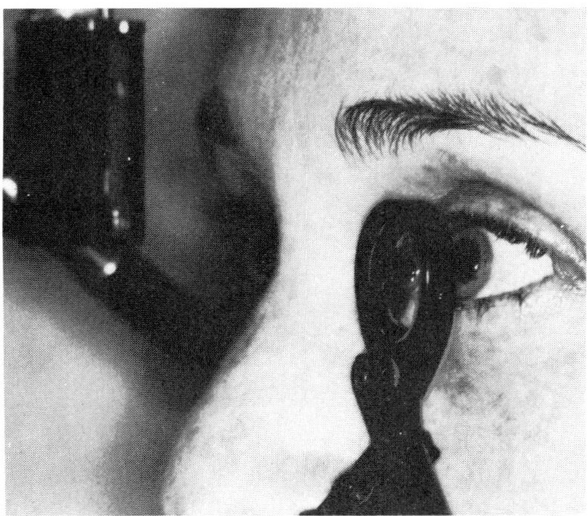

Fig. 27-10. Hruby lens used to examine the fundus under magnification.

I

indentation tonometer: a tonometer that uses a variable weight and plunger to indent the cornea an amount depending on the intraocular pressure. It is widely used because it is simple, inexpensive, and portable. It tends to distort the outer coats of the eye.

Ishihara's test: a test for defects in recognizing colors, based on the tracing of numbers or patterns in a series of multicolored charts or plates (Fig. 27-11).

J

Jaeger's test: a test for near vision, in which lines of reading matter are printed in a series of sizes of type. J1 is the smallest type. The number indicates the print size.

K

keratometer (ophthalmometer): an instrument that measures the central 3.3 mm of the anterior curvature of the cornea in its two meridians. The readings are called K readings. The measurement is in diopters, with the average cornea having a power of 42 to 48 D.

Kestenbaum's rule: measurement in which the numerator of the patient's distant visual acuity is divided into the denominator. The result should equal the magnification for seeing J5 on a near-vision chart. It is used as a guide for people with limited vision who need a reading aid.

Krimsky's prism test: a test in which light is shone into the eyes and its position in the pupil is noted; a prism is placed over the deviating eye until the light reflection is centered. The amount of prism requiried for this centering is a measure of the deviation.

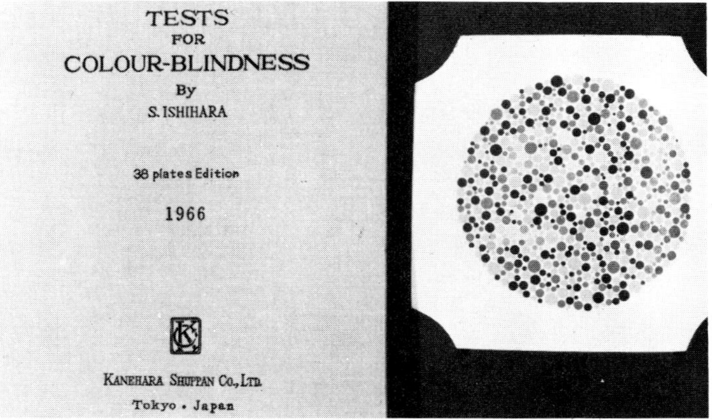

Fig. 27-11. Ishihara's test for color blindness.

L

lensometer: an instrument used to measure the dioptric power and the optical center of a lens, the presence of prisms, and the direction of the base of a prism. It can be manual or automatic, with or without a device for recording.

light-stress test: a test of macular function. A bright light is shone into the macula of the eye, and the time for recovery of visual acuity is noted. A person with macular disease will have a delayed visual recovery time.

Lloyd stereocampimeter: a device consisting of two charts, one visible to each eye, which are combined stereoscopically in such a manner that the central field of one eye can be examined while fixation is maintained by the other.

Luedde exophthalmometer: see *exophthalmometer*.

M

Maddox rod: a group of red or colorless parallel glass rods that together act as a cylinder. The purpose of the Maddox rod is to disassociate the eyes and prevent them from fusing. It does this by changing a point of light to a line or streak of light for the eye and viewing the line target behind the rod (Fig. 27-12). It uses prisms to detect and measure the presence and amount of phorias.

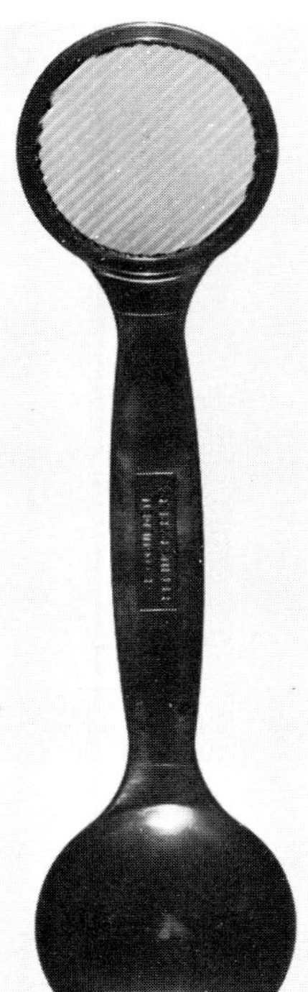

Fig. 27-12. Hand-held Maddox rod combined with occluder.

Maddox wing test: a device used to detect the presence of heterophoria in near vision and to measure its magnitude (Fig. 27-13).

major amblyoscope: a device used to measure strabismus and assess binocular vision; also used to treat suppression and amblyopia.

Mecholyl test: test for Adie's tonic-pupil syndrome, in which the pupil is hypersensitive to Mecholyl. The pupil does not respond to direct light, but will respond to one drop of fresh Mecholyl.

N

night-vision goggles: lenses that can intensify light up to 15,000 times; used as an aid for people with retinitis pigmentosa who cannot see in the dark.

O

occluder: an opaque or translucent device placed before an eye to obscure or block vision.

ophthalmodynamometry: measurement of the ophthalmic artery pressure by viewing retinal vessels of the eye. Pressure is applied to the eye while the observer notes the first pulsation of the central retinal artery (diastolic) and then with further pressure, the total absence of a pulsation (systolic reading).

ophthalmometer: an instrument to measure the corneal curvature by using the cornea as a front-surface mirror. It is commonly called a keratometer.

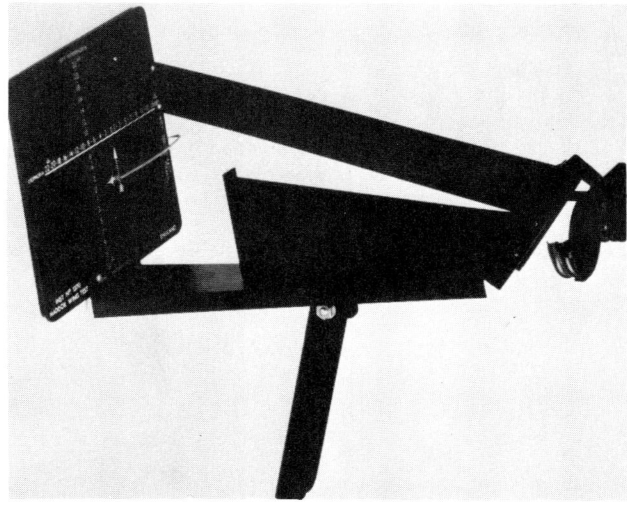

Fig. 27-13. Maddox wing test.

ophthalmoscope, direct (Fig. 27-14): an instrument used to see the retina and the optic nerve at ×15 magnification. Additional devices on the ophthalmoscope include the following:

red filters: red filters are used to define melanin pigment because it absorbs red rays and thereby contrasts strongly with the rest of the fundi.

polarized light: the light leaving the ophthalmoscope is polarized so that irritating reflections from the patient's cornea are reduced.

slit illumination: a slit beam of light is helpful in evaluating the level of various areas of the retina.

aperture discs: the smaller aperture is useful in looking through a miotic pupil such as is frequently found in glaucoma patients.

cobalt blue filters: cobalt blue filters provide the best method to study fluorescein angiography of fundus and to look at the stained tear film in contact lens work.

ophthalmoscope, indirect:

binocular indirect ophthalmoscope: instrument that enables a broad examination of the retina right to the ora serrata, which is not possible with a direct ophthalmoscope. A real inverted image is seen at approximately ×4 to ×5 magnification with stereoscopic vision.

monocular indirect ophthalmoscope: an instrument that allows broad inspection of the fundi but yields an erect image. Depth perception is not possible with this device because only one eye is used for inspection. The beam of light can be reduced in aperture so that visualization through a small pupil is possible.

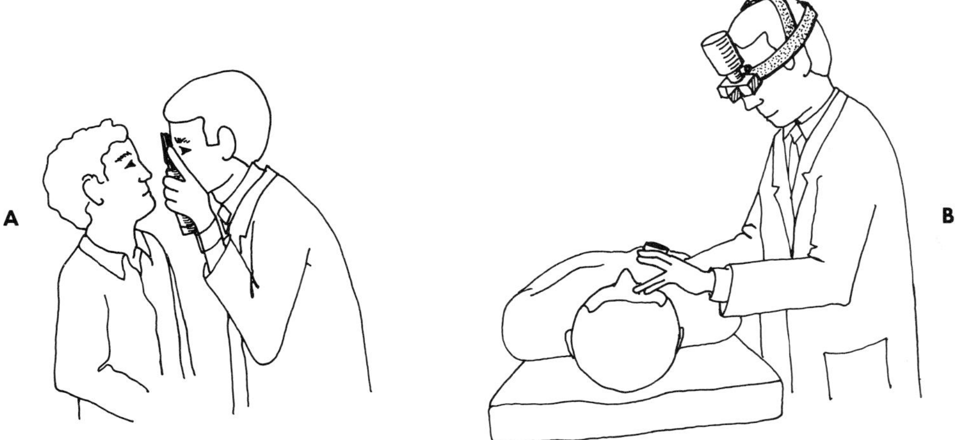

Fig. 27-14. **A,** direct ophthalmoscopy. **B,** indirect ophthalmoscopy.

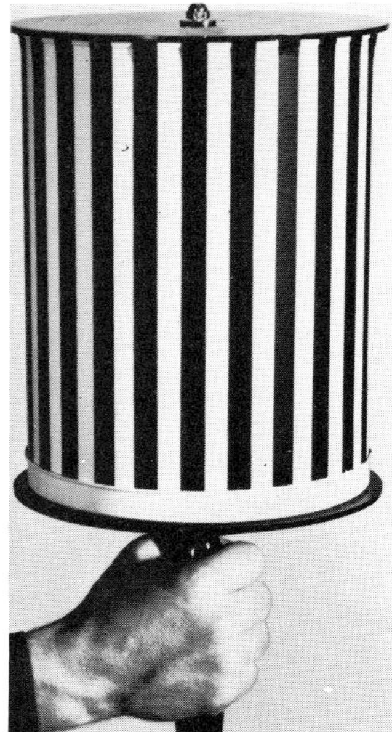
Fig. 27-15. Optokinetic drum.

optokinetic drum: a drum covered with white and black vertical strips; when rotated at a distance of 1 foot from the patient, the revolving stripes induce a jerky nystagmus. Used to test neurological function and visual function in infants (Fig. 27-15).

optokinetic tape: a strip of small squares or lines that can elicit jerk nystagmus when pulled in front of a fixating individual (Fig. 27-16).

P

pachometer: a device used to measure the thickness of the cornea and the depth of the anterior chamber.

Paredrine test: sympathomimetic test used in the diagnosis of postganglionic Horner's syndrome.

perimeter: an instrument for measuring the peripheral field of vision.

phoropter: an entire set of trial lenses mounted on a circular wheel so that each lens can be brought before the aperture of the viewing system by merely turning a dial.

pinhole disc: a black disc with one or multiple openings that allow only central rays to pass through. Vision that is improved with a pinhole disc can be aided by spectacle lenses.

Placido's disc: a flat disc with white and black rings that encircle a central round aperture; used to detect early keratoconus and to measure the topography of

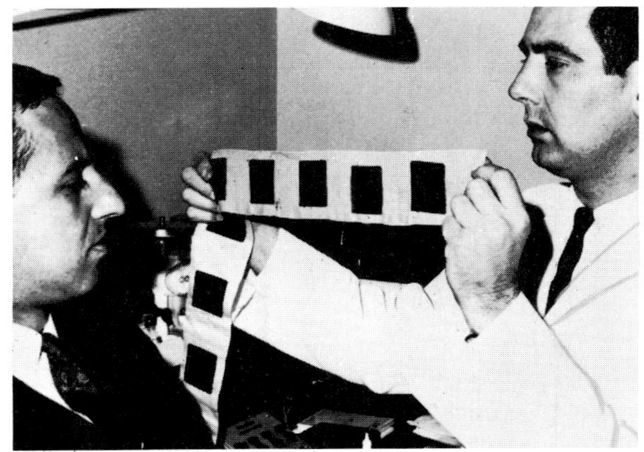

Fig. 27-16. Optokinetic tape.

the cornea. This measurement is often used with a computer technique in designing contact lenses. The reflections of the rings on the cornea indicate the regularity of the central corneal contours, as well as its periphery.

pneumatic tonometer: instrument providing an air blast, which works on the principle of an interval timer, measuring the time it takes from the generation of a puff of air to the point where the cornea is flat.

prism: a triangular piece of glass or plastic that changes the pathway of light and bends it to its base. A prism placed in front of an eye will cause the object of regard to be shifted to its apex. The following prisms are available: (1) loose prisms; (2) horizontal and vertical prism bars; and (3) Risley rotary prisms. Two prisms are mounted in rings, one in front of the other, and are rotated by a dial. When the bases of each prism lie behind one another, the power is additive. The Risley prism offers a rapid and strong increase in prism power.

prism cover test: a test in which the image of the deviating eye is displaced by a prism so that the image falls on the macula. At that point, covering one eye will not cause a refixation movement of the other eye.

profile analyzer: an instrument to evaluate the blend of the junction zone of hard contact lenses.

provocative test: a test to artificially provoke an elevation of intraocular pressure as a diagnostic test for glaucoma.

pseudoisochromatic plates: color plates, such as the Ishihara plates, used to detect color blindness.

R

Radiuscope: a quality-controlled instrument used to detect contact lens warpage and to measure the base curve of a contact lens.

reading rectangle: a low-vision aid in which the rectangular opening shows only a few lines of type.

retinoscope: an instrument for determining the refractive error of the eye. Two types are the *spot retinoscope*, which produces a circular image in the pupil, and the *streak retinoscope*, which produces a straight-line image in the pupil. The streak retinoscope is often referred to as the Copeland retinoscope, with respect to its inventor.

S

Schirmer's test: filter-paper test to measure tear flow. Wetting at least 10 mm of the filter paper in 5 minutes is regarded as adequate tear function.

Seidel's test: a test using fluorescein to detect the presence of a leaking wound communicating externally from the anterior chamber.

shadowgraph: an instrument used to examine a contact lens for defects and to check its diameter, the width of the peripheral curve, and the blend of the curve.

slit lamp: an instrument that provides a narrow slit beam of strong light; used with a corneal microscope for examination of the front portions of the eye.

spot retinoscope: see *retinoscope*.

stereocampimeter: see *Lloyd stereocampimeter*.

streak retinoscope: see *retinoscope*.

T

tangent screen: a field device designed to measure the central 30 degrees of visual field; is used to detect central field loss, especially in glaucoma (Fig. 27-17).

tomography: form of radiological investigation (x-ray films) in which good definition can be obtained with tissue sections slightly less than 1 mm in thickness. An example is computerized transverse axial tomography (CT scan).

tonography: a test used to determine the outflow of aqueous humor under the continuous pressure exerted by the weight of a tonometer over a 4- or 5-minute period.

Tonomat: a type of applanation tonometer consisting of a standard weight with a variable flattened area. At its base is a small, flat, disposable footplate that is lightly stained with a coating material supplied with the instrument. The footplate is momentarily lowered onto the cornea. It is removed and then printed onto dampened filter paper, resulting in a permanent imprint of the cornea.

tonometer: instrument for measuring the pressure of the eye.

topogometer: an instrument designed to measure the size of the optic cap, the spherical apex of the cornea. The point at which the cornea loses its spherical shape and becomes flatter is usually regarded as the limit of the corneal cap. This has a radius of 4 to 6 mm in most eyes.

transilluminator: a low-heat, high-intensity light source that permits retro-illumination studies of the retina and vitreous when the media are cloudy. If a solid mass is in the vitreous cavity, it will not yield a red glow in the pupillary area when light is presented behind the mass.

U

ultrasonography: a method that uses high-frequency sound waves to penetrate tissues opaque to light; can be used to detect solid masses in the retina or choroid. It also can delineate the axial length of the globe and anterior chamber for intraocular lens calculations. There are *A scan* and *B scan* ultrasonographic techniques.

V

Visuscope (Cüppers): an instrument designed to determine the presence of eccentric fixation.

W

water-drinking test: a glaucoma-provocative test based on drinking 1000 ml of cold tap water after a fasting period of 3 hours. The rapid ingestion of a large quantity of water increases the aqueous production in the eye resulting in an abnormally elevated intraocular pressure in a patient with glaucoma.

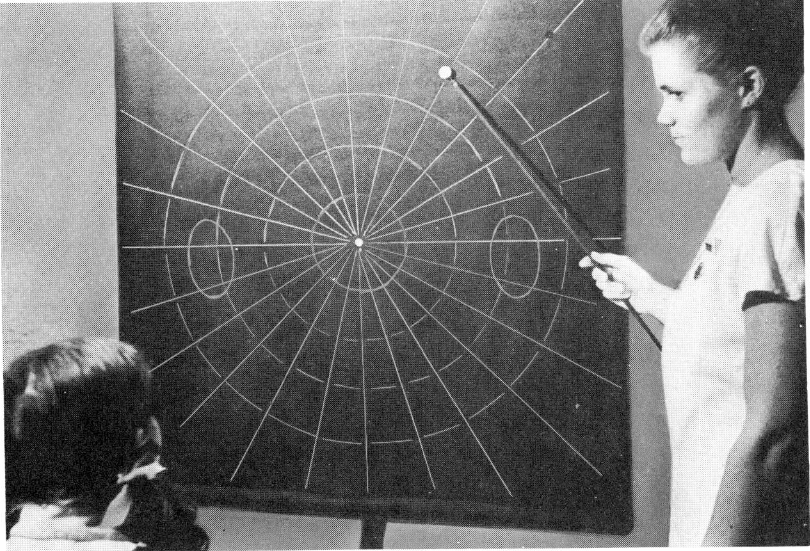

Fig. 27-17. Tangent screen examination measures the central field only.

Wirt stereo test: a depth perception test. For a child three lines of animals are shown from which to make a selection. If all three lines are correctly selected, the child has stereopsis of approximately 100 seconds of arc. For adults there are nine frames of raised rings, the first being the most obvious, the last, the most difficult. If all are read correctly, stereopsis of 40 seconds of arc is present (see Fig. 27-7).

Worth four-dot test: a test to detect amblyopia. The patient wears spectacles with a green lens and a red lens and looks at a target of one white, one red, and two green discs. If four discs are seen, there is no suppression of either eye. If three discs are seen, there is suppression; if five discs are seen, fusion is absent.

CHAPTER 28

MISCELLANEOUS TERMS

In previous chapters we listed words according to clinically useful categories. A number of common words, particularly words relating to trauma and inflammation, affect many categories and many parts of the eye, eyelid, and orbit. They are grouped together in this chapter.

A

ablepharon: the absence of an eyelid.

abscess: localized area of inflammation.

achromia: absence of color; lack of normal pigmentation.

achromate: one who is totally color blind and perceives colors as black, white, and grays.

actinomycosis: unicellar filamentous organisms occupying a position intermediate between bacteria and mold that may cause conjunctivitis, keratitis, and uveitis, as well as blockage of lacrimal passages.

adaptation: adjustment to an environment or a stimulus, especially the ability of the eye to adjust on exposure to different intensities of light.

adenovirus: a virus comprising a large group of 31 different serotypes. Types 3, 7, 8, 11, and 19 are those most commonly associated with eye infections. Types 8 and 19 are associated with epidemic keratoconjunctivitis (EKC), and types 3 and 7 with pharyngoconjunctival fever (PCF).

anoxia: a diminished supply of oxygen to the body tissues.

Ascaris lumbricoides: a nematode or worm that may invade the conjunctival sac.

asepsis: absence of microorganisms.

Aspergillus: a fungus that may cause infection of the conjunctiva, lacrimal passages, sclera, and corneal ulcer.

Ault's line: linear scar seen on the tarsal conjunctiva near the lid margin in patients with trachoma.

avirulent: lack of infectiousness.

avulsion: a tearing out of a part, such as avulsion of an eyelid.

B

Bell's phenomenon: upward-and-outward deviation of the eyes occurring in sleep or with forcible closure of the eyelids.

blennorrhea: a mucoid discharge from various parts of the body, including the external eye, caused by an inflammatory process.

blue sclera: abnormality in which the sclera is thin and has a blue appearance because the underlying pigmented choroid shows through the thin sclera.

Brushfield's spots: transient whitish areas in the iris at birth. They are common in children with Down's syndrome and in many normal children.

C

calipers, surgical: a tonglike instrument with a scale at the wide end to make internal or external measurements.

canaliculitis: inflammation of the lacrimal canaliculi, often caused by fungus infection.

cellulitis, orbital: inflammation of the tissues surrounding the eye.

Chlamydia: an organism larger than viruses but smaller than bacteria which causes inclusion conjunctivitis and trachoma.

cobblestone conjunctivitis: a papillary hypertrophy of the tarsal conjunctiva as seen after contact lens wear or allergic conjunctivitis.

corectopia: displacement of pupil from its normal position.

craniotomy: a surgical exploration of the brain to identify and localize areas interrupting function.

cryptophthalmos: congenital absence of eyelids.

cyclectomy: an excision of part of the ciliary body.

cyclitic membrane: sheet of inflammatory scar tissue in front of or behind the lens of the eye.

cyclitis: inflammation of the ciliary body.

D

denervation supersensitivity: sensitivity to neural effector substance that follows postganglionic interruption of the nerve supply of organs innervated by the autonomic nervous system.

deuteranomaly: mild form of red-green color blindness, with reduced sensitivity to green.

deuteranopia: severe form of red-green color blindness, with greatest loss of sensitivity for green.

distichiasis: lashes growing from openings of meibomian glands.

Down's syndrome: mongolism, a form of arrested physical and mental development characterized by slanting eyes, cataracts, white spots of the iris, and blepharitis.

E

ectasia of sclera: a localized bulging of the sclera lined with uveal tissue; a staphyloma.

emphysema, orbital: air in the orbit tissues; generally follows traumatic rupture of a nasal sinus, particularly the lamina papyracea of the ethmoid bone.

endogenous uveitis: inflammation of the uveal tract arising from causes within the body in contrast to those introduced from outside the body, as in injuries (exogenous).

endophthalmitis: inflammation of most of the internal tissues of the eyeball.

epiblepharon: congenital redundant skin fold overlying the inner portion of the lower lid.

episcleritis: inflammation in the tissues overlying the sclera.

erysipelas: acute infection of the skin and subcutaneous tissues.

erythema multiforme: disease characterized by typical skin lesions that are bright red centrally with a pale peripheral zone surrounded by a red ring that progresses to a bulla; mucosal lesions, especially of the eyes and mouth; fever; and severe toxemia.

exotoxins: toxins that are released by bacteria and thereby produce a toxic reaction. For example, in a patient with marginal blepharitis caused by *Staphylococcus aureus*, the exotoxins produced by the bacteria may cause a marginal infiltrate or ulcer.

G

gonorrheal ophthalmia: blinding infectious eye disease of newborn infants acquired in the birth canal from gonorrhea.

granuloma: a benign nodule that occurs as a result of a localized inflammation surrounded by epithelioid cells.

granulomatous uveitis: inflammation of the iris, ciliary body, or choroid.

H

Herbert's peripheral pits: small depressed scars near limbus visible with the slit lamp in patients with trachoma.

histoplasmosis: fungal inflammation affecting the eye.

hypopyon: the presence of a purulent matter in the anterior chamber of the eye. Usually seen in the inferior part of the anterior chamber as a whitish mass.

I

injection: the congestion of ciliary or conjunctival blood vessels causing redness of the eye.

iridescent vision: halos around lights, particularly in corneal edema.

K

keloid: hypertrophic scar that may follow ocular injury or skin surgery. Most common in black people.

keratitis punctata (KP): white deposits found against the endothelium of the cornea occurring in cyclitis, caused by the circulation of inflammatory debris in the aqueous.

Koeppe nodule: accumulation of epitheloid cells at the pupillary margin as occurs in granulomatous uveitis.

L

lid lag: a lag in following movement of the upper lid as the eye moves from upward to downward gaze; seen most frequently in thyroid disease.

lobotomy: removal of a lobe of the brain.

M

Marfan's syndrome: widespread defects of elastic tissue associated with long fingers and toes, cardiovascular defects, and dislocated or sublocated crystalline lens of the eye.

metamorphopsia: condition in which objects appear distorted because of retinal edema or damage.

micronystagmus: very fine movements of the eyes normally present at all times.

microphthalmos: a developmental defect in which the eyeball is abnormally small.

micropsia: a condition in which objects are seen as smaller than they really are.

migraine: a vascular headache characterized by an aura, one-sided head pain, and a positive family history.

Mikulicz's syndrome: chronic lymphocytic infiltration with enlargement of lacrimal and salivary glands.

molluscum contagiosum: a disease caused by a virus that produces a wartlike lesion on the skin. If a lesion occurs on the eyelid, this may cause a follicular conjunctivitis or a keratitis.

mongolism: see *Down's syndrome*.

N

neovascular: refers to any newly formed blood vessels as may occur in the retina of diabetics and those with other disorders.

neovascularization: recent formation of new blood vessels in a part, such as the cornea or retina.

neurectomy: an incision of a nerve either peripheral or central in origin.

neuritis: inflammation of a nerve or nerves.

Newcastle disease virus: virus that causes a follicular conjunctivitis in people who work with poultry.

O

ophthalmia: inflammation of the eye or of the conjunctiva.

opsin: protein constituent of the visual pigment rhodopsin.

orbital cellulitis: see *cellulitis, orbital.*

orbital emphysema: see *emphysema, orbital.*

osteogenesis imperfecta: a hereditary dominant disorder characterized by brittle bones, multiple fractures, blue sclera, and deafness.

P

panophthalmitis: an inflammatory process involving the entire inner eye plus the outer ocular membranes (i.e., the cornea and sclera).

paracentesis: surgical drainage of the aqueous humor of the eye from the anterior chamber.

Parinaud's oculoglandular syndrome: a group of clinical findings in which there is a unilateral granulomatous conjunctivitis often associated with an enlarged preauricular or submandibular lymph node.

pars planitis: exudative edema on anterior portion of the retina.

penetrating injury: a penetration through tissue that disrupts the entire structure.

peritomy: the surgical separation of the conjunctiva from the limbus.

phlyctenule: localized lymphocytic infiltration of the conjunctiva.

pituitary ablation: destruction of pituitary gland.

poliosis: condition characterized by the absence of pigment in the hair resulting in the white eyelashes. Poliosis of the eyelashes occurs in sympathetic ophthalmia, syphilis, and Vogt-Koyanagi bilateral uveitis.

probing: a probe is passed through the tear outflow system to create patency of the congenitally blocked nasolacrimal duct.

prolapse of iris: herniation of iris tissue through a penetrating wound.

pseudomembranous conjunctivitis: see *membranous conjunctivitis.*

purulent: characterized by production of pus.

pyocyaneus *(Pseudomonas aeruginosa):* a bacterium commonly found in the intestinal tract and frequently in the skin, ear, and nose and capable of producing a devastating infection when it invades broken corneal epithelium.

R

reflex, oculocardiac: a slowing of the rhythm of the heart following compression of the eyes; if ocular compression produces acceleration of the heart, the reflex is called inverted.

S

sarcoidosis: disease of unknown cause affecting almost all systems of body and frequently the eye.

scleritis: inflammation of the sclera.

skew deviation: vertical nonparalytic deviation of the eyes as a result of cerebellar disease.

Soemmering's ring: a peripheral ring of lens capsule and cortex remaining after injury to the lens.

staphyloma: see *ectasia of sclera.*

Stevens-Johnson syndrome: a form of erythema multiforme characterized by inflammation and later by scarring of the conjunctiva and oral mucosa.

sympathetic ophthalmia: inflammation of one eye caused by an inflammation in the other eye, without infection.

T

thromboendarterectomy: surgical removal of clot from inner lining of blood vessel.

total hyphema (eight ball or black ball hyphema): the anterior chamber becomes totally filled with dark-colored blood.

traumatic aniridia: the root of the iris is totally torn from its attachment to the ciliary body.

traumatic mydriasis: a result of a hard blow to the eye that produces rupture of the iris sphincter and causes a permanent dilation of the pupil.

trichiasis: inversion of the eyelashes, resulting in irritation and abrasion of the cornea.

tuberculosis: an acute or chronic infectious disease caused by the tubercle bacillus that may affect any organ or tissue in the body.

U

uveoparotid fever: the condition of sarcoidosis with involvement of the uvea and the parotid gland.

V

vaccinia: viral disease that occasionally produces pustules on the eyelids of a child who has been vaccinated against smallpox.

vernal catarrh: type of allergic conjunctivitis occurring commonly in the spring. It may cause large inflammatory cobblestone plaques under the upper eyelid.

virulence: the disease-producing properties of a microorganism.

Vogt-Koyanagi bilateral uveitis: disease associated with absent lashes, baldness, and disturbance in hearing.

Vossius' ring: a ring of pigment visible on the front surface of the lens after trauma to the eye.

APPENDIX A

SHORT FORMS IN CLINICAL USE

Acc.	accommodation
add	addition
o.d.	right eye *(oculus dexter)*
o.s.	left eye *(oculus sinister)*
o.u.	both eyes *(oculi unitas)*
RE	right eye
LE	left eye
NV	near vision
PH	pinhole
V	vision or visual acuity
mm	millimeter
mg	milligram
SC	without correction
CC	with correction
HM	hand movements
LP	light perception
MR	Maddox rod
L & A	light and accommodation
EOMB	extraocular muscle balance
EOM	extraocular movements
CF	counting fingers
XP	exophoria
XT	exotropia
W	wearing
IOP	intraocular pressure
T	tension
ung.	ointment
A	applanation tensions
KP	keratic precipitates
PSC	posterior subcapsular cataract
ASC	anterior subcapsular cataract
ET	esotropia
°	degree
Δ	prism diopter
D	diopter
RH	right hyperphoria
LH	left hyperphoria
P.D. or I.P.D.	interpupillary distance
NPA	near point of accommodation
NPC	near point of convergence
MR	medial rectus (muscle)
LR	lateral rectus (muscle)
SR	superior rectus (muscle)
IR	inferior rectus (muscle)
SO	superior oblique (muscle)
IO	inferior oblique (muscle)
BO	base out
BI	base in
BD	base down
BU	base up
NRC	normal retinal correspondence
ARC	abnormal retinal correspondence
J1, J2, J3, etc.	test types for reading vision
N5, N6, etc.	test types for near vision
b.i.d. or b.d.	twice daily
t.i.d. or t.d.	three times daily
q.i.d.	four times daily
a.c.	before meals
p.c.	after meals
i.c.	between meals
ne rep. or non rep.	do not repeat
oculent	eye ointment
per os	orally, by mouth
p.r.n.	when required, as necessary
q.h.	every hour
q.2h.	every 2 hours
q.s.	quantity sufficient
stat.	at once

□ Modified from Stein, H.A., and Slatt, B.J.: The ophthalmic assistant, ed. 3, St Louis, 1983, The C.V. Mosby Co.

The following abbreviations may sometimes be found on ophthalmic charts:

VA	visual acuity
VAc or VAcc	visual acuity with correction
VAs or VAsc	visual acuity without correction
VA	visual acuity with the unaided eye
OT	ocular tension
AT or Appl	applanation tension
ST	Schiötz tension
EOM	extraocular muscle

E_1	esophoria for distance
E^1	esophoria for near
ET_1	esotropia for distance
ET^1	esotropia for near
X_1	exophoria for distance
X^1	exophoria for near
E(T)	intermittent esotropia
X(T)	intermittent exotropia
dd	disc diameters

APPENDIX B

METRIC CONVERSION

	When you know	Multiply by	To find
Length	inches (in)	2.5	centimeters (cm)
	feet (ft)	30.4	centimeters
	miles (mi)	1.6	kilometers (km)
Area	square inches (in^2)	6.5	square centimeters (cm^2)
	square miles (mi^2)	2.6	square kilometers (km^2)
Weight	ounces (oz)	28.3	grams (g)
	pounds (lb)	0.45	kilograms (kg)
Volume and capacity	teaspoons (tsp)	4.6	milliliters (ml)
	tablespoons (Tbsp)	14.0	milliliters
	fluid ounces (fl oz)	28.0	milliliters
	cups (c)	0.227	liters (L)
	pints (pt)	0.568	liters
	quarts (qt)	1.1	liters
	gallons (gal)	4.5	liters
	cubic inches (cu in)	16.3872	cubic centimeters (cc)
Speed and velocity	miles per hour (mph)	1.609	kilometers per hour (km/h)
	feet per seconds (fps)	30.4	centimeters per second (cm/s)
Temperature	Fahrenheit temperature (°F)	5/9 (after subtracting 32)	Celsius temperature (°C)

Mass

1 lb = 0.454 kg
1 kg = 2.205 lb
½ oz = 14.17 g
1 oz = 28.35 g

Length

1 in = 2.540 cm
1 ft = 0.3048 m
1 mi = 1.609 km
10 millimeters (mm) = 1 cm = 0.3937 in
100 cm = 1 m = 39.37 in
1000 m = 1 km = 0.62137 mi

Volume

1 q = 1.1366 L
1 gal = 4.4561 L
½ oz = 15 ml
1 oz = 30 ml
10 ml = 1 cc = 0.338 fl oz
10 cl = 1 deciliter (dl) = 6.1025 in^2
10 dl = 1 L = 1.0567 liquid qt
100 L = 1 hectoliter (hl) = 26.418 gal

Temperature

0° Celsius = 32° Fahrenheit
0° Fahrenheit = −17.8° Celsius
100° Celsius = 212° Fahrenheit

APPENDIX C

ESTIMATING VISUAL LOSS

LOSS OF CENTRAL VISION IN ONE EYE

Visual acuity for distance (Snellen)	Snellen	Meters (D)	Jaeger	Percent visual efficiency*	Percent visual loss
20/20	14/14	0.35	1−	100	0
20/25	14/18	0.44	2−	96	4
20/30	14/21	0.59	—	91	9
20/40	14/28	0.71	3	84	16
20/50	14/35	0.88	6	77	23
20/60	14/42	1.08	—	70	30
20/70	14/49	1.30	7	64	36
20/80	14/56	—	8	59	41
20/100	14/70	1.76	11	49	51
20/160	14/112	—	14−	29	71
20/200	14/140	3.53	—	20	80
20/400	14/280	7.06	—	3	97

*The percentage of visual efficiency of the two eyes may be determined by the following formula:

$$\frac{(3 \times \%\text{Visual efficiency of better eye}) + \%\text{Visual efficiency of poorer eye}}{4} = \%\text{Binocular visual efficiency}$$

☐ From Stein, H.A., and Slatt, B.J.: The ophthalmic assistant, ed. 3, St Louis, 1983, The C.V. Mosby Co.

Estimating loss of visual field

A visual field test is performed on the perimeter with a 3-mm test object in each of the eight 45-degree meridians. The sum of each of these meridians is added and the percentage of visual efficiency arrived at by dividing by 485, the total of a normal field. For example:

Normal field	Degrees	Constricted field	Degrees
Temporally	85	Temporally	45
Down and temporally	85	Down and temporally	25
Down	55	Down	30
Nasally	55	Down and nasally	25
Up and nasally	55	Nasally	25
Down and nasally	50	Up and nasally	25
Up	45	Up	25
Up and temporally	55	Up and temporally	35
TOTAL	485	TOTAL	235

%Visual efficiency $\frac{235 \times 100}{485} = 46\%$

APPENDIX D

VERTEX CONVERSION TABLE*

Spectacle lens power	Plus lenses							
	Effective power at corneal plane of spectacles at designated distance from cornea (vertex distance/millimeters)							
	8 mm	9 mm	10 mm	11 mm	12 mm	13 mm	14 mm	15 mm
4.00	4.12	4.12	4.12	4.12	4.25	4.25	4.25	4.25
4.50	4.62	4.75	4.75	4.75	4.75	4.75	4.75	4.87
5.00	5.25	5.25	5.25	5.25	5.25	5.37	5.37	5.37
5.50	5.75	5.75	5.75	5.87	5.87	5.87	6.00	6.00
6.00	6.25	6.37	6.37	6.37	6.50	6.50	6.50	6.62
6.50	6.87	6.87	7.00	7.00	7.00	7.12	7.12	7.25
7.00	7.37	7.50	7.50	7.62	7.62	7.75	7.75	7.75
7.50	8.00	8.00	8.12	8.12	8.25	8.25	8.37	8.50
8.00	8.50	8.62	8.75	8.75	8.87	8.87	9.00	9.12
8.50	9.12	9.25	9.25	9.37	9.50	9.50	9.62	9.75
9.00	9.75	9.75	9.87	10.00	10.12	10.25	10.37	10.37
9.50	10.25	10.37	10.50	10.62	10.75	10.87	11.00	11.12
10.00	10.87	11.00	11.12	11.25	11.37	11.50	11.62	11.75
10.50	11.50	11.62	11.75	11.87	12.00	12.12	12.25	12.50
11.00	12.00	12.25	12.37	12.50	12.75	12.87	13.00	13.12
11.50	12.62	12.87	13.00	13.12	13.37	13.50	13.75	13.87
12.00	13.25	13.50	13.62	13.87	14.00	14.25	14.50	14.62
12.50	13.87	14.12	14.25	14.50	14.75	15.00	15.25	15.37
13.00	14.50	14.75	15.00	15.25	15.50	15.62	16.00	16.12
13.50	15.12	15.37	15.62	15.87	16.12	16.37	16.62	16.87
14.00	15.75	16.00	16.25	16.50	16.75	17.12	17.50	17.75
14.50	16.50	16.75	17.00	17.25	17.50	17.87	18.25	18.50
15.00	17.00	17.37	17.75	18.00	18.25	18.62	19.00	19.37
15.50	17.75	18.00	18.25	18.75	19.00	19.37	19.75	20.25
16.00	18.25	18.75	19.00	19.37	19.75	20.25	20.50	21.00
16.50	19.00	19.37	19.75	20.25	20.50	21.00	21.50	21.87
17.00	19.75	20.25	20.50	21.00	21.50	22.00	22.25	22.87
17.50	20.50	20.75	21.25	21.75	22.25	22.75	23.25	23.75
18.00	21.00	21.50	22.00	22.50	23.00	23.50	24.00	24.62
18.50	21.75	22.25	22.75	23.25	23.75	24.50	25.00	25.62
19.00	22.50	23.00	23.50	24.00	24.75	25.25	26.00	26.50

*Spectacle lens power worn at various distance to equivalent contact lens power.

☐ From Stein, H.A., and Slatt, B.J.: The ophthalmic assistant, ed. 3, St Louis, 1983, The C.V. Mosby Co.

Minus lenses							
Effective power at corneal plane of spectacles at designated distance from cornea (vertex distance/millimeters)							
8 mm	9 mm	10 mm	11 mm	12 mm	13 mm	14 mm	15 mm
3.87	3.87	3.87	3.87	3.87	3.75	3.75	3.75
4.37	4.37	4.25	4.25	4.25	4.25	4.25	4.25
4.75	4.75	4.75	4.75	4.75	4.75	4.62	4.62
5.25	5.25	5.25	5.12	5.12	5.12	5.12	5.12
5.75	5.62	5.62	5.62	5.62	5.50	5.50	5.50
6.12	6.12	6.12	6.00	6.00	6.00	6.00	5.87
6.62	6.62	6.50	6.50	6.50	6.37	6.37	6.37
7.12	7.00	7.00	6.87	6.87	6.87	6.75	6.75
7.50	7.50	7.37	7.37	7.25	7.25	7.25	7.25
8.00	7.87	7.87	7.75	7.75	7.62	7.62	7.50
8.37	8.37	8.25	8.25	8.12	8.00	8.00	8.00
8.87	8.75	8.62	8.62	8.50	8.50	8.37	8.37
9.25	9.12	9.12	9.00	8.87	8.87	8.75	8.75
9.62	9.62	9.50	9.37	9.37	9.25	9.12	9.12
10.12	10.00	9.87	9.75	9.75	9.62	9.50	9.50
10.50	10.37	10.37	10.25	10.12	10.00	9.87	9.87
11.00	10.87	10.75	10.62	10.50	10.37	10.25	10.12
11.37	11.25	11.12	11.00	10.87	10.75	10.62	10.50
11.75	11.62	11.50	11.37	11.25	11.12	11.00	10.87
12.25	12.00	11.87	11.75	11.62	11.50	11.37	11.25
12.62	12.50	12.25	12.12	12.00	11.87	11.75	11.50
13.00	12.75	12.62	12.50	12.37	12.25	12.00	11.87
13.37	13.25	13.00	12.87	12.75	12.50	12.37	12.25
13.75	13.62	13.50	13.25	13.00	12.87	12.75	12.62
14.25	14.00	13.75	13.62	13.50	13.25	13.00	12.87
14.50	14.37	14.12	14.00	13.75	13.62	13.50	13.25
15.00	14.75	14.50	14.25	14.12	14.00	13.75	13.50
15.37	15.12	14.87	14.75	14.50	14.25	14.00	13.87
15.75	15.50	15.25	15.00	14.75	14.62	14.37	14.12
16.12	15.87	15.62	15.37	15.12	14.87	14.75	14.50
16.50	16.25	16.00	15.75	15.50	15.25	15.00	14.75

APPENDIX E

DIOPTERS OF CORNEAL REFRACTING POWER*

Diopters	Radius (mm)		Diopters	Radius (mm)	
	Curvature			Curvature	
Drum reading	Convex	Concave	Drum reading	Convex	Concave
52.00	6.49	6.51	47.87	7.05	7.07
51.87	6.50	6.53	47.75	7.07	7.09
51.75	6.52	6.54	47.62	7.08	7.11
51.62	6.54	6.56	47.50	7.10	7.13
51.50	6.55	6.57	47.37	7.12	7.15
51.37	6.57	6.59	47.25	7.14	7.17
51.25	6.58	6.61	47.12	7.16	7.19
51.12	6.60	6.62	47.00	7.18	7.21
51.00	6.62	6.64	46.87	7.20	7.23
50.87	6.63	6.66	46.75	7.22	7.25
50.75	6.65	6.67	46.62	7.24	7.27
50.62	6.66	6.69	46.50	7.26	7.29
50.50	6.68	6.71	46.27	7.28	7.31
50.37	6.70	6.72	46.25	7.30	7.33
50.25	6.73	6.75	46.12	7.32	7.35
50.12	6.73	6.75	46.00	7.34	7.37
50.00	6.75	6.77	45.87	7.36	7.39
49.87	6.76	6.79	45.75	7.38	7.41
49.75	6,80	6.82	45.62	7.40	7.43
49.62	6.80	6.82	45.50	7.42	7.45
49.50	6.82	6.84	45.37	7.44	7.47
49.37	6.83	6.85	45.25	7.46	7.49
49.25	6.85	6.87	45.12	7.48	7.51
49.12	6.87	6.89	45.00	7.50	7.53
49.00	6.89	6.91	44.87	7.52	7.55
48.87	6.90	6.93	44.75	7.55	7.57
48.75	6.92	6.95	44.62	7.57	7.58
48.62	6.94	6.96	44.50	7.59	7.60
48.50	6.96	6.98	44.37	7.61	7.62
48.37	6.97	7.00	44.25	7.63	7.65
48.25	6.99	7.02	44.12	7.65	7.67
48.12	7.01	7.03	44.00	7.67	7.70
48.00	7.03	7.05			

□ From Stein, H.A., and Slatt, B.J.: Fitting guide for rigid and soft contact lenses, ed. 2, St. Louis, 1984, The C.V. Mosby Co.

Diopters	Radius (mm)		Diopters	Radius (mm)	
	Curvature			Curvature	
Drum reading	Convex	Concave	Drum reading	Convex	Concave
43.87	7.67	7.72	39.87	8.47	8.50
43.75	7.72	7.74	39.75	8.49	8.52
43.62	7.74	7.77	39.62	8.52	8.55
43.50	7.76	7.79	39.50	8.54	8.58
43.37	7.78	7.81	39.37	8.57	8.61
43.25	7.80	7.84	39.25	8.60	8.63
43.12	7.83	7.86	39.12	8.63	8.66
43.00	7.85	7.88	39.00	8.65	8.69
42.87	7.88	7.90	38.87	8.68	8.72
42.75	7.90	7.92	38.75	8.71	8.75
42.62	7.92	7.95	38.62	8.74	8.78
42.50	7.95	7.97	38.50	8.77	8.80
42.37	7.97	8.00	38.37	8.80	8.84
42.25	8.00	8.02	38.25	8.82	8.86
42.12	8.01	8.05	38.12	8.85	8.89
42.00	8.04	8.07	38.00	8.88	8.92
41.87	8.06	8.10	37.87	8.91	8.95
41.75	8.09	8.12	37.75	8.94	8.98
41.62	8.11	8.15	37.62	8.97	9.01
41.50	8.13	8.17	37.50	9.00	9.04
41.37	8.16	8.19	37.37	9.03	9.07
41.25	8.18	8.22	37.25	9.06	9.10
41.12	8.20	8.24	37.12	9.09	9.13
41.00	8.23	8.27	37.00	9.12	9.16
40.87	8.26	8.29	36.87	9.14	9.19
40.75	8.28	8.32	36.75	9.19	9.23
40.62	8.31	8.34	36.62	9.22	9.26
40.50	8.34	8.37	36.50	9.25	9.29
40.37	8.36	8.39	36.37	9.28	9.32
40.25	8.39	8.42	36.25	9.31	9.35
40.12	8.41	8.44	36.12	9.35	9.38
40.00	8.44	8.47	36.00	9.38	9.42
			34.00	9.93	9.97

*Conversion table relating diopters of corneal refracting power to millimeters of radius of curvature for an assumed index of refraction of 1.3375. The column under convex curvature should be used when the keratometer is used to measure the cornea, and the third column is used to measure concave surfaces such as the CPC of a corneal contact lens in terms of its equivalent corneal refracting power in diopters.

APPENDIX F

COMPENSATION FOR EFFECT OF VERTEX DISTANCES (USED WHEN PLUS LENS IS MOVED FROM THE EYE)

℞ power (D)	Distance moved (mm)									
	1	2	3	4	5	6	7	8	9	10
7.00	6.95	6.90	6.86	6.81	6.76	6.72	6.67	6.63	6.59	6.54
7.25	7.20	7.15	7.10	7.05	7.00	6.95	6.90	6.85	6.81	6.76
7.50	7.44	7.39	7.43	7.28	7.23	7.18	7.13	7.08	7.03	6.98
7.75	7.69	7.63	7.57	7.52	7.46	7.41	7.35	7.30	7.24	7.19
8.00	7.94	7.87	7.81	7.75	7.69	7.63	7.58	7.52	7.46	7.41
8.25	8.18	8.12	8.05	7.99	7.92	7.86	7.80	7.74	7.68	7.62
8.50	8.43	8.36	8.29	8.22	8.15	8.09	8.02	7.96	7.90	7.83
8.75	8.67	8.60	8.53	8.45	8.38	8.31	8.24	8.18	8.11	8.05
9.00	8.92	8.84	8.76	8.69	8.61	8.54	8.47	8.40	8.33	8.26
9.25	9.17	9.08	9.00	8.92	8.84	8.76	8.69	8.61	8.54	8.47
9.50	9.41	9.32	9.24	9.15	9.07	8.99	8.91	8.83	8.75	8.68
9.75	9.66	9.56	9.47	9.38	9.30	9.21	9.13	9.04	8.96	8.88
10.00	9.90	9.80	9.71	9.62	9.52	9.43	9.35	9.26	9.17	9.09
10.25	10.15	10.04	9.94	9.85	9.75	9.66	9.56	9.47	9.38	9.30
10.50	10.39	10.28	10.18	10.08	9.98	9.88	9.78	9.69	9.59	9.50
10.75	10.64	10.52	10.41	10.31	10.20	10.10	10.00	9.90	9.80	9.71
11.00	10.88	10.76	10.65	10.54	10.43	10.32	10.21	10.11	10.01	9.91
11.25	11.12	11.00	10.88	10.77	10.65	10.54	10.43	10.32	10.22	10.11
11.50	11.37	11.24	11.12	10.99	10.87	10.76	10.64	10.53	10.42	10.31
11.75	11.61	11.48	11.35	11.22	11.10	10.98	10.86	10.74	10.63	10.51
12.00	11.86	11.72	11.58	11.45	11.32	11.19	11.07	10.95	10.83	10.71
12.25	12.10	11.96	11.82	11.68	11.54	11.41	11.28	11.16	11.03	10.91
12.50	12.35	12.20	12.05	11.90	11.76	11.63	11.49	11.36	11.24	11.11
12.75	12.59	12.43	12.28	12.13	11.99	11.84	11.71	11.57	11.44	11.31
13.00	12.83	12.67	12.51	12.36	12.21	12.06	11.92	11.78	11.64	11.50
13.25	13.08	12.91	12.74	12.58	12.43	12.27	12.13	11.98	11.84	11.70
13.50	13.32	13.15	12.97	12.81	12.65	12.49	12.33	12.18	12.04	11.89
13.75	13.56	13.38	13.21	13.03	12.87	12.70	12.54	12.39	12.24	12.09
14.00	13.81	13.62	13.44	13.26	13.08	12.92	12.75	12.59	12.43	12.28
14.25	14.05	13.86	13.67	13.48	13.30	13.13	12.96	12.79	12.63	12.47

☐ From Stein, H.A., and Slatt, B.J.: Fitting guide for rigid and soft contact lenses, ed. 2, St. Louis, 1984, C.V. Mosby, Co.

℞ power (D)	Distance moved (mm)									
	1	2	3	4	5	6	7	8	9	10
14.50	14.29	14.09	13.90	13.70	13.52	13.34	13.16	12.99	12.83	12.66
14.75	14.54	14.33	14.12	13.93	13.74	13.55	13.37	13.19	13.02	12.85
15.00	14.78	14.56	14.35	14.15	13.95	13.76	13.57	13.39	13.22	13.04
15.25	15.02	14.80	14.58	14.37	14.17	13.97	13.78	13.59	13.41	13.23
15.50	15.26	15.03	14.81	14.60	14.39	14.18	13.98	13.79	13.60	13.42
15.75	15.51	15.27	15.04	14.82	14.60	14.39	14.19	13.99	13.79	13.61
16.00	15.75	15.50	15.27	15.04	14.81	14.60	13.39	14.18	13.99	13.79
16.25	15.99	15.74	15.49	15.25	15.03	14.81	14.59	14.38	14.18	13.98
16.50	16.23	15.97	15.72	15.48	15.24	15.01	14.79	14.57	14.37	14.16
16.75	16.47	16.21	15.95	15.70	15.45	15.22	14.99	14.77	14.56	14.35
17.00	16.72	16.44	16.18	15.92	15.67	15.43	15.19	14.96	14.74	14.53
17.25	16.96	16.67	16.40	16.44	15.88	15.63	15.39	15.16	14.93	14.71
17.50	17.20	16.91	16.63	16.36	16.09	15.84	15.59	15.35	15.12	14.89
17.75	17.44	17.14	16.85	16.57	16.30	16.04	15.79	15.54	15.31	15.07
18.00	17.68	17.37	17.08	16.79	16.51	16.25	15.99	15.73	15.49	15.25
18.25	17.92	17.61	17.30	17.01	16.72	16.45	16.18	15.92	15.68	15.43
18.50	18.16	17.84	17.53	17.23	16.93	16.65	16.38	16.11	15.86	15.61
18.75	18.40	18.07	17.75	17.44	17.14	16.85	16.57	16.30	16.04	15.79
19.00	18.65	18.30	17.98	17.66	17.35	17.06	16.77	16.49	16.23	15.97
19.25	18.89	18.54	18.20	17.87	17.56	17.26	16.96	16.68	16.41	16.14
19.50	19.13	18.77	18.42	18.09	17.77	17.46	17.16	16.87	16.59	16.32
19.75	19.37	19.00	18.65	18.30	17.97	17.66	17.35	17.06	16.77	16.49
20.00	19.61	19.23	18.87	18.52	18.18	17.86	17.54	17.24	16.95	16.67
20.25	19.85	19.46	19.09	18.73	18.39	18.06	17.74	17.43	17.13	16.84
20.50	20.09	19.69	19.31	18.95	18.59	18.25	17.93	17.61	17.31	17.01
20.75	20.33	19.92	19.53	19.16	18.80	18.45	18.12	17.80	17.48	17.18
21.00	20.57	20.15	19.76	19.37	19.00	18.65	18.31	17.98	17.66	17.36
21.25	20.81	20.38	19.98	19.59	19.21	18.85	18.50	18.16	17.84	17.53
21.50	21.05	20.61	20.20	19.80	19.41	19.04	18.69	18.34	18.01	17.70
21.75	21.29	20.84	20.42	20.01	19.62	19.24	18.88	18.53	18.19	17.87

APPENDIX G

COMPENSATION FOR EFFECT OF VERTEX DISTANCES (USED WHEN PLUS LENS IS MOVED TOWARD THE EYE)

℞ power (D)	Distance moved (mm)									
	1	2	3	4	5	6	7	8	9	10
7.00	7.05	7.10	7.15	7.20	7.25	7.31	7.36	7.42	7.47	7.53
7.25	7.30	7.36	7.41	7.47	7.52	7.58	7.64	7.70	7.76	7.82
7.50	7.56	7.61	7.67	7.73	7.79	7.85	7.92	7.98	8.04	8.11
7.75	7.81	7.87	7.93	8.00	8.06	8.13	8.19	8.26	8.33	8.40
8.00	8.06	8.13	8.20	8.26	8.33	8.40	8.47	8.55	8.62	8.70
8.25	8.32	8.39	8.46	8.53	8.60	8.68	8.76	8.83	8.91	8.99
8.50	8.57	8.56	8.72	8.80	8.88	8.96	9.04	9.12	9.20	9.29
8.75	8.83	8.91	8.99	9.07	9.15	9.23	9.32	9.41	9.50	9.59
9.00	9.08	9.16	9.25	9.34	9.42	9.51	9.61	9.70	9.79	9.89
9.25	9.34	9.42	9.51	9.61	9.70	9.79	9.89	9.99	10.09	10.19
9.50	9.59	9.68	9.78	9.88	9.97	10.07	10.18	10.28	10.39	10.50
9.75	9.85	9.94	10.04	10.15	10.25	10.36	10.46	10.58	10.69	10.80
10.00	10.10	10.20	10.31	10.42	10.53	10.64	10.75	10.87	10.99	11.11
10.25	10.36	10.46	10.58	10.69	10.80	10.92	11.04	11.17	11.29	11.42
10.50	10.61	10.73	10.84	10.96	11.08	11.21	11.33	11.46	11.60	11.73
10.75	10.87	10.99	11.11	11.23	11.36	11.49	11.62	11.76	11.90	12.04
11.00	11.12	11.25	11.38	11.51	11.64	11.78	11.92	12.06	12.21	12.36
11.25	11.38	11.51	11.64	11.78	11.92	12.06	12.21	12.36	12.52	12.68
11.50	11.63	11.77	11.91	12.05	12.20	12.35	12.51	12.67	12.83	12.99
11.75	11.89	12.03	12.18	12.33	12.48	12.64	12.80	12.97	13.14	13.31
12.00	12.15	12.30	12.45	12.61	12.77	12.93	13.10	13.27	13.45	13.64
12.25	12.40	12.56	12.72	12.88	13.05	13.22	13.40	13.58	13.77	13.96
12.50	12.66	12.82	12.99	13.16	13.33	13.51	13.70	13.89	14.08	14.29
12.75	12.91	13.08	13.26	13.44	13.62	13.81	14.00	14.20	14.40	14.61
13.00	13.17	13.35	13.53	13.71	13.90	14.10	14.30	14.51	14.72	14.94
13.25	13.43	13.61	13.80	13.99	14.19	14.39	14.60	14.82	15.04	15.27
13.50	13.68	13.87	14.07	14.27	14.48	14.69	14.91	15.13	15.37	15.61
13.75	13.94	14.14	14.34	14.55	14.77	14.99	15.21	15.45	15.69	15.94
14.00	14.20	14.40	14.61	14.83	15.05	15.28	15.52	15.77	16.02	16.28
14.25	14.46	14.67	14.89	15.11	15.34	15.58	15.83	16.09	16.35	16.62

☐ From Stein, H.A., and Slatt, B.J.: Fitting guide for rigid and soft contact lenses, ed. 2, 1984, C.V. Mosby Co.

℞ power (D)	Distance moved (mm)									
	1	2	3	4	5	6	7	8	9	10
14.50	14.71	14.93	15.16	15.39	15.63	15.88	16.14	16.41	16.88	16.96
14.75	14.97	15.20	15.43	15.67	15.92	16.18	16.45	16.73	17.01	17.30
15.00	15.23	15.46	15.71	15.96	16.22	16.48	16.76	17.05	17.34	17.65
15.25	15.49	15.73	15.98	16.24	16.51	16.79	17.07	17.37	17.68	18.00
15.50	15.74	16.00	16.26	16.52	16.80	17.09	17.39	17.69	18.01	18.35
15.75	16.00	16.26	16.53	16.81	17.10	17.39	17.70	18.02	18.35	18.70
16.00	16.26	16.53	16.81	17.09	17.39	17.70	18.02	18.35	18.69	19.05
16.25	16.52	16.80	17.08	17.38	17.69	18.01	18.34	18.68	19.03	19.40
16.50	16.78	17.06	17.36	17.67	17.98	18.31	18.65	19.01	19.38	19.76
16.75	17.04	17.33	17.64	17.95	18.28	18.62	18.97	19.34	19.72	20.12
17.00	17.29	17.60	17.91	18.24	18.58	18.93	19.30	19.68	20.07	20.48
17.25	17.55	17.87	18.19	18.53	18.88	19.24	19.62	20.01	20.42	20.85
17.50	17.81	18.13	18.47	18.82	19.18	19.55	19.94	20.35	20.77	21.21
17.75	18.07	18.40	18.75	19.11	19.48	19.86	20.27	20.69	21.12	21.58
18.00	18.33	18.67	19.03	19.40	19.78	20.18	20.59	21.03	21.48	21.95
18.25	18.59	18.94	19.31	19.69	20.08	20.49	20.92	21.37	21.84	22.32
18.50	18.85	19.21	19.59	19.98	20.39	20.81	21.25	27.71	22.20	22.70
18.75	19.11	19.48	19.87	20.27	20.69	21.13	21.58	22.06	22.56	23.08
19.00	19.37	19.75	20.15	20.56	20.99	21.44	21.91	22.41	22.92	23.46
19.25	19.63	20.02	20.43	20.86	21.30	21.76	22.25	22.75	23.28	23.81
19.50	19.89	20.89	20.71	21.15	21.61	22.08	22.58	23.10	23.65	24.22
19.75	20.15	20.56	20.99	21.44	21.91	22.40	22.92	23.46	24.02	24.61
20.00	20.41	20.83	21.28	21.74	22.22	22.73	23.26	23.81	24.39	25.00
20.25	20.67	21.10	21.56	22.03	22.53	23.05	23.59	24.16	24.76	
20.50	20.82	21.38	21.84	22.33	22.84	23.38	23.93	24.52		
20.75	20.91	21.65	22.13	22.63	23.15	23.70	24.28			
21.00	21.45	21.92	22.41	22.93	23.46	24.03				
21.25	21.71	22.19	22.70	23.22	23.78					
12.50	21.97	22.47	22.98	23.52						
21.75	22.23	22.74	23.37							

APPENDIX H

DIOPTRIC CURVES FOR EXTENDED RANGE OF KERATOMETER

High power (with +1.25 D lens over aperture)				Low power (with −1.00 D lens over aperture)			
Drum reading (D)	True dioptric curvature (D)	Drum reading (D)	True dioptric curvature (D)	Drum reading (D)	True dioptric curvature (D)	Drum reading (D)	True dioptric curvature (D)
52.00	61.00	46.87	55.87	42.00	36.00	36.87	30.87
51.87	60.87	46.75	55.75	41.87	35.87	36.75	30.75
51.75	60.75	46.62	55.62	41.75	35.75	36.62	30.62
51.62	60.62	46.50	55.50	41.62	35.62	36.50	30.50
51.50	60.50	46.37	55.37	41.50	35.50	36.37	30.37
51.37	60.37	46.25	55.25	41.37	35.37	36.25	30.25
51.25	60.25	46.12	55.12	41.25	35.25	36.12	30.12
51.12	60.12	46.00	55.00	41.12	35.12	36.00	30.00
51.00	60.00			41.00	35.00		
		45.87	54.87				
50.87	59.87	45.75	54.75	40.87	34.87		
50.75	59.75	45.62	54.62	40.75	34.75		
50.62	59.62	45.50	54.50	40.62	34.62		
50.50	59.50	45.37	54.37	40.50	34.50		
50.37	59.37	45.25	54.25	40.37	34.37		
50.25	59.25	45.12	54.12	40.25	34.25		
50.12	59.12	45.00	54.00	40.12	34.12		
50.00	59.00			40.00	34.00		
		44.87	53.87				
49.87	58.87	44.75	53.75	39.87	33.87		
49.75	58.75	44.62	53.62	39.75	33.75		
49.62	58.62	44.50	53.50	39.62	33.62		
49.50	58.50	44.37	53.37	39.50	33.50		

Courtesy Bausch & Lomb, Inc.

☐ From Stein, H.A., and Slatt, B.J.: Fitting guide for rigid and soft contact lenses, ed. 2, 1984, C.V. Mosby, Co.

High power (with +1.25 D lens over aperture)				Low power (with −1.00 D lens over aperture)			
Drum reading (D)	True dioptric curvature (D)	Drum reading (D)	True dioptric curvature (D)	Drum reading (D)	True dioptric curvature (D)	Drum reading (D)	True dioptric curvature (D)
49.37	58.37	44.25	53.25	39.37	33.37		
49.25	58.25	44.12	53.12	39.25	33.25		
49.12	58.12	44.00	53.00	39.12	33.12		
49.00	58.00			39.00	33.00		
		43.87	52.87				
48.75	57.75	43.75	52.75	38.87	32.87		
48.62	57.62	43.62	52.62	38.75	32.75		
48.50	57.50	43.50	52.50	38.62	32.62		
48.37	57.37	43.37	52.37	38.50	32.50		
48.25	57.25	43.25	52.25	38.37	32.37		
48.12	57.12	43.12	52.12	38.25	32.25		
48.00	57.00	43.00	52.00	38.12	32.12		
				38.00	32.00		
47.87	56.87						
47.75	56.75			37.87	31.87		
47.62	56.62			37.75	31.75		
47.50	56.50			37.62	31.62		
47.37	58.37			37.50	31.50		
47.25	56.25			37.37	31.37		
47.12	56.12			37.25	31.25		
47.00	56.00			37.12	31.12		
				37.00	31.00		

BIBLIOGRAPHY

1. Brunner, T.F., and Berkowitz, L.: Elements of scientific and specialized terminology, Minneapolis, 1967, Burgess Publishing Co.
2. Cassin, B., and Solomon, S.: Dictionary of eye terminology, Gainesville, Fla., 1984, Triad Publishing Company.
3. Cline, D., et al.: Dictionary of visual science, ed. 3, Radnor, Pa., 1980, Chilton Book Co.
4. Duke-Elder, S.: The practice of refraction, ed. 8, St. Louis, 1969, The C.V. Mosby Co.
5. Fell, P.J., and Skees, W.D.: The doctor's computer handbook, Belmont, Calif., 1984, Lifetime Learning Publications.
6. Franks, R., and Swartz, H.: Simplified medical dictionary, Oradell, N.J., 1977, Medical Economics Co.
7. Funk & Wagnalls standard dictionary, international ed., vols. 1 and 2, New York, 1966, Funk & Wagnalls Publishing Co.
8. Gordon, B.L., et al.: Current medical terminology, Chicago, 1966, American Medical Association Publishers.
9. Havener, W.H.: Synopsis of ophthalmology, ed. 4, St. Louis, 1975, The C.V. Mosby Co.
10. Henkind, P., Priest, R.S., and Schiller, G.: Compendium of ophthalmology, Philadelphia, 1982, J.B. Lippincott Company.
11. Jaffe, N.S.: Cataract surgery and its complications, St. Louis, 1972, The C.V. Mosby Co.
12. Klein, E.: A comprehensive etymological dictionary of the English language, New York, 1967, Elsevier Publishing Co.
13. Lewis, C., and Short, C.: A Latin dictionary, 1962, Oxford-Clarendon Press.
14. Liddell, H.G., and Scott, R.: A Greek English lexicon, 1961, Jones and Makenzie, Oxford-Clarendon Press.
15. Lindberg, D.C.: Theories of vision from Al-Kindi to Kepler, Chicago, 1976, University of Chicago Press.
16. May, M.T., tr. and ed.: Galen on usefulness of the parts of the body, 2 vols., Ithaca, N.Y., 1968, Cornell University Press.
17. Minckler, J.: Pathology of the nervous system, 1968, McGraw-Hill Book Co.
18. Murray, J.A., et al.: The Oxford English dictionary, 13 vols., 1961, Oxford-Clarendon Press.
19. Newell, F.W.: Ophthalmology—principles and concepts, ed. 4, St. Louis, 1978, The C.V. Mosby Co.
20. Reinecke, R.D., Stein, H.A., and Slatt, B.J.: Introductory manual for ophthalmic assistants, St. Louis, 1972, The C.V. Mosby Co.
21. Skinner, H.A.: The origin of medical terms, ed. 2, Baltimore, 1961, The Williams & Wilkins Co.
22. Stedman's medical dictionary, ed. 23, Baltimore, 1976, The Williams & Wilkins Co.
23. Stein, H.A., and Slatt, B.J.: The ophthalmic assistant, ed. 3, St. Louis, 1976, The C.V. Mosby Co.
24. Stein, H.A., and Slatt, B.J.: Fitting guide for hard and soft contact lenses, St. Louis, 1979, The C.V. Mosby Co.
25. Thompson, W.A.R., and Wolfers, M.: Black's medical dictionary, ed. 21, London, 1976, A. & C. Black Publishers.
26. Young, C.G., and Austrin, M.G.: Student's workbook for learning medical terminology step by step, St. Louis, 1979, The C.V. Mosby Co.

ALPHABETIC LISTING OF OPHTHALMIC TERMINOLOGY

A

B

D

E

G

H

I

J

N

O

Y

Z